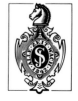

Since 1973 the Royal College of
Obstetricians and Gynaecologists has
regularly convened Study Groups to
address important growth areas within
obstetrics and gynaecology. An
international group of eminent scientists
and clinicians from various disciplines is
invited to present the results of recent
research and take part in in-depth
discussion. The resulting volume
containing the papers presented and also
edited transcripts of the discussions is
published within a few months of the
meeting and provides a summary of the
subject that is both authoritative and up
to date.

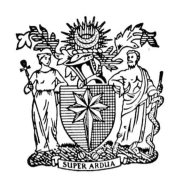

*Previous Study Group publications
available from Springer-Verlag:*

Early Pregnancy Loss
Edited by R. W. Beard and F. Sharp

AIDS in Obstetrics and Gynaecology
Edited by C. N. Hudson and F. Sharp

Fetal Growth
Edited by F. Sharp, R. B. Fraser and
R. D. G. Milner

Micturition
Edited by J. O. Drife, P. Hilton and
S. L. Stanton

*The Royal College of Obstetricians and
Gynaecologists gratefully acknowledges
the sponsorship of the Study Group by
Ciba-Geigy Pharmaceuticals; The
Department of Health; Duphar
Laboratories Limited; The National
Dairy Council; Organon Laboratories
Limited; Roussel Laboratories Limited;
Schering Health Care Limited; Syntex
Pharmaceuticals Limited; Wyeth
Laboratories*

HRT and Osteoporosis

Edited by
J. O. Drife and J. W. W. Studd

With 65 Figures

Springer-Verlag
London Berlin Heidelberg New York
Paris Tokyo Hong Kong

James O. Drife, MD, FRCS Ed, FRCOG
Professor of Obstetrics and Gynaecology, Clarendon Wing, Leeds
General Infirmary, Leeds LS1 3EX

John W. W. Studd, MD, BS, FRCOG
Consultant Obstetrician and Gynaecologist, King's College Hospital,
London SE5 9RS and Director, The Menopause Clinic, Dulwich
Hospital, East Dulwich Grove, London SE22 8PT

ISBN 3–540–19628–5 Springer-Verlag Berlin Heidelberg New York
ISBN 0–387–19628–5 Springer-Verlag New York Berlin Heidelberg

British Library Cataloguing in Publication Data
HRT and osteoporosis.
1. Women. Bones. Osteoporosis. Drug therapy. Oestrogens
I. Drife, James O. (James Owen) 1947– II. Studd, John W.W.   616.71
ISBN 3–540–19628–5

Library of Congress Cataloging-in-Publication Data
HRT and osteoporosis/ edited by James O. Drife and John W. W. Studd.
p.   cm. Based on the 22nd Study Group of the Royal College of Obstetricians and
Gynaecologists held in January 1990: sponsored by Ciba–Geigy Pharmaceuticals and
others.   Includes index.
ISBN 0–387–19628–5 (alk. paper). — ISBN 3–540–19628–5 (alk. paper)
1. Osteoporosis—Hormone therapy—Congresses.   2. Osteoporosis—Hormone
therapy—Complications and sequelae—Congresses.   3. Aged women—Diseases—
Congresses.   I. Drife, James O., 1947– II. Studd, John.   III. Geigy Pharmaceuticals.
IV. Royal College of Obstetricians and Gynaecologists (Great Britain). Study Group
(22nd: 1990)
[DNLM: 1. Estrogen Replacement Therapy—congresses.   2.Menopause—congresses.
4. Osteoporosis—etiology—congresses.   5. Osteoporosis—prevention & control—
congresses.   WE 250 H873 1990]   RC931.073H77   1990   616.7′16–dc20
DNLM/DLC
for Library of Congress   90–10029
                                                                                    CIP

Typeset by Flairplan Limited, Ware
Printed by The Alden Press, Osney Mead, Oxford
2128/3916–543210   Printed on acid-free paper

Preface

For many years the fact that older women are susceptible to fractures was dismissed as a natural consequence of ageing. Now, both doctors and the general public are becoming increasingly aware that ovarian failure is an important cause of osteoporosis and that much of the bone loss after the menopause can be prevented by oestrogen treatment. This has raised important questions about the safety and acceptability of long-term treatment with sex hormones, about the economic costs and benefits of such treatment, and about the role of specialists and general practitioners in promoting and monitoring hormone replacement therapy (HRT).

These questions have far-reaching implications involving many medical disciplines and they have revealed serious gaps in our knowledge. Nevertheless, practical guidance is urgently needed by women and their doctors and by those responsible for public health policies. The Royal College of Obstetricians and Gynaecologists made osteoporosis the subject of its 22nd Study Group, held in January 1990. An international panel of leading researchers was invited to participate in a three-day workshop, allowing time for in-depth discussion as well as the presentation of papers.

The participants included epidemiologists, endocrinologists and a geriatrician as well as gynaecologists, scientists and physicians specialising in bone disease. The meeting began with discussions on benefits and risks of oestrogen treatment before focusing on the problems of screening for osteoporosis and the place of HRT in the community. The interaction between leading authorities from different disciplines was intensely stimulating and the meeting provided a rare opportunity for comprehensive discussion. It was not possible to refer all material back to the authors or discussants; it is hoped that the proceedings have been reported fairly and accurately.

The Editors are very grateful to Miss Sally Barber, Postgraduate Secretary of the RCOG, for her pleasant efficiency in supervising the production schedule for this book. They also wish to thank the participants who gave so much of their time and expertise to the meeting, and whose constructive co-operation produced a series of practical conclusions and recommendations. We hope these will make a helpful contribution to the development of this important aspect of preventive medicine.

London 1990   James Drife
                                                           John Studd

Contents

SECTION III: RISKS AND BENEFITS OF HRT

SECTION IV: THERAPEUTIC POTENTIAL

SECTION V: HRT AND THE COMMUNITY

Participants

Professor D. C. Anderson
Professor of Endocrinology, University of Manchester, Department of Medicine, Hope Hospital, Salford M6 8HD, UK

Professor D. T. Baird
MRC Clinical Research Professor of Reproductive Endocrinology, Department of Obstetrics and Gynaecology, University of Edinburgh, Centre for Reproductive Biology, 37 Chalmers Street, Edinburgh EH3 9EW, UK

Dr D. H. Barlow
Clinical Reader, Nuffield Department of Obstetrics and Gynaecology, University of Oxford, John Radcliffe Hospital, Oxford OX3 9DU, UK

Professor A. Boyde
Department of Anatomy and Developmental Biology, University College London, Gower Street, London WC1E 6BT, UK

Dr M. Brincat
Consultant, Department of Obstetrics and Gynaecology, St Luke's Hospital Medical School, G'mangia, Malta

Miss L. D. Cardozo
Consultant Obstetrician and Gynaecologist, King's College Hospital, Denmark Hill, London SE5 9RS, UK

Dr M. P. Cust
Lecturer in Obstetrics and Gynaecology, Department of Obstetrics and Gynaecology, University Hospital, Nottingham NG7 2UH, UK

Dr J. O. Drife
Convener of Study Groups, RCOG and Honorary Consultant, Professor of Obstetrics and Gynaecology, Clarendon Wing, Leeds General Infirmary, Leeds LS1 3EX, UK

Mrs L. K. Edwards
The Director, National Osteoporosis Society, Barton Meade House, PO Box 10, Radstock, Bath BA3 3YB, UK

Dr I. Fogelman
Consultant Physician, Director of Nuclear Medicine, Department of Nuclear Medicine, Guy's Hospital, London SE1 9RT, UK

Dr R. M. Francis
Senior Lecturer in Medicine (Geriatrics), Department of Medicine (Geriatrics), University of Newcastle upon Tyne, Newcastle General Hospital, Newcastle upon Tyne NE4 6BE, UK

Dr T. J. Garnett
Research Assistant, The Menopause Clinic, Dulwich Hospital, East Dulwich Grove, London SE22 8PT, UK

Dr D. H. Gath
Clinical Reader in Psychiatry, University Department of Psychiatry, Warneford Hospital, Oxford OX3 7JX, UK

Dr N. P. Halliday
Senior Principal Medical Officer, Department of Health, Eileen House, 80–94 Newington Causeway, London SE1 6YX, UK

Dr D. McK. Hart
Consultant Gynaecologist and Honorary Clinical Lecturer, Stobhill Hospital, Glasgow G21 3UW and Western Infirmary, Glasgow G11 6NT, UK

Dr J. A. Kanis
Reader and Consultant Physician, Department of Human Metabolism and Clinical Biochemistry, Medical School, Beech Hill Road, Sheffield S10 2RX, UK

Dr R. Lindsay
Professor of Clinical Medicine and Chief of Internal Medicine, Helen Hayes Hospital, Route 9W, West Haverstaw, New York 10993, USA

Dr T. W. Meade
Director, MRC Epidemiology and Medical Care Unit, Northwick Park Hospital, Harrow HA1 3UJ, UK

Miss J. C. Montgomery
Senior Registrar in Obstetrics and Gynaecology, University College
Hospital, Gower Street, London WC1, UK

Dr M. Notelovitz
President and Medical Director, Women's Medical and Diagnostic
Center and The Climacteric Clinic, Office Park West, 222 S.W. 36th
Terrace, Suite C, Gainesville, Florida 32607, USA

Professor I. Persson
Associate Professor, Department of Obstetrics and Gynaecology,
University Hospital, S–751 85 Uppsala, Sweden

Professor D. W. Purdie
Director of Postgraduate Medical Education, Postgraduate Centre,
Hull Royal Infirmary, Hull HU3 2JZ, UK

Dr M. F. Roche
Senior Registrar in Public Health Medicine, Department of Community
Medicine and General Practice, Gibson Building, Radcliffe Infirmary,
Oxford OX2 6HE, UK

Professor R. K. Ross
Department of Preventive Medicine, Norris Cancer Hospital #803,
University of Southern California, 2025 Zonal Avenue, Los Angeles,
California 90033, USA

Dr D. Rothman
Senior Medical Officer, Department of Health, Eileen House, 80–94
Newington Causeway, London SE1 6YX, UK

Dr P. L. Selby
Lecturer in Medicine, Department of Medicine, University of
Manchester, Manchester Royal Infirmary, Oxford Road, Manchester
M13 9WL, UK

Dr J. C. Stevenson
Consultant Endocrinologist, Wynn Institute for Metabolic Research,
21 Wellington Road, London NW8 9SQ, UK

Mr J. W. W. Studd
Consultant Obstetrician and Gynaecologist, King's College Hospital,
London SE5 9RS and Director, The Menopause Clinic, Dulwich
Hospital, East Dulwich Grove, London SE22 8PT, UK

Professor M. P. Vessey
Professor of Social and Community Medicine, Department of
Community Medicine and General Practice, Gibson Building,
Radcliffe Infirmary, Oxford OX2 6HE, UK

Mr M. I. Whitehead
Senior Lecturer/Consultant Gynaecologist, Academic Department of
Obstetrics and Gynaecology, King's College School of Medicine and
Dentistry, London SE5 9PJ, UK

Additional Contributors

Dr J. Aaron
Department of Human Metabolism and Clinical Biochemistry,
University of Sheffield Medical School, Beech Hill House, Sheffield
S10 2RX, UK

Dr H. O. Adami
Department of Surgery, University Hospital, S–751 85, Uppsala,
Sweden

Dr L. Bergkvist
Department of Surgery, University Hospital, S–751 85, Uppsala,
Sweden

Dr F. Cosman
Instructor in Medicine, Columbia University, College of Physicians
and Surgeons, USA

Dr D. Crook
Laboratory Director, Wynn Institute for Metabolic Research, 21
Wellington Road, London NW8 9SQ, UK

Mr M. C. Ellerington
Wynn Institute for Metabolic Research, 21 Wellington Road,
London NW8 9SQ, UK

Dr K. S. Eyres
Department of Human Metabolism and Clinical Biochemistry,
University of Sheffield Medical School, Beech Hill House, Sheffield
S10 2RX, UK

Mr K. F. Ganger
Research Fellow, Academic Department of Obstetrics and
Gynaecology, King's College School of Medicine and Dentistry,
London SE5 9PJ, UK

Dr A. Henderson
Department of Obstetrics and Gynaecology, Dulwich Hospital, London SE22 8PT, UK

Dr B. E. Henderson
Kenneth Norris Jr Cancer Center, University of Southern California, 1441 Eastlake Avenue, Los Angeles, California 90033, USA

Mr T. C. Hillard
Wynn Institute for Metabolic Research, 21 Wellington Road, London NW8 9SQ, UK

Dr A. Horsman
Director, MRC Bone Mineralisation Group, The General Infirmary at Leeds, Leeds LS1 3EX, UK

Dr S. A. Iles
Wellcome Research Fellow in Mental Health, University Department of Psychiatry, Warneford Hospital, Oxford OX3 7JX, UK

Dr T. M. Mack
Professor, PMB–B105, 2025 Zonal Avenue, Los Angeles, California 90033, USA

Dr E. V. McCloskey
Department of Human Metabolism and Clinical Biochemistry, University of Sheffield Medical School, Beech Hill House, Sheffield S10 2RX, UK

Dr C. Moniz
Consultant Chemical Pathologist, Department of Clinical Biochemistry, King's College Hospital, London SE5 9RS, UK

Dr D. V. O'Doherty
Department of Human Metabolism and Clinical Biochemistry, University of Sheffield Medical School, Beech Hill House, Sheffield S10 2RX, UK

Dr M. C. Pike
Professor and Chairman, PMB–A201, 1420 San Pablo Street, Los Angeles, California 90033–9987, USA

Dr A. Rodin
Senior Registrar in Obstetrics and Gynaecology, Department of Obstetrics and Gynaecology, Guy's Hospital, London SE1 9RT, UK

Mr M. Savvas
Senior Registrar, Department of Obstetrics and Gynaecology,
Dulwich Hospital, London SE22 8PT, UK

Sister A. M. Sutcliffe
Research Co-ordinator, Bone Diseases, Department of Geriatric
Medicine, Newcastle General Hospital, Westgate Road, Newcastle
upon Tyne NE4 6BE, UK

Dr N. R. Watson
Research Assistant, The Menopause Clinic, Dulwich Hospital, East
Dulwich Grove, London SE22 8PT, UK

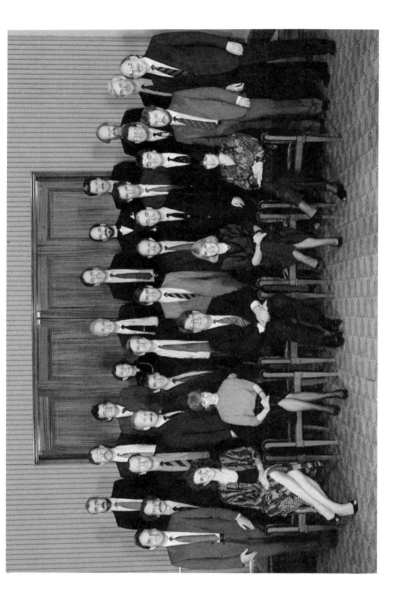

Back row (left to right): Dr R. Lindsay, Dr D. McK. Hart, Dr R. M. Francis, Dr D. Rothman, Dr N. P. Halliday, Dr T. W. Meade, Dr J. O. Drife, Mr M. I. Whitehead, Professor A. Boyde, Mr D. H. Barlow.
Middle Row: Dr I. Fogelman, Professor R. K. Ross, Professor D. W. Purdie, Dr I. Persson, Dr J. A. Kanis, Professor M. P. Vessey, Professor D. C. Anderson, Dr P. L. Selby, Dr M. Brincat, Professor D. T. Baird, Mr M. P. Cust, Dr T. Garnett, Dr J. C. Stevenson, Dr M. Notelovitz.
Front row: Ms L. Edwards, Dr M. F. Roche, Mr J. W. W. Studd, Dr J. C. Montgomery, Miss L. D. Cardozo.

Section I
Pathophysiology of the Menopause

Chapter 1

Biology of the Menopause

D. T. Baird

Introduction

The average life expectancy of women in Western countries is now about 75 years and at least 90% will reach 65 years. Thus the majority of women will spend approximately one-third of their life in the menopausal state. By definition the menopause is the last menstrual period and its timing can only be determined in retrospect; by convention if there has been no spontaneous period for 12 months, ovarian failure with consequent lack of menstrual bleeding is deemed to have occurred. Ovarian failure is an integral part of the menopause; amenorrhoea due to lack of pituitary gonadotrophins or removal of the uterus with conservation of the ovaries is not usually included in the menopausal state.

The last menstrual period is a definite event which is indicative of a series of changes in function of the ovaries which has been termed the menopausal transition. Changes in the pituitary–ovarian axis which are manifest by changes in the pattern of menstrual cycles have been termed "premenopause". The ovaries do not cease functioning immediately after the last menstrual period and in many women there is infrequent development of follicles during the early postmenopausal years. This chapter outlines the biological basis of the menopause, the endocrine changes associated with ovarian failure and their role in the aetiology of menopausal symptoms.

Ovarian Failure

The essential feature of the menopause is the failure of follicular development which hitherto had occurred continuously. Normal ovarian activity is totally dependent on an adequate stock of oocytes. Although steroid hormones are produced by the somatic cells of the ovary, germ cells are involved in the development and differentiation of the theca and granulosa cells. In reproductive life a number of primordial follicles start to develop, the number being related to the total number of ovarian oocytes. A finite number of oocytes are laid down in fetal life (about 7 million) and once this number has been exhausted in adult life irreversible ovarian failure occurs [1].

The factors regulating the number of oocytes formed during fetal life and their subsequent recruitment are unknown. The quality of the oocytes appears to play some role in the rate of atresia; in chromosome abnormalities like Turner's syndrome there are a normal number of oocytes in fetal life but they have usually all undergone atresia by the time of puberty [2]. The timing of ovarian failure, therefore, will be a function of the total number of oocytes, and the rate at which they are recruited and undergo atresia. In certain breeds of sheep and mice this varies between different genetic strains [3]. There may be genetic factors in women because the age of onset of the menopause is much closer in monozygotic than in dizygotic twins [4].

The median age of the menopause in most societies is remarkably constant at around 50 years [5]. Unlike the age of menarche, there is no convincing evidence that this age has altered in the last 100 years. Very few factors are known to influence the onset of ovarian failure other than those which damage and/or destroy oocytes, i.e. radiation or cytotoxic drugs. There is reasonably good evidence that the menopause occurs at a younger age in women who smoke although the mechanism by which this occurs is unknown [6].

Endocrine Changes and the Menopause

The cessation of menstrual periods is due to a lack of stimulation of the endometrium by ovarian steroids. In the reproductive years the uterus is subject to cyclical fluctuations in the secretion of oestradiol and progesterone which occur as a result of growth and regression of the Graafian follicle and corpus luteum. In premenopausal women the follicle is the source of over 90% of oestradiol produced in the body and when folliculogenesis ceases at the menopause, the levels of oestradiol fall markedly. Associated with the marked decline in the concentration of oestradiol, the secretion of FSH and LH by the anterior pituitary rises and, hence, the characteristic feature of the menopause is hypergonadotrophic hypogonadism (Fig. 1.1).

However, the postmenopausal woman is not totally devoid of oestrogen. The concentration of oestrone is much less than that of oestradiol, suggesting an extraovarian source of oestradiol [7]. Although both the adrenal and the postmenopausal ovary secrete some oestrogen, the contribution to the total production rate is insignificant compared to that produced by extraglandular conversion of androgen precursors [8]. The most important androgen used for production of oestrogens by the postmenopausal woman is androstenedione. This C_{19} steroid, which has little, if any, intrinsic androgenic activity, is converted in the liver and fat tissue to oestrone, which is the major oestrogen in peripheral plasma. Although the extent of extraglandular conversion is influenced

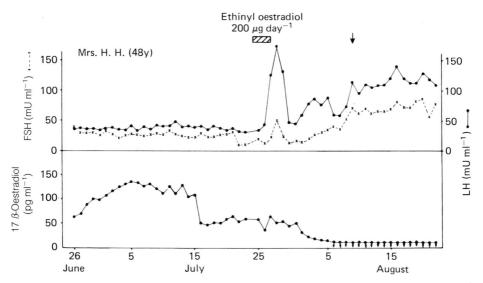

Fig. 1.1 Concentration of oestradiol, LH and FSH in a woman (48 years) during the menopausal transition. Note the anovulatory cycle which preceded the last menstrual period. (▨). Ethinyl oestradiol 200 μg/day for 3 days provoked a normal positive feedback of LH. The arrow indicates the onset of hot flushes. (Data from Van Look et al. 1977 [19].)

by age and obesity, the amount of oestrone produced is mainly dependent on the quantity of secreted androstenedione. Although the postmenopausal ovary secretes some androstenedione, the major source is the adrenal and is responsive to ACTH. The adrenal source of androstenedione is clearly illustrated by the fact that its concentration in postmenopausal women shows a diurnal variation, with its concentration coinciding with that of cortisol (and presumably ACTH) [9]. The production of adrenal androgens is related to body weight and it is likely, therefore, that the higher amount of oestrogen produced in fat women is due to higher production of androgen precursor as well as its higher rate of aromatisation in fat tissue.

The postmenopausal ovary secretes testosterone, contributing approximately 50% of the total blood production rate [10]. After oophorectomy there is little change in the concentration of androstenedione but that of testosterone falls significantly. Testosterone is probably mainly produced by stroma cells of the ovary which are stimulated by the raised levels of LH. Dehydroepiandrosterone (DHA) and its sulphate (DHAS) are also secreted by the adrenal in large amounts but their contribution to oestrogen production by extraglandular conversion into androstenedione and subsequently into oestradiol is negligible except in pregnancy.

In summary, in postmenopausal women the production of oestrogen drops markedly and leads, in many women, to signs of oestrogen deficiency. However, the levels of oestrone and oestradiol vary greatly between women and in some the production of oestrogens from extraglandular sources may be sufficient to stimulate endometrial hypertrophy and bleeding.

Gonadotrophins

A characteristic of the menopausal state is the marked rise in the concentration of both FSH and LH [11]. In some women who are still having regular menstrual cycles the concentration of FSH (but not LH) may rise several years before the menopause [12]. This is most apparent in the early and mid-follicular phase of the cycle, often returning to within the normal range during the luteal phase. The concentration of oestradiol and progesterone in these cycles is usually normal.

Recent research has offered some insight into this apparent paradox. The ovary secretes inhibin, a glycoprotein which has the property of suppressing the secretion of FSH selectively. During the follicular phase of the cycle, inhibin is secreted by antral follicles but during the luteal phase virtually all the inhibin is secreted by the corpus luteum. It is possible, therefore, that during the menopausal transition as the total number of follicles in the ovary declines, the basal secretion of inhibin by the ovary is reduced and, hence, the level of FSH rises (Fig. 1.2). However, after ovluation the corpus luteum may secrete normal amounts of inhibin, which, together with oestradiol, suppress FSH levels to normal. Recent preliminary data show a siginificant decline in the concentration of inhibin in women aged between 40 and 50 years (E. A. Lenton, D. Woodward, D. deKrester, D. Robertson, personal communication).

The rise in the concentration of FSH is not solely due to increased secretion. It has become apparent that many heterogeneous forms of FSH are produced by the anterior pituitary, differing with respect to their charge and electrophoretic mobility [13]. At the menopause the pituitary secretes more negatively charged forms of FSH which have a longer half-life. Thus part of the rise in the concentration of FSH is due to its slower clearance (and hence increased biopotency when measured in an in vivo bioassay) as well as to increased rate of

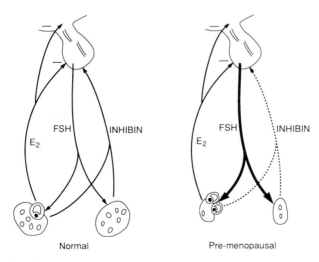

Normal   Pre-menopausal

Fig. 1.2.   Suggested hypothalamic–pituitary–ovarian relationships in menopausal transition. As the number of oocytes declines the secretion of inhibin falls and hence the basal level of FSH rises.

secretion due to removal of negative feedback effect of oestradiol and inhibin [14]. These differences in clearance are due to different subtypes of the same hormone, because when sialic acid is removed by treatment with neuraminidase, the residual molecules have identical electrophoretic mobility. These changes are a result of the hypo-oestrogenic state because they can be reversed by administration of exogenous oestrogen [15].

The rise in concentration of FSH in the premenopausal years may account for the shortening of the follicular phase [16] and the higher incidence of dizygotic twinning which occurs in late reproductive life [17]. The level of FSH is maintained above the threshold required to activate small antral follicles into the preovulatory phase, with the result that although the total number of antral follicles is diminished, two or more large antral follicles are selected for ovulation (Fig. 1.2). Thus with more than one preovulatory follicle the secretion of oestradiol reaches the level necessary to provoke an LH surge sooner and, hence, the follicular phase is shortened.

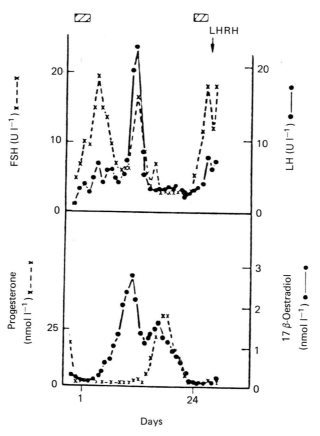

Fig. 1.3. Short follicular phase in a woman (49 years) during the menopausal transition. Cross-hatched bars indicate menstruation. Note the monotropic elevation of FSH in the follicular phase which is suppressed during the luteal phase. (From Van Look et al. 1977 [19].)

The pattern of menstrual cycles prior to the menopause is very variable [18]. Some women have short cycles due to shortened follicular phase whereas many will have prolonged intermenstrual intervals (Fig. 1.3). In these women there may be several weeks without any evidence of follicular activity as indicated by low oestrogen levels, during which time the concentration of FSH rises progressively and may reach the menopausal range [19]. Eventually the levels of oestrogen rise and the concentration of FSH falls although it may take several weeks before it reaches the normal range. Although there is no direct information about ovarian morphology in these women, it is tempting to speculate that the number of follicles has fallen below that necessary to ensure that at least one small antral follicle is available each month for development as a preovulatory follicle.

Menopausal Symptoms

A number of symptoms occur in women at the time of the menopause and are therefore thought by women to be due to "the change of life". More specifically because the menopause is due to ovarian failure, it has been assumed by many that these symptoms are due to oestrogen deficiency. In a carefully conducted survey of nearly 300 women in general practice in Aberdeen, Barbara Thompson and her colleagues conclude that only hot flushes and night sweats were specifically related to menopausal status itself rather than age, social circumstance, etc. [20]. Certainly these two symptoms are consistently relieved by administration of oestrogen.

Hot flushes are associated with a generalised discharge of the sympathetic system with resulting vasodilation of skin blood vessels, increased heart rate and palpitations. The increased skin temperature has been shown to coincide in most instances with a pulse of LH in blood, suggesting that the two events are interrelated [21]. It is presumed that pulses of LH are due to stimulation of the anterior pituitary by GnRH secreted in association with a co-ordinated discharge of hypothalamic GnRH neurons. The hot flush is not due to either LH or GnRH because it occurs in hypophysectomised women [22]. It seems more likely that change in the synthesis of neurotransmitters, such as dopamine, noradrenaline, prostaglandins and/or serotonin, which are involved in release of GnRH is also involved in neuroendocrine mechanisms responsible for hot flushes. Although hot flushes are associated with hypo-oestrogenism, they occur only in women with an intact hypothalamus following withdrawal of oestrogen. Thus, women with primary gonadal failure do not experience hot flushes unless they have previously been treated with oestrogen. Withdrawal of oestrogen in women with hypothalamic amenorrhoea following psychological stress or weight loss does not result in hot flushes, in contrast to those with idiopathic gonadotrophin deficiency (Kallmann's syndrome) [23]. These studies clearly indicate that whereas the hypothalamic events which lead to hot flushes occur coincidentally with LH and therefore presumably GnRH pulses, the instability of the thermoregulating centre is still apparent in the absence of GnRH neurons. However, even when GnRH neurons are present, if there is a suppression of hypothalamic function associated with a disturbance in the pattern of neutrotransmitters, hot flushes do not occur even following withdrawal of oestrogens.

In addition to hot flushes there are a number of symptoms and signs directly due to deficiency of oestrogen which may occur in postmenopausal women. Vaginal atrophy may result in senile vaginitis and the complaint of dyspareunia. Atrophy of the breasts, thinning of vulvar skin (kraurosis vulvae) and cystitis are all amenable to treatment with oestrogens. Osteoporosis due to accelerated loss of bone mineral will be discussed in following chapters. Many of the other symptoms which women complain of at this time, e.g. insomnia, loss of memory etc., may not be due directly to withdrawal of oestrogen but are certainly aggravated by the troublesome physical symptoms of oestrogen deficiency.

Conclusions

In the last 90 years fundamental changes have taken place in the demography of all countries of the world. For example, the average life expectancy of a British woman has risen from 50 years in 1900 to over 75 years at the present time. At the same time the average number of children has fallen progressively so that in 1990 a women is likely to be pregnant or breast feeding for only two or three years during reproductive life. This change in life expectancy and pattern of reproduction has profound effects on the factors influencing women's health. Thus, there has been a dramatic reduction in the maternal mortality and the debility caused by repeated childbearing but a marked rise in the morbidity associated with menstrual disorders. The deferment of the age of first pregnancy is one of the important factors associated with the high incidence of carcinoma of the breast in Western society. Nearly all methods of contraception result in repeated ovarian cycles which are thought to play some role in the aetiology of endometriosis, uterine fibroids and ovarian cancer.

It is paradoxical that at the menopause, the burden of menstruation is replaced by the problems of ovarian failure. Very few other mammals live long enough in the natural state to exhibit a menopause, although ovarian failure has been reported in rhesus monkeys in captivity [24]. There would appear to be no biological advantage in prolonging life expectancy beyond the time when reproduction is no longer possible and, hence, the menopausal state is probably a consequence of man's "unnatural" extension of life expectancy. As 90% of women will survive at least to 65 years the majority will spend a significant proportion of their lives in the postmenopausal state. It is clearly important that we should have information about the consequences of ovarian failure so that advice can be given as to the management which will result in optimal health.

References

1. Baker TG. Radiosensitivity of mammalian oocytes with particular reference to the human female. Am J Obstet Gynecol 1971; 110:746–61.
2. Carr DHL, Haggar RA, Hart AG. Germ cells in the ovaries of 40 female infants. Am J Clin Pathol 1968; 49:521–6.
3. Faddy MJ, Gosden RG, Edwards RG. Ovarian follicle dynamics in mice; a comparative study of three inbred strains and an F1 hybrid. J Endocrinol 1983; 96:23–33.
4. Goecke H. Die Klinik des Klimakteriums. Arch Gynak 1959; 193:33–49.

5. Gosden RG. Biology of menopause; the causes and consequences of ovarian ageing. London, Academic Press, 1985; 8.
6. Kaufman DW, Slone D, Rosenberg L, Miettinen OS, Shapiro S. Cigarette smoking and age at natural menopause. Am J Public Health 1980; 70:420–2.
7. Baird DT. Steroids in blood reflecting ovarian function. In: Baird DT, Strong JA, eds. Control of gonadal steroid secretion. Edinburgh: Edinburgh University Press, 1971; 176–187.
8. Siiteri PK, MacDonald PC. The role of extraglandular estrogen in human endocrinology. In: Greep RO, Ashwood EB, eds. Handbook of physiology, Section 7, Endocrinology Vol II, Part 1. Washington, American Physiological Society, 1973:615–29.
9. Vermeulen A. The hormonal activity of the postmenopausal ovary. J Clin Endocrinol Metab 1976; 42:247–53.
10. Judd HL, Judd GE, Lucas WE, Yen SSC. Endocrine function of the postmenopausal ovary: concentration of androgens and estrogens in ovarian and peripheral vein blood. J Clin Endocrinol Metab 1974; 39:1020–4.
11. Wide L. Radioimmunoabsorbent assay of follicle stimulating hormone and luteinizing hormone in serum and urine of men and women. Acta Endocrinol (Copenh) 1973; Suppl. 174.
12. Sherman BM, Wallace RB. Menstrual patterns: menarche through menopause. In: Baird DT, Michie EA, eds. Mechanism of menstrual bleeding, vol 25. New York: Raven Press, 1985; 157–63.
13. Wide L. Follicle-stimulating hormones in anterior pituitary glands from children and adults differ in relation to sex and age. J Endocrinol 1989; 123:519–29.
14. Wide L, Wide M. Higher plasma diasappearance rate in the mouse for pituitary follicle stimulating hormone of young women compared to that of men and eldery women. J Clin Endocrinol Metab 1984; 58:426–9.
15. Wide L. Male and female forms of human follicle stimulating hormone in serum. J Clin Endocrinol Metab 1982; 55:682–8.
16. Sherman BM, Wallace RB, Treloar AE. The menopausal transition: endocrinological and epidemiological considerations. J Biosoc Sci [Suppl] 1979; 6:19–35.
17. Parkes AS. Multiple births in women. J Reprod Fertil [Suppl] 1969; 6:105–16.
18. Trelaor AE, Boynton RE, Benn BG, Brown BW. Variation of the human menstrual cycle throughout reproductive life. Int J Fertil 1967; 12:77–126.
19. Van Look PFA, Lothian H, Hunter WM, Michie EA, Baird DT. Hypothalmic–pituitary–ovarian function in perimenopausal women. Clin Endocrinol 1977; 7:13–31.
20. Thompson B, Hart SA, Durno D. Menopausal age and symptomatology in a general practice, J Biosoc Sci 1973; 5:71–82.
21. Tataryn IV, Meldrum DR, Lu KH, Frumar AM, Judd HL. LH, FSH and skin temperature during the menopausal hot flush. J Clin Endocrinol Metab 1979; 49:152–4.
22. Mulley G, Mitchell JRA, Tattersall RB. Hot flushes after hypophysectomy. Br Med J 1977; 2:1062.
23. Gambone J, Meldrum DR, Laufer L, Chang RJ, Lu JKH, Judd HL. Further delineation of hypothalamic dysfunction responsible for menopausal hot flushes. J Clin Endocrinol Metab 1984; 59:1097–102.
24. van Wagenen G. Vital statistics from a breeding colony: reproduction and pregnancy outcome in Macaca mulatta. J Med Primatol 1972; 1:3–28.

Chapter 2

The Biology of Bone

D. C. Anderson

In this volume there is a danger that, because such an important condition as osteoporosis is being considered, bones may be viewed solely in terms of this degenerative disease. Yet of course we cannot hope to understand the process of degeneration of bone, whether through osteoporosis or any other bone disease, without first considering how and why the bone developed in the first place. This chapter therefore, briefly outlines five important aspects of bone which relate to its normal development and function.

Classification of Bone Types

Bone can be classified in a number of different ways. Three such classifications relate respectively to development, location, and microscopic structure.

Classification by Development

The two main categories are endochrondrial (or cartilaginous) and intra-membranous. Long bones for example form upon a cartilaginous structure which provides the initial anatomical form of the bone, in a cartilaginous mould which grows as the organism grows. At a particular stage the cartilage cells in certain parts of the bone, initially the central diaphysis, undergo terminal differentiation which involves their eventual death. Before dying they make matrix components different from the normal glycosaminoglycans of cartilage. These include the production of type 1 collagen in place of type 2 and type 10 collagens, and production of matrix vesicles, which are necessary for mineralisation. The cartilaginous matrix around the dying hypertrophic chondrocytes calcifies, and in so doing obtains the properties which allow osteoclasts to resorb it, a process which is immediately followed by formation of true histological bone. In children and adolescents who are still growing, this process is confined to the epiphyseal growth plates. This process of growth at the ends of the long bone is complemented by the increasing diameter of the cortex of the bone, as a result of deposition of lamellar bone by the periosteal cells. The long bone expands and remodels progressively as this process is complemented by reabsorption in the endosteum. It is evident that the hypertrophic cartilaginous cells provide the initial structure upon which trabecular bone, seen for example at the ends of the femur, is ultimately formed.

Intramembranous bone, in contrast, does not require a pre-existing cartilaginous matrix. An example is the calvaria (vertex of the skull). As the bone is developing the sutures are composed of highly proliferative cells, and between them are calcifying plates of bone. These plates have formed close to blood vessels by de novo differentiation of osteoblast precursors present in the mesenchyme overlying the membranes, probably in association with endothelial cells. The structure of these plates is more complicated than would first appear to be the case, their growth being partly dictated by the underlying brain, which is expanding rapidly in early fetal life, and partly by the location within them of blood vessels that drain into the venous sinuses. It is evident therefore that when the bone is first being formed, factors other than the classical bone cells discussed below are of great importance in determining the final structure of the bone. In the calvaria laterally plates of cartilaginous and membranous bone are closely apposed. As with cartilaginous bone, as soon as intramembranous bone forms it becomes invaded by bone-resorbing osteoclasts; these facilitate expansion of the plates, in part by keeping open the channels around blood vessels which are then filled in concentrically as they expand.

Classification by Location

Bone can also be classified into cortical bone (which could be thought of as either periosteal or true cortical (Haversian) bone), and trabecular or cancellous bone. The relative proportions of cortical and trabecular bone vary enormously within an anatomical bone such as the femur or the radius. Thus the shaft of the femur consists almost entirely of cortical bone (Fig. 2.1), whereas the proximal femur consists of a thin rim of cortical bone and underlying this is a large amount of densely packed cancellous bone. These considerations are clearly important in relation to osteoporosis, when we come to consider the application of diagnostic methods and their interpretation at different sites.

Classification According to Microscopic Structure

Bone may be woven or lamellar, and may be considered to be primary (the bone is first laid down), or secondary (bone that is laid down after undergoing a process of bone resorption). Viewed with cross-polarised light, woven bone appears amorphous; furthermore the osteocytes in woven bone are rounded and do not appear compressed. Lamellar bone, by contrast, has an ordered array of

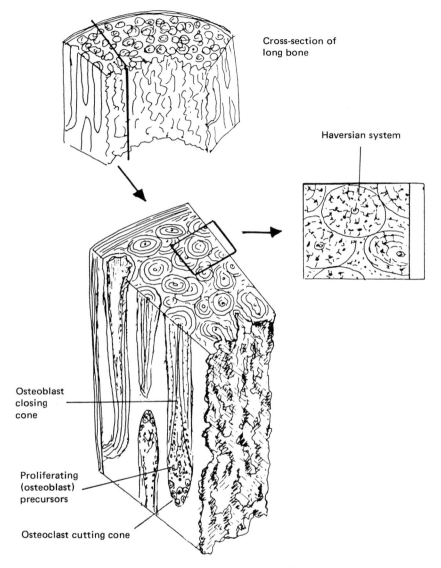

Cross-section of
long bone

Haversian system

Osteoblast
closing
cone

Proliferating
(osteoblast)
precursors

Osteoclast cutting cone

Fig. 2.1. Diagram to illustrate the overall structure of cortical bone, and the formation of Haversian systems.

collagen fibres and the osteocytes contained among them are much more flattened. What dictates whether woven or lamellar bone is produced is not entirely clear. In many diseases where bone is laid down extremely rapidly, however, such as in Paget's disease (Fig. 2.2), it appears to be principally woven bone. In lamellar bone the collagen fibres are laid down parallel to the bone surface; their orientation in that plane varies in a regular way, giving rise to the

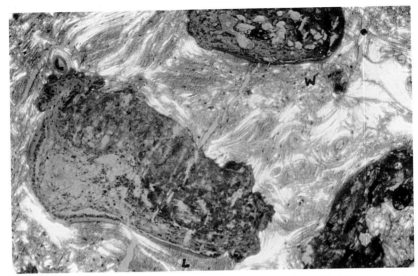

Fig. 2.2.   Bone from a case of Paget's disease, viewed with cross-polarised light to show a mixture of lamellar (L) or woven (W) bone. Bone turnover is greatly increased due to uncontrolled osteoclastic activity.

appearance of banded lamellae. The primary periosteal bone is lamellar as is that normally laid down on trabecular surfaces.

The structure of the (secondary) Haversian systems is important because they probably contribute greatly to the final strength, particularly of the long bones. They are lined up principally parallel to the long axis, and their stucture can be best understood by appreciating the process whereby they have been formed. They are initiated by the onset of osteoclastic resorption, which in cortical bone is tunnelling in nature; a phalanx of osteoclasts enters the bone from blood vessels or the underlying marrow cavity and cores out a tunnel of bone some 50–100 μm across and up to several millimetres in length. For reasons that are not understood there is a strong preference for these tunnels to be orientated along the long axis of the bone. In the wake of this advancing resorption cone and at a much more leisurely pace, the space is filled in, by a process which involves the establishment of a central blood supply, proliferation of osteoblast precursors and their subsequent filling-in of the cavity (except its central core) with lamellar bone. This bone encases as expected a lattice-work of intercommunicating osteocytes, in cytoplasmic contact through their canalicular processes. The final product in longitudinal and cross-section is illustrated in Fig. 2.1. On the surface of trabecular bone this process is not seen in such stark form, and it is interesting that many talks concerning osteoporosis imply that this is a two-dimensional process. It is true that the scalloping-out and subsequent filling-in of a Howship's lacuna does lead to the production of a relatively flat disc of new bone; the orderly three-dimensional nature of the whole process is much more dramatic in the cortex.

The Origin of Bone Cells (Fig. 2.3)

The osteogenic cells are chondroblasts (which become chrondrocytes) and osteoblasts (which become osteocytes). For the sake of clarity it is important that the term "osteoblast" is reserved for a cell that is actively laying down bone. These cells vary in overall shape from plump to rather flattened, and they are metabolically highly active. They produce both the organic matrix and the mechanism for it to mineralise. Ultimately the mature osteoblast may either die or become entombed as a viable osteocyte, or it may finish as a surface osteocyte (the so-called lining cell). In an Haversian system, and probably in a trabecular packet too, all the proliferation of osteoblast precursors occurs before they start to lay down bone [1]. These precursors evidently are organised so that those nearest to the bone surface complete their differentiation and/or maturation first, followed progressively by more superficial cells, until the process is completed and a new Haversian system or trabecular bone packet is formed (Fig. 2.1).

What is known about the origin of these cells is summarised diagrammatically in Fig. 2.3. The evidence for this sort of lineage is now very strong, based on isolation of cloning of cells and their implantation into special chambers in animals in vivo [2–4]. It is evident there is a pluripotential osteogenic stem cell, and going further back probably a general stromal cell precursor, the precursor of marrow fibroblastic, adipocytic reticular and osteogenic cells. The bifurcation point to cartilage- or bone-forming cells probably occurs quite late in this process of differentiation.

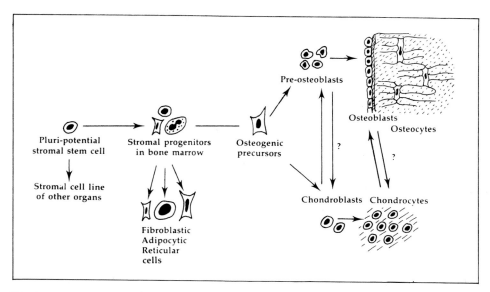

Fig. 2.3. Summary of current evidence concerning the lineage of osteogenic cells. (Reproduced from [4] with permission.)

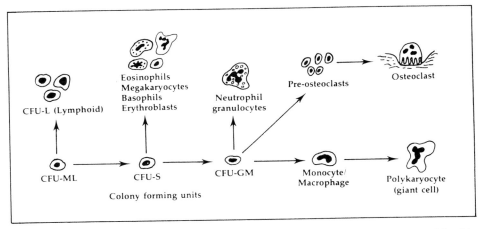

Fig. 2.4. Proposed origin of the osteoclast: see text for details. (Reproduced from [4] with permission.)

Origin and Structure of Osteoclasts (Fig. 2.4)

The osteoclast is an extremely interesting and complicated cell that is multi-nucleated and forms by fusion of precursor cells. It is characterised by a clear (sealing) zone round its perimeter, by numerous mitochondria and vacuoles, and a so-called ruffled border which overlies an acid and proteolytic lake into which are secreted protons which dissolve the mineral and hydrolytic enzymes which destroy collagen (Fig. 2.5). The cells are motile, at least while not resorbing bone, and their bone-resorbing properties have been extensively studied in vitro.

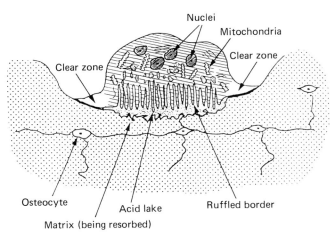

Fig. 2.5. Diagram to illustrate the structure of a bone-resorbing osteoclast.

Concerning the origin of the osteoclasts, a number of transplant experiments, for example between quail and chick, and more recently cloning studies have demonstrated quite clearly that the osteoclast is a bone marrow-derived cell (see ref. 4 for review). It would appear that there are various branch points as with the stromal cell, the product being committed progressively to more and more specialised options.

Bone Matrix and its Mineral Mineralisation

The mature osteoblast lays down matrix which consists of collagen (almost entirely type 1 collagen) and non-collagen proteins which include osteocalcin, osteonectin and osteopontin. The process involves first formation of a tropo-collagen matrix which then becomes cross-linked to form mature type 1 collagen. Osteoporosis is a feature of osteogenesis imperfecta where there is a failure of production of normal type 1 collagen. Matrix vesicles are important and act as the nucleation site for mineralisation between the collagen bundles. This is then followed by orderly hydroxyapatite crystal formation. After the matrix has been laid down, by a process that it not fully understood, matrix vesicles which contain the enzyme alkaline phosphatase (thought to act by breaking down pyrophosphate) act as nucleation sites for formation of hydroxy-apatite crystals. Osteoblasts also pump calcium ions into the bone space, thereby facilitating a deposition of calcium hydroxyapatite.

Bone Cell "Coupling"

Frost [5] has been responsible for many of the concepts loosely described as bone cell coupling. He described the phases of activation, where osteoclasts come into an area to initiate the process, resorption, reversal and formation. These events (as illustrated in Fig. 2.1) are in fact a continuous process. A good analogy may be to think of the Channel Tunnel: at the advance end is osteoclast machinery cutting into the bone and this process is closely linked to the process behind it of tidying up the surface of the tunnel and producing a lining. The only difference is that in the case of the Haversian system the tunnel is virtually completely filled apart from a small space containing the blood vessel down the middle. Very little is known of the mechanism of this coupling process. My own suspicion is that the coupling results from mature osteoclasts in the process of resorbing bone producing sufficient of a growth factor or factors to promote replication, both of their own precursors and of osteoblast precursors. Coupling is necessary to maintain the former process particularly in gouging out a Haversian canal, because it is known from experimental work in animals that the average life span of an osteoclast nucleus is in the region of 5–10 days [6] and yet the process of the resorption of the Haversian system may go on for several months. This is an area of active research and also one of considerable lack of clarity in the literature.

Bone Active Hormones and Growth Factors

The classical hormones are parathyroid hormone (PTH), calcitonin, 1,25-dihydroxyvitamin D_3 and, certainly in terms of an action following growth plate, insulin related growth factor 1, which is the mediator of many of the actions of growth hormone. What do we know of the actions of hormones on bone? [7,8]. PTH appears to act via osteoblasts, and possibly on the mature lining cell, to cause that cell to lose contact with its neighbours, thereby exposing the bone surface to a greater chance of interaction with a roving osteoclast. Calcitonin acts directly on osteoclasts (which possess calcitonin receptors and are switched off by this hormone). 1,25-Dihydroxyvitamin D_3 acts both on the mature osteoblasts and also on the osteoclast precursor. It also acts on bone indirectly by its intestinal action, which controls the prevailing level of serum calcium and phosphate and therefore the calcium×phospate product. Oestradiol appears to act directly on the osteoblasts and more recently the existence of androgen receptors in bone has also been shown. What was a very contentious issue seems now to have been resolved and it is generally agreed that oestrogens can act directly upon bone, although whether or not this is their only action remains to be seen.

Mechanism of Action

Some hormones, for example the steroids and 1,25-dihydroxyvitamin D_3, have soluble receptors which act on the nucleus – the so-called zinc finger receptors, which allow transcription and translation of certain parts of the genome. Other cells and other hormones and growth factors, for example parathyroid hormone and probably parathyroid hormone-related peptide, act through a cell surface receptor that is linked via a coupling protein to the enzyme adenylate cyclase. When the hormone binds, this alters the confirmation of the various coupling-protein subunits, and the alpha subunit (having bound to GTP) now disassociates and then binds to the catalytic subunit of adenlyate cyclase, which is activated as a consequence. Calcitonin is thought to act on the osteoclasts by a similar mechanism. Other hormones and growth factors, for example insulin, insulin-related growth factor 1, and probably platelet-derived growth factor, also act through cell surface receptors that are coupled to a tyrosine protein kinase. In the case of insulin there appears to be a two subunit receptor while in others it is a single unit which spans the cell membrane and possesses both hormone-binding and kinase activity.

Another important group of hormones acts via receptors which are also enzymes which break down phospholipids to form diacylglycerol and inositol trisphosphates; the latter in turn leads to the release of calcium from intracellular stores and activation of an enzyme protein kinase C and activation of calmodulin. Yet another method of action is illustrated by gonadotrophin-releasing hormone, which appears to act by opening up cell surface calcium channels, again leading to an increase in intracellular calcium and calmodulin activation. This mechanism is believed to operate for some of the growth factors.

There is no point yet in discussing which are the important growth factors in bone because in many cases this is not yet established. Indeed, in an area where much more is known, namely the control of conventional bone marrow cells, we know that the growth factors act rather like letters of an alphabet – different combinations of letters coding for different paths of differentiation – and it is probably wrong to think in terms of action of a single growth factor. Furthermore, almost certainly the growth factors that are active in bone, derangements of which may be responsible for certain bone diseases, are also important at many other stages in development – first in embryonic life, and for inducing alterations in bone structure, as for example repair of microfractures and remodelling in response to mechanical forces applied to particular bones.

Although at present many of these processes seem far removed from such common diseases as osteoporosis, they should not be ignored if we are to understand the pathophysiology of these disorders.

References

1. Jaworski ZFG, Hooper C. Study of cell kinetics within evolving Haversian systems. J Anat 1980; 131:91–102.
2. Owen M. Lineage of osteogenic cells and their relationship to the stromal systems. J Bone Miner Res 1988; 3:1–25.
3. Bab I, Passi-Even L, Gazit D et al. Osteogenesis in in vivo diffusion chamber cultures of human marrow cells. J Bone Miner Res 1988; 4:373–86.
4. Gordon MT, Anderson DC. The origin of bone cells. Bone 1990; 7:57–60.
5. Frost HM. Dynamics of bone remodelling. In: Bone biodynamics. Boston: Little, Brown, 1964; 315.
6. Ash P, Loutit, JF, Townsend KM. Osteoclasts derived from haematopoietic stem cells. Nature 1980; 283:669–70.
7. Anderson DC. Hormone and the skeleton. In: Smith R, ed. Osteoporosis 1990. London: Royal College of Physicians, 1990; 79–90.
8. Mundy GR. Hormonal factors which influence calcium homeostasis. In: Calcium homeostasis: hypercalcaemia and hypocalcaemia. London: Martin Dunitz, 1989.

Discussion

Anderson: Professor Baird said that inhibin was produced from the antral follicles. Is it really the antral follicles or is it the others in the cohort that are maturing during that cycle?

Baird: It is not the dominant follicle.

Anderson: But my understanding is that as the woman approaches the menopause, a small population of follicles is maturing, one of which will be selected to be the dominant follicle. If it is the antral follicles, is that not incompatible with it coming mainly from the corpus luteum in the luteal phase?

Baird: No, because so much more comes from the corpus luteum in relation to the amount that is produced in the follicular phase. The corpus luteum is producing 90% of the inhibin at any stage, but the production from the two ovaries in the follicular phase is identical. So one can assume that the smaller antral follicles are producing as much as the dominant ones.

Anderson: But the cohort of other follicles which become atretic is equally distributed between the two ovaries?

Baird: Yes.

Stevenson: Could Professor Anderson comment on the role of osteocytes? It has been suggested that these cells, which seem to communicate with each other and communicate with the surface of the bone, might be important as acting as strain gauges.

Anderson: I do not think I am the right person to ask. I suspect that there is no real difference between a surface lining cell, which is probably just an osteocyte that has not been completely buried, and the deep cells that it is communicating with which are classically called osteocytes. I do not know whether they act as strain gauges or not but it would be nice if they did.

Boyde: The theory just mentioned by Dr Stevenson is coupled with the concept that the osteocytes are able to read the strain deformation put into the bone proteoglycans by strain events in the preceding 24-hour period, for example. I can say that from the methodological point of view there is a large amount of room for doubt about the basic observation concerning the possibility of altering the orientation of the bone proteoglycan components. I suspect that we will be back to looking for the cytoskeleton of the osteocyte, the bone lining cell being extremely important in this respect.

Anderson: But the orientation of the osteones in cortical bone (we do not know much about it in trabecular bone) must be dictated by where the osteoclasts have cut out bone. Therefore the question we should be asking is what makes an osteoclast boring into cortical bone know to travel north–south rather than east–west or sideways, or to turn its orientation. Does Professor Boyde disagree?

Boyde: No. I think that is the most profoundly interesting thing about cortical bone structure. We have to remember that the canals in cortical bone are nothing other than the capillary bed in that bone and that although the major axis of the capillary bed is the longitudinal grain axis, it is in fact like any other capillary bed and there are lots of oblique directions.

That the osteoclast should know that it should continue to maintain this longitudinal capillary bed axis is extremely interesting. But we could work on the *reductio ad absurdum* principle, that if the osteoclasts bored in the wrong direction they would bore back into an existing canal and would not have any bone to bore into.

Purdie: Could I ask about the postmenopausal ovarian stroma? The data from the Chelsea Hospital I thought very interesting. They switched off the high tonic levels of FSH and LH in postmenopausal women and showed that this resulted in reduced levels of circulating androstenedione and oestrone downstream in the plasma.

Does the postmenopausal ovarian stroma make a significant contribution to health and should the present gynaecological practice of oophorectomy in postmenopausal women during hysterectomy be retained?

Baird: The data are somewhat conflicting. My data of concentrations in plasma in intact women and in women of the comparable age group who have had their postmenopausal ovaries removed is a mean of perhaps seven papers. I think it is compatible with the data from ovarian vein blood in that the difference in concentration of oestrogens is really not enough to account for much secretion of either oestrone or oestradiol. However, the difference in concentration of testosterone between the peripheral blood and the ovarian vein blood is quite considerable, and that would fit in with the fact that the testosterone concentration in postmenopausal women tends to be altered by removing the ovaries, whereas the concentration of androstenedione does not change that much.

Probably the stroma makes androgens and it makes mainly testosterone. I think this is because the activity of 5α-reductase and the 17-keto-reductase is in the direction of testosterone in the stroma.

Studd: Gynaecologists tend to have monocular vision about osteoporosis and treatment in that they feel that the effect of oestrogens is greater than many other treatments, including the classical hormones that Professor Anderson spoke about. Do we know what happens to the new bone formed with oestrogens? Is it normally calcified? Is it normal bone?

Anderson: As far as I know it is normally mineralised bone.

Studd: And the corollary is, if women are producing new bone with oestrogens should they have supplementary calcium as well?

Anderson: Obviously calcium is needed to mineralise bone, but provided one is on a reasonable intake, I doubt if adding supplement makes much difference.

A problem which will be discussed later is, how do they put back the scaffolding? Even if a lot of bone can be laid down with conventional hormones there is a big problem in restoring the scaffolding. That is the big problem with just using oestrogens or more or less anything else in established osteoporosis.

Kanis: I suspect that Professor Baird would not really want to go down in history as saying that the postmenopausal state is "unbiological". Was he implying that a woman's work is done at age 50? Does he not think that there may be a biological function of the menopause in a teleological sense perhaps for rearing children rather than producing children? If not then when does a man's life become "unbiological"?

Baird: It is the dominant male passing on his genes that matters to the species, and as long as he is able to serve women and is allowed to do so in the biological sense that is all that matters for evolution. Whereas the restriction on biology in the female is the ability to first of all get pregnant and second carry that baby through the pregnancy and rear it to the point where it will survive.

In a biological sense we could say there might be some advantage in surviving for some five or six years after the menopause, but in any case the fertility rates between the ages of 40 and 50 years are so low that it really makes very little difference. I suspect that is why in other mammalian species we do not see menopausal animals; they have already passed on their genes to the next generation.

Chapter 3

Symptoms and Metabolic Sequelae of the Menopause

J. W. W. Studd, N. R. Watson and A. Henderson

The endocrinological and metabolic changes which accompany the climacteric produce a multitude of symptoms and have profound effects on the emotional, psychological and physical well-being of women. With increased longevity the vast majority of British women experience the menopause and subsequently spend more than a third of their lives in a state of oestrogen deficiency. Many of the associated symptoms and long-term metabolic disadvantages can be prevented with oestrogen therapy. Thus women receiving oestrogen replacement therapy suffer fewer strokes, fewer heart attacks, and less depression, and their life expectancy is increased by more than 3 years compared to untreated women. It is thus appropriate, when screening for prevention of osteoporosis is considered, that cognizance is made of the fact that women are not merely "skeletons" and the general benefits of oestrogen therapy must be considered.

Vasomotor Symptoms

The most characteristic symptoms of the climacteric are the hot flushes, night sweats, palpitations and headaches which occur due to vasomotor instability and affect 80% of women. The possibility of a link between pituitary hormones and hot flushes was first suggested by Caspar et al. [1]. They reported a one to one correlation between objectively measured flushes and the pulsatile release of luteinising hormone (LH) into the peripheral circulation. However, further research has shown that LH is not the direct cause of hot flushes but that its release is precipitated by an event which also produces hot flushes. This is clear for three reasons. First, hypophysectomised women who secrete virtually no LH experience flushes with the menopause [2]. Second, preventing LH pulses by long-term treatment with a potent gonadotrophin releasing hormone (GnRH) agonist does not stop and may in fact worsen hot flushes [3]. Third, with hormone replacement therapy the elimination of hot flushes occurs before suppression of gonadotrophins to premenopausal levels [4].

It is also unlikely that GnRH is necessary for the triggering of hot flushes. Women with isolated gonadotrophin deficiency representing a defect in GnRH production still experience hot flushes which are indistinguishable objectively from those of menopausal women [5]. Further research on the neurotransmitter input into the hypothalamic GnRH releasing neurons is therefore required to elucidate the exact mechanism of flushing.

Thermal entrainment studies measure the changes in peripheral capillary blood flow with changes in temperature and indicate excellent control of temperature and skin blood flow in the premenopausal woman. This balance is achieved by the thermoregulatory centre of the hypothalamus, which controls the autonomic nervous system and which breaks down after the menopause with the decline in oestrogen levels, resulting in hot flushes [6,7]. In a study by Brincat et al. [8] all the postmenopausal women had poor vascular control at rest which showed a dose-related correction with oestrogen therapy. Thus treatment with oestrogens produced a brisker blood-flow response of smaller magnitude with little change in the overall blood flow from one stimulus to the next. Erlik et al. [9] in their "sleepgram" studies have shown that these vasomotor attacks occurring at night in menopausal and postmenopausal women are associated with recurrent waking periods. Thus insomnia, chronic fatigue and to some extent depression may also be a direct result of vasomotor instability.

Winner et al. [10] have also shown that women between the ages of 50 and 60 years have more falling attacks than men of the same age (Fig. 3.1), in part due

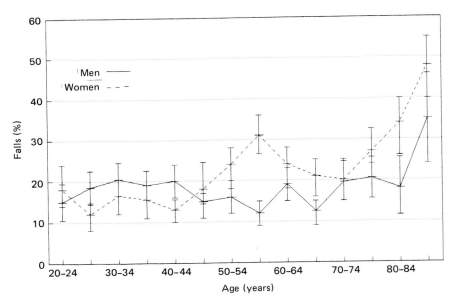

Fig. 3.1. Proportion of falls with age. (Modified from Winner et al. [10].)

to the giddiness produced by these vasomotor symptoms. As fractures are a result of changes in bone density and the forward force of falling it is certain that the giddiness and locomotor instability of the climacteric are major factors in the increased incidence of fractures in the older woman.

Vasomotor symptoms are simple to treat with a small dose of oestrogens by any route, and will usually disappear within 10 days of commencing therapy. By doing so the physician removes not only the discomfort of facial flushing and body sweats, but also the exhaustion resulting from interrupted sleep, and the giddiness and subsequent falls occurring in women who may, unknowingly, have an osteoporotic skeleton.

Local Atrophy

The symptoms of local atrophy affecting target organs are also classical complaints related to oestrogen deficiency. Vaginal dryness, dyspareunia and atrophic vaginitis are virtually universal menopausal problems which are easy to treat with systemic or local oestrogens. Fragmentation of elastic fibres, fusion of collagen fibres and diminution of cell volume all occur, resulting in involution of the uterus and non-calcified fibroids. The cervix similarly decreases in size, becoming flush with the narrowed vaginal vault. The glycogen content of vaginal epithelial cells falls in proportion to declining oestrogen levels. Subsequently commensal lactobacilli decrease in number with loss of the protective acidic pH of the vagina allowing an exudative overgrowth of streptococci, staphylococci and coliforms. Vaginal skin thickness decreases, vaginal walls lose their rugosity and are characteristically pale pink and more fragile, and numerous tiny red punctate points of capillary loops can be seen through the thin vaginal skin, revealing the clinical picture of atrophic vaginitis. A vaginal swab even on an unstained saline preparation will reveal few superficial pyknotic cells and many round large nucleated parabasal and basal cells. This indicates a low maturation index as a result of declining oestrogen exposure.

The lower urinary tract also suffers from this process of generalised atrophy. This will be discussed in more detail in Chapter 6 but the importance of the "urethral syndrome" and recurrent symptoms of dysuria, urgency and incontinence should not be overlooked. These symptoms are probably due to loss of collagen from the bladder and urethral sphincter, and urinary tract atrophy. Versi et al. [11] showed that various urethral pressure parameters correlate well with skin collagen content. Predictably these troublesome symptoms do not respond to antibiotics or antispasmodics but transitional epithelial cells of the urinary tract respond well to oestrogen therapy, which successfully alleviates symptoms.

Generalised Atrophy

Women frequently complain of dry, thin skin, brittle nails and increasing hair loss after the menopause. These symptoms should not be dismissed as imaginary or cosmetic consequences of disturbed self-image. They are due to a generalised loss of collagen which gives the skin of postmenopausal women its typically thin, dry, inelastic and translucent appearance. This is discussed in greater depth in Chapter 5.

There are also systemic symptoms and changes due to loss of collagen. It is likely that the muscle, bone and joint pain which occur in this age group and respond to oestrogen therapy are a result of collagen loss from these tissues.

Most important of all is the hypothesis by Albright et al. [12], that postmenopausal osteoporosis is essentially a disorder of connective tissue associated with thin skin and low oestrogen levels. The collagen of the bone matrix is lost, with demineralisation occurring as a secondary effect. This view is a logical one as osteoporotic bone in fact shows normal calcification: overall, however, there is an inadequate amount of bone tissue present. Collagen is the scaffolding of bone and gives bone its strength: calcium determines the brittle nature of bone. Further support for this theory comes from the fact that most of the clinical risk factors for osteoporosis, i.e. caucasian race, anorexia [13] and corticosteroid therapy [14,15], are also associated with thin skin. Afro-Caribbean patients have a much lower incidence of osteoporosis and correspondingly greater skin collagen, and a greater incidence of disorders linked to excess connective tissue, such as fibromyomata and keloid formation.

There is good evidence that oestrogen therapy increases skin thickness [16] and skin collagen [17] but currently there are no data on the effects of equivalent doses of oestrogen on the collagenous bone matrix. This will require a long-term prospective bone biopsy study investigating histomorphometric changes in bone structure.

Peak bone density occurs around the age of 40 years and bone mass is then lost at the rate of about 1% per annum until the menopause. Thus up to 10%–15% of bone mass can be lost before the accelerated bone loss occurs as a consequence of the profound hypo-oestrogenism of the postmenopausal years. This insidious decline in ovarian function ten years before the menopause is also revealed by progressive loss of fertility, an increase in follicle-stimulating hormone (FSH) levels and the appearance of oestrogen-responsive climacteric symptoms in the perimenopausal years.

There is evidence that ovaries conserved at the time of hysterectomy fail prematurely. Siddle at al. [18] showed that in these patients the age of ovarian failure was advanced by a mean of 6 years from the time of the normal menopause. This occurred at whatever age the hysterectomy had been performed and was not merely a feature of the older premenopausal patients. Twenty-five per cent of women developed endocrinological evidence of ovarian failure within two years of a hysterectomy. Several age-related studies of bone density have shown a decreased vertebral and femoral neck bone density in hysterectomised women compared with controls, regardless of whether the ovaries were conserved or not. In a cross-sectional study relating bone density to age, Watson et al. [19] have also shown that the decrease in bone density which occurs following hysterectomy and bilateral oophorectomy shows little difference from that in patients in whom the ovaries are conserved.

The considerable risk of premature pathology suffered by women after oophorectomy is well recognised and all would agree that these patients need prompt and prolonged oestrogen replacement therapy. It may be that those patients who have had a hysterectomy with ovarian conservation run a similar risk of long-term involutional disease.

Psychological

Depression, irritability and fatigue, together with loss of energy and loss of self-confidence, have a complex origin not only related to oestrogen deficiency but also involving a period of psychosocial transition with important domestic stresses [20,21] and feelings of loss of youth and feminity [22]. Such psychological symptoms are common: Montgomery et al. [23] showed an 86% incidence of psychological pathology in menopause clinics studying these selected patients. This compares with a 52% incidence in general gynaecology clinics and 20% in general outpatient clinics, and was even higher than that found in psychiatric outpatients.

There is an excess of depression in women which is found whether figures for hospital admissions, community statistics or suicide attempts are studied [24]. The traditional view of psychiatrists is that this depression is entirely environmental – a view strongly supported by contemporary feminism. There is no doubt that the "empty nest syndrome" [25], death of parents [26], inadequate career opportunities, coupled with an intrinsic loss of self-value around the time of the menopause are substantial causes for depression, but the possibility of a hormonal component to depression in this age group has largely been denied by current psychiatric wisdom.

We believe that this view is wrong. The probability of a hormonal component is suggested by the finding that the excess of depression in women over men occurs only from the age of puberty and is most noticeable at times of rapid hormonal change, i.e. premenstrual depression, postnatal depression and climacteric depression. Conversely, during the last trimester of pregnancy cases of depression are reduced and suicide is rare.

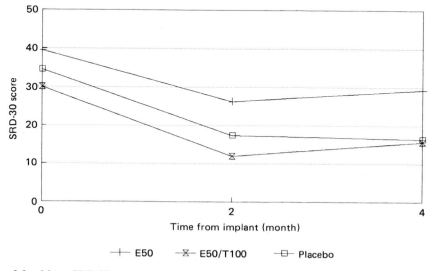

Fig. 3.2. Mean SRD-30 score in postmenopausal patients treated with implants/placebo, using the Kellner and Sheffield Self-rating Scale of Distress. (From Montgomery et al. [23].)

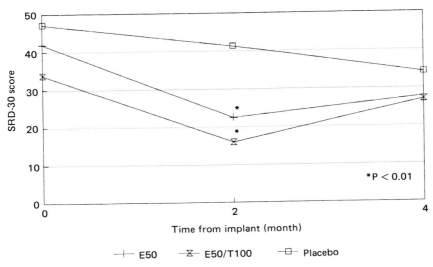

Fig. 3.3. Mean SRD-30 score in perimenopausal patients treated with implants/placebo, using the Kellner and Sheffield Self-rating Scale of Distress. (From Montgomery et a. [23].)

In a randomised placebo-controlled study of oestradiol or oestradiol plus testosterone implants, Montgomery et al. [23] showed a significant improvement in depression and anxiety using the Kellner and Sheffied Self-rating Scale of Distress (SRD–30 scores) in 60 climacteric women. However, this improvement was not demonstrated in those women who were postmenopausal (Fig. 3.2) but was seen only in patients who were symptomatic with regular periods (Fig. 3.3). This supports the view that climacteric women with hormonally responsive depression are likely to be menstruating perimenopausal women. Depression in these women is usually cyclical and is essentially premenstrual depression. Cyclical depression of premenstrual syndrome (PMS) becomes worse with age and blends with the additional psychological symptoms of the climacteric. The tragedy is that the hormonal aetiology of the depression in these women is not recognised because they are still menstruating. Despite the results of the above study and epidemiological studies which have shown that climacteric depression is most common and severe in the 2–3 years preceding cessation of periods [27], up to 30%–40% of women in this age group will be prescribed antidepressants and tranquillisers to which they may become habituated and which may have few beneficial effects.

Magos et al. [28] demonstrated the efficacy of oestradiol implants in the treatment of the cyclical depression of PMS. Watson et al. [29] subsequently showed that oestradiol patches in an anovulatory dose were also an effective treatment for the condition (Figs. 3.4 and 3.5). The addition of sufficient progestogen to prevent endometrial hyperplasia did, however, reproduce some of the cyclical symptoms of the syndrome (Fig. 3.6).

It would seem that the psychological symptoms of the climacteric are a continuum of similar symptoms characteristic of PMS. With time these symptoms become more severe and less cyclical until the patient no longer

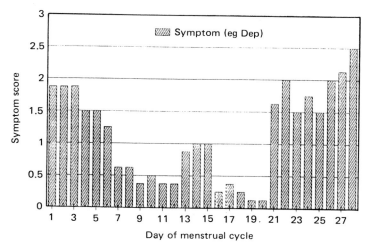

Fig. 3.4. Pretreatment assessment of patients with premenstrual syndrome. (From Watson et al. [29].)

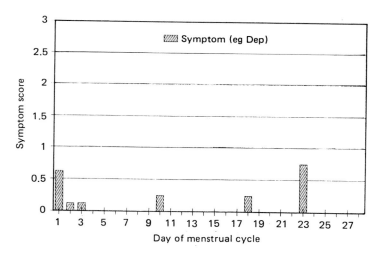

Fig. 3.5. Post-treatment assessment of patients with premenstrual syndrome following treatment with 2 mg oestradiol patch. (From Watson et al. [29].)

experiences even two symptom-free weeks each month. She then suffers almost continuous depression, anxiety and irritability with less cyclical mastalgia but more headaches, vasomotor symptoms, and loss of energy and libido. Recognition that these oestrogen-responsive symptoms may occur for up to 10 years before the menopause and may last for many years after the cessation of periods will be a major advance in the alleviation of menopausal pathology.

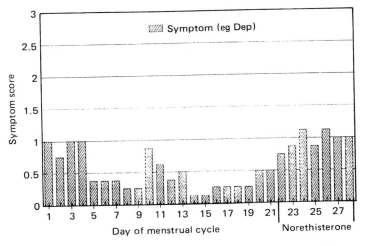

Fig. 3.6. Post-treatment assessment of patients with premenstrual syndrome following treatment with 2 mg oestradioal patch and cyclical norethisterone. (From Watson et al. [29].)

Cardiovascular System

Ischaemic heart disease is the commonest cause of death in both men and women [30]. Premenopausal women have well-documented inherent protection against this condition compared to their male counterparts and epidemiological studies have shown that onset of the disease is delayed by 10–12 years in women. The plasma lipid profiles of such women are consistent with this protective effect and show higher HDL-cholesterol (and particularly HDL_2 subfraction) levels with lower LDL-cholesterol levels than equivalent males [31]. This protection appears to be mediated by oestrogens, which when given after the menopause produce a dramatic reduction of up to 50% in mortality from ischaemic heart disease [32].

Characteristic increase in HDL-cholesterol and decrease in LDL-cholesterol with exogenous oestrogen administration was first shown by Barr et al. in 1952 [33] and has been confirmed by more recent studies [34]. Population studies also indicate that postmenopausal women taking hormone replacement therapy have higher levels of HDL-cholesterol than age-matched controls [35,36]. This increase in HDL is associated particularly with the HDL_2 subfraction [37]. In addition to plasma lipid changes, oestrogen has numerous other effects on the cardiovascular system which may exert a beneficial influence on cardiovascular disease (Table 3.1) [38].

Most long-term studies of oestrogen therapy and the risk of ischaemic heart disease relate to unopposed oestrogen therapy. The effect of supplementary cyclical administration of a progestogen, which is current practice in patients with a uterus, is uncertain and remains of particular concern in view of the possible deleterious effects on plasma lipids. Both natural progesterone and synthetic progestogens produce a fall in plasma triglyceride levels. However, progestogens with moderate or high androgenic activity (norethisterone, levo-norgestrel) lower HDL and HDL_2 subfractions [39] and this change appears to be maintained even with combined oestrogen and progestogen therapy, thus theoretically offsetting the beneficial influence of oestrogen [40]. This action appears to be related to the androgenic and not the progestogenic properties of progestogens. Thus progestogens with mild androgenic activity such as med-oxyprogesterone acetate, or the newer progestins with no androgenic activity such as desogestrel, have not been shown to exert any adverse effects on plasma lipid profiles either in oral contraceptive users [41] or in postmenopausal women [42].

Table 3.1.   Effects of ovarian hormones on the cardiovascular system

Direct effects
Increases arterial blood flow
Stabilises blood flow

Indirect effects
Changes in lipids
   Increases HDL
   Decreases LDL

Changes in chemical mediators
   Catecholamines
   Vasoactive peptides
   Prostaglandins
   Neurotransmitters
   Renin substrate

Conclusion

Oestrogen deficiency commences before cessation of periods and creates generalised physical and psychological pathology. The facts that these problems can be prevented and that useful life can be prolonged for approximately three years with oestrogen replacement therapy should be acknowledged when we are considering the prevention of osteoporosis in postmenopausal women. Our aims should be to make safe and inexpensive oestrogen replacement therapy available to all climacteric women who need it. Targeting resources on the identification of skeletal problems only confounds the real health care challenge.

References

1. Caspar RF, Yen SSC, Wilkes MM. Menopausal flushes: a neuroendocrine link with pulsatile luteinizing hormone secretion. Science 1979; 205:823–5.
2. Meldrum DR, Erlik Y, Lu JKH et al. Objective recorded hot flushes in patients with pituitary insufficiency. J Clin Endocrinol Metab 1981; 52:684–7.
3. Casper RF, Yen SSC. Menopausal flushes: effect of pituitary gonadotrophin desensitisation by a potent luteinizing hormone-releasing factor agonist. J Clin Endocrinol Metab 1981; 53:1056–8.
4. Studd JWW, Chakravarti S, Oram D. The climacteric. In: Greenblatt R, Studd JWW, eds. The menopause, clinics in obstetrics and gynaecology. Philadelphia: W.B. Saunders, 1977; 4:3–29.

5. Gambone J, Meldrum DR, Laufer L et al. Further delineation of hypothalamic dysfunction responsible for menopausal hot flushes. J Clin Endocrinol Metab 1984; 59:1097–102.

6. Tataryn IV, Lomax P, Bajorek JG, Chesarek W, Meldrum DR, Judd HL. Postmenopausal hot flushes: a disorder of thermoregulation. Maturitas 1980; 2:101–7.

7. Kronenberg F, Cote LJ, Linkie DM, Dyrenfurther I, Downey JA. Menopausal hot flushes: thermoregulatory, cardiovascular and circulating catecholamine and LH changes. Maturitas 1984; 6:31–43.

8. Brincat M, de Trafford JC, Lafferty K, Studd JWW. Peripheral vasomotor control and menopausal flushing – a preliminary report. Br J Obstet Gynaecol 1984; 91:1107–10.

9. Erlik Y, Tataryn I, Meldrum D et al. Association of waking episodes with menopausal hot flushes. JAMA 1981; 245:1741–7.

10. Winner ST, Morgan CA, Grimley Evans J. Perimenopausal risk of falling and incidence of distal forearm fracture. Br Med J 1989; 298:1486–8.

11. Versi E, Brincat M, Cardozo LD, O'Dowd T, Cooper D, Studd JWW. Correlation of urethral phsiology and skin collagen in postmenopausal women. Br J Obstet Gynaecol 1988; 2:147–52.

12. Albright F, Bloomberg E, Smith PH. Postmenopausal osteoporosis. Trans Assoc Am Physicians 1940; 55:298–305.

13. Savvas M, Treasure J, Studd J. Fogelman I, Moniz C, Brincat M. The effect of anorexia nervosa on skin thickness, skin collagen and bone density. Br J Obstet Gynaecol 1989; 96:1392–4.

14. Kirby JD, Munro DD. Steroid induced atrophy in an animal and human model. Br J Dermatol 1976; 94:111–19.

15. Arho P. Skin thickness and collagen content in some endocrine and connective tissue diseases Acta Derm Venerol 1972: 69 (Suppl):1–48.

16. Brincat M, Studd JWW, Moniz CF, Parsons V, Darby AJ. Skin thickness and skin collagen mimic an index of osteoporosis in the postmenopausal woman. In: Christiansen C, et al. eds. Osteoporosis. Proceedings of the Copenhagen international symposium on osteoporosis, 1984; 353–5.

17. Brincat M, Moniz CF, Studd JWW, Darby AJ, Magos AL, Cooper D. Sex hormones and skin collagen content in postmenopausal women. Br Med J 1983; 287:1337–8.

18. Siddle N, Sarrel P, Whitehead M. The effect of hysterectomy on the age at ovarian failure: identification of a subgroup of women with premature loss of ovarian function and literature review. Fertil Steril 1987; 47:94–100.

19. Watson NR, Studd JWW, Henderson AF. The effect of simple hysterectomy on bone density in premenopausal women. Proceedings of the second congress of the international society of gynaecological endocrinology, Jerusalem, Israel, 18–23 March 1990 (in press).

20. Dominion J. The role of psychiatry in the menopause. Clin Obstet Gynecol 1977; 4:241–58.

21. Schneider M, Brotherton P. Physiological, psychological and situation stresses in depression during the climacteric. Maturitas 1979; 1:153–8.

22. Kaufert PA. Myth and menopause. Soc. Health Ill 1982; 4:141–66.

23. Montgomery JC, Brincat M, Tapp A, Appleby L, Versi E, Fenwick PBC, Studd JWW. Effect of oestrogen and testosterone implants on psychological disorders in the climacteric. Lancet 1987; i:297–9.

24. Studd JWW, Watson NR. Estrogens and depression in women. In: Belfort P, Pinotti JA, Eskes TKAB, eds. Proceedings of the 12th world congress of gynecology and obstetrics, Rio, 1988; 297–301.

25. Van Keep PA, Kellerhals JM. The impact of socio-cultural factors on symptom formation. Psychother Psychosom 1974; 23:251–63.

26. Brown GW, Harris T. Social origins of depression. London: Tavistock Publications, 1978.

27. Jaszmann L. Epidemiology of climacteric and post-climacteric complaints. In: Van Keep PA, Lauritzen C, eds. Ageing and oestrogens. Basel: Karger, 1973; 22–5.

28. Magos AL, Brincat M, Studd JWW. Treatment of the pre-menstrual syndrome by subcutaneous oestradiol implants and cyclical oral norethisterone – a placebo controlled study. Br Med J 1986; 1:1629–33.

29. Watson NR, Studd JWW, Riddle AF, Savvas M. Suppression of ovulation by transdermal oestradiol patches. Br Med J 1988; 297:900–1.

30. Castelli W. Epidemiology of coronary heart disease: The Framingham study. Am J Med 1984; 76:4–12.

31. Gordon T, Castelli WP, Hjortland MC, Kannel WB, Dawber TR. High density lipoprotein as a protective factor against coronary heart disease: The Framingham Study. Am J Med 1977; 62:707–14.

32. Bush TL, Barrett-Connor E, Cowan LD et al. Cardiovascular mortality and non-contraceptive use of oestrogen in women. Circulation 1987; 75:1102–9.
33. Barr DP, Russ EM, Elder HA. The influence of estrogens on lipoproteins in atherosclerosis. Trans Assoc Am Physicians 1952; 65:102–11.
34. Jensen J, Rio BJ, Strom V, Nilas L, Christiansen C. Long-term effects of percutaneous oestrogens and oral progesterone on serum lipoproteins in postmenopausal women. Am J Obstet Gynecol 1987; 156:66–71.
35. Knopp RH, Walden CE, Wahl PW et al. Oral contraceptive and post-menopausal estrogen effects on lipoprotein, triglyceride and cholesterol in an adult female population relationship to estrogen and progestin potency. J Clin Endocrinol Metab 1981; 53:1123–32.
36. Wilson PWF, Garrison RJ, Castelli WP. Post-menopausal estrogen use, cigarette smoking and cardiovascular morbidity in women over 50. The Framingham Study. N Engl J Med 1985; 313:1038–43.
37. Tikkanen MJ, Nikkila EA, Kuusi T, Sipinen S. High density lipoprotein-2 and hepatic lipase: reciprocal changes produced by estrogen and norgestrel. J Clin Endocrinol Metab 1982; 54:1113–17.
38. Sarrel PM. Estrogen replacement therapy. Obstet Gynecol 1988; 72:Suppl 3s-5s.
39. Tikkanen MJ, Nikkila EA, Kuusi T, Sipinen S. Reduction of plasma high-density lipoprotein cholesterol and increase of post-heparin plasma hepatic lipase activity during pregostin treatment. Clin Chim Acta 1981; 115:63–71.
40. Hirvonen E, Malkonen M, Manninen V. Effects of different progestogens on lipoproteins during post-menopausal replacement therapy. N Engl J Med 1981; 304:560–5.
41. Kloosterboer HJ, van Wayjen RGA, van den Ende A. Effects of the oral contraceptive combination 0.150 mg desogestrel and 0.02 mg ethinyloestradiol on serum lipids including the HDL subfraction. Acta Obstet Gynecol Scand 1987; 144:33–6.
42. Kuusi T, Nikkila EA, Tikkanen MJ, Sipinen S. Effects of two progestins with different androgenic properties on hepatic endothelial lipase and high density lipoprotein-2. Atherosclerosis 1985; 54:251–62.

Chapter 4

Psychological Effects of the Menopause

D. Gath and S. Iles

Introduction

The menopause may have several psychological effects, but this chapter will focus solely on depression, which is generally regarded as the most common effect. Depression at the menopause is often said to have three distinctive features. First, it is said that the risk of a woman becoming depressed at the menopause is exceptionally high. Second, menopausal depression is said to have special causes, notably lack of oestrogen. Third, the treatment of menopausal depression is said to be special, particularly in relation to the indications for hormone replacement therapy. The aim of this chapter, therefore, is to examine three questions:

1. Is depression more frequent at the menopause than at other times in a woman's life?
2. Does such depression have special causes, whether physical or psychological?
3. Does it have special treatment needs?

The first point to stress is that the evidence on these questions can be only as good as the research methods used to investigate them. It has to be said that some published studies have not had convincing results because of limitations of method. Examples will be given of two common shortcomings.

The first is the failure to distinguish between depressed mood and depressive disorder. Depressed mood is a symptom which can be variously called sadness, low spirits, despondency or demoralisation. It is a common symptom which everyone experiences from time to time. It can occur independently of depressive disorder, and in itself is not particularly serious. On the other hand, depressive disorder is a syndrome; it is less common than depressed mood, but much more serious and disabling. A full description of the depressive syndrome can be found in a standard textbook of psychiatry [1]. For present purposes it is sufficient to say that the syndrome consists of depressed mood plus other features. The latter include "loss" symptoms, notably loss of energy, loss of interest, and loss of the capacity to enjoy things that would normally be enjoyable. Concentration is poor, and thoughts are gloomy in their content, dwelling on ideas of guilt, worthlessness, pessimism and sometimes suicide. Speech is slow, laboured and reduced in amount. Similarly, physical movements are slow and reduced. Important for the diagnosis are features sometimes called "biological", namely early morning waking (waking in the early hours of the morning, filled with gloom and apprehension at the prospect of the coming day, mulling over passed failures, and completely unable to get to sleep again); diurnal variation of mood; loss of sex drive; loss of appetite and loss of weight. In the most severe cases, delusions and hallucinations may occur, but these psychotic features are not common.

For research purposes, it is essential to use standardised measures for detecting such symptoms, for rating their severity, and for deciding whether or not the diagnosis is depressive syndrome. Two kinds of measure are available, interview and self-rated. Interview measures make use of a glossary of psychiatric symptoms which are precisely defined. These symptoms are then rated, usually on the basis of intensity, frequency and persistence over a defined period of time, for example, the past four weeks. The Present State Examination (PSE) [2] is a well-known example of a standardised interview for detecting and rating a range of psychiatric symptoms, including depressive symptoms. The Hamilton Depression Scale [3] and the Montgomery Asberg Depression Scale [4] specify methods for rating depressive symptoms at interview. The other type of scale, the self-rated scale, is completed by the patient; an example of a useful scale is the Beck Depression Inventory [5]. Standardised measures such as these are mandatory nowadays, but are not always used.

The second shortcoming is inaccurate specification of the term "menopause". Some studies simply define patients as being "of menopausal age" without reference to their actual menopausal status; but this method of definition is not justified, because the menopause is not closely correlated with age. The only satisfactory method is to use precise operational definitions. For example, McKinlay et al. [6] proposed the following: premenopausal, having menstruated in the past three months; menopausal, having menstruated in the past year but not in the past three months; postmenopausal, not having menstruated in the past 12 months. (For a more elaborate scheme see reference [7].)

The Frequency of Depression at the Menopause

The answer to whether depression is more frequent at the menopause than at other times in a woman's life depends on the population studied, and how it is studied. For example, high rates of depression have been reported among unrepresentative samples, namely middle-aged women attending gynaecological outpatient clinics [8,9], and those attending menopause clinics [10]. These findings are only to be expected, since rates of psychiatric disorder are raised among attenders at all hospital outpatient clinics.

The risk of depression at the menopause can only be properly assessed by community surveys, that is, surveys of women in the general population. Postal surveys of the general population have given conflicting results; for example, depression at the menopause was found to be increased in Dundee [11], but not in London [7]. However, postal surveys are not generally as sensitive as interview surveys.

Four major interview surveys have used large, random samples, precise definitions and standardised methods for case detection. In Sweden, 899 middle-aged women in the community were interviewed on two occasions six years apart [12]. Using DSMIIIR psychiatric diagnostic criteria [13] no association was found between depressive disorder and the menopause. Two surveys were based on interviews but used a self-report scale, the CES-D [14], to diagnose depressive disorder. In the first study, over 2000 women in the USA were studied [15] and in the second, 477 women in Canada were studied [16]. Neither study found any association between depressive disorder and menopausal status. In a survey of 521 women in Oxford, the Present State Examination [12] and the General Health Questionnaire [17] were used to detect psychiatric disorder; again no association was found between psychiatric state and the menopause.

Therefore, it seems from interview surveys using standardised measures that the risk of depressive disorder at the menopause is not raised. This finding is at variance with popular beliefs.

The Causes of Depression at the Menopause

The question as to whether depression at the menopause has special causes is important because of its implications for treatment.

The causes of depression at the menopause can be of two kinds, psychological and physical.

The Menopause as a Psychological Cause of Depression

The question here is: can depression be induced psychiatrically by the meno-pause, in the same way as it can be induced by a bereavement, broken engagement, loss of job, or similar loss events? In the case of the menopause, this reaction might occur through regrets at lost fertility or a subjective sense of lost femininity.

Evidence from research on "artificial" menopause suggests that such emo-tional reactions to the normal menopause are unlikely to be particularly frequent. For example, research in Oxford found that regrets for lost fertility or femininity were not particularly common after "surgical" menopause resulting from hysterectomy alone or from hysterectomy plus bilateral ovariectomy [18]; nor were such reactions common after elective interval sterilisation [19,20].

Although it seems unlikely that depressive reactions to the menopause are specially common in the general population, it should be borne in mind that individual women may have such reactions. Therefore, appropriate enquiry should always be made when assessing a depressed menopausal woman.

Whilst the menopause may be depressing to some women, to others it may be welcome because it brings freedom from menstruation and from the possibility of childbearing. Thus the menopause can be experienced as positive, and as bringing a new lease of life.

Women's reactions to the menopause are likely to be influenced by cultural attitudes. Such attitudes vary widely. For example, in Islamic and certain African societies, postmenopausal women are freed from seclusion taboos associated with menstruation; thus, the menopause brings about a positive change in status [21]. Similarly, Sikh women in a Canadian community see the menopause as a cleansing and liberating event, and enjoy the transition to being an "elder" [22]. However, in other societies (for example, Greek peasants) postmenopausal women are regarded as being out of the main stream of life; they have to wear dark clothes, and see themselves as growing old and declining [21].

Middle-age Adversities as Psychological Causes of Depression

In clinical practice it is essential to bear in mind that a menopausal woman may be depressed not because of the menopause, but because of various adversities that are common in middle-life.

Middle-age commonly brings events which are potential causes of depression; for example, a woman's parents may become ill or die, or her children may leave home and move to another continent. Careful research has shown that such events (sometimes called "exit events") are particularly frequent in the six months before the onset of depressive disorders at any age [23].

Apart from stressful events, it has been suggested that women may become depressed in middle-age because they feel there is nothing useful left to do – the so-called redundancy syndrome. Another important factor may be an awareness that the husband shows less affection than in the past.

There is some evidence that stressful events and adverse circumstances may be more important that the menopause as determinants of depression. Thus, it has been reported that life stress contributes more to depressive symptoms in middle-aged women than menopausal status [24]. McKinlay et al. [15] found that depressive illness in middle-aged women was related less to the menopause than to the events and situations of mid-life. Examples of the latter were marital separation or divorce, widowhood, chronic physical illness and worry over a family member.

Thus it seems that the events and circumstances of middle-life may be important determinants of depression in some women. However, there is no reason to suppose that such events are any more frequent or stressful than those occurring in other epochs of life. For example, problems of infant-rearing may be very stressful to young mothers, whereas social isolation may be a great problem in old age.

Even so, the events of middle-life should always be borne in mind in the assessment of the individual woman of middle-age.

The Menopause as a Physical Cause of Depression

If lack of oestrogen influences mood, it may do so directly as a biochemical effect, or indirectly by causing physical symptoms (flushes or sweats) which in turn induce depression.

It is difficult to establish direct biochemical mechanisms whereby oestrogen influences mood, but one conceptual approach is to work out possible pathways. In general, these are based on prevailing hypotheses of the aetiology of affective illness, namely that depressive syndrome is caused by a functional deficiency of noradrenaline or 5-hydroxytryptamine (5HT). In one possible pathway, oestrogen may reduce the availability of plasma tryptophan for brain 5HT synthesis and hence reduce 5HT neurotransmission which in turn may influence mood [25,26]. However, the probability of an association between brain 5HT and depression remains controversial [27]. Another possibility is that oestrogen may influence mood by enhancement of central noradrenergic functioning via an inhibitory effect on the degradation of monoamine transmitters [28]. A third possibility is that oestrogen may alter the sensitivity of central monoamine receptors [29], perhaps via an action on the cell nucleus. It is stressed that although these effects of oestrogen on monoamine mechanisms can be demonstrated experimentally, there is no firm evidence linking changes in mono-aminergic function to menopausal depression, or indeed other kinds of affective illness.

There is also no conclusive evidence for the possible indirect effects of oestrogen. In postal surveys, it has been found that psychological symptoms such as depression peaked at an age before the peaking of vasomotor symptoms such as flushes and sweats [11,30]. However, an interview survey of over 500 middle-aged women in Oxford found a significant association between flushes/sweats and psychiatric symptoms [31] – though of course this does not prove a causal connection between the two.

Since there is no firm evidence as to whether lack of oestrogen causes depression either directly as a biochemical effect or indirectly through physical symptoms, it is interesting to consider whether the administration of oestrogen alleviates depression.

Does Oestrogen Alleviate Depression?

Here the distinction between depressive disorder and depression as a symptom is important.

For depressive disorder, the evidence is scanty. Klaiber et al. [28] carried out a double-blind study of women with severe depressive disorder, which had not responded to standard antidepressant medication. High doses of oestrogen (5–25 mg daily) were found to be more effective than placebo in reducing depressive symptoms on the Hamilton Rating Scale [3]. The overall reduction was not great for the group as a whole, and the effect did not seem to vary according to whether or not the woman was postmenopausal. Nevertheless, a subgroup of the oestrogen-treated women showed a marked improvement. This finding raises the possibility that oestrogen may be of some benefit for some depressed women who do not respond to antidepressant medication, but at present there are no means of identifying such women. Also, the risks associated with such high dosage of oestrogen must be borne in mind.

Among women with depressed mood (but not depressive disorder), oestrogen has been reported as beneficial by several investigators. For example, after surgical menopause, oestrogen was more effective than placebo in improving mood [32], and mood covaried with circulating oestrogen levels in the physiological range [33]. In another study, mixed mood symptoms in postmenopausal women were helped more by oestrogen–testosterone implants than by placebo [34].

Against this positive evidence, some investigators have reported that psychological symptoms (not the depressive syndrome) responded no better to oestrogen than to placebo (for example, reference [35]).

Overall, however, the literature suggests that oestrogen can alleviate the mood and induce a general sense of well-being.

The Treatment of Menopausal Depression

Finally: Does menopausal depression require special treatment?

If a women presents in the clinic with physical symptoms of oestrogen lack (flushes or sweats), and if she appears to be depressed, careful assessment is required so that treatment of the depression can be rationally planned.

Several questions need to be asked. Does the patient have physical symptoms of oestrogen lack, for example, flushes, sweats or vaginal dryness? If so, how severe are these symptoms? Is she suffering solely from depressed syndrome? (To make this distinction, reference can be made to the definition of the depressive syndrome on p. 36. If the patient does have the depressive syndrome, how severe and disabling is it? When was the onset in relation to the onset of flushes and sweats?

Apart from the menopause, are there any adverse events or circumstances that are common in middle-age? If so, do these factors appear to have induced the depression?

The treatment plan will depend on whether the patient seems to have depressed mood or the depressive syndrome. If she has solely depressed mood, and if this mood seems to be clearly secondary to severe flushes or sweats, then oestrogen replacement therapy may be appropriate. On the other hand, if the depressed mood seems to result from adverse events or circumstances, then psychological or social help may be appropriate.

If the patient has the full depressive syndrome, then oestrogen therapy should not be the first line of treatment. Instead the patient should be treated with antidepressant medication or with psychological treatment, or with both (a decision which could be referred to the general practitioner or a psychiatrist). If the patient with depressive syndrome also has vasomotor symptoms which are prominent and distressing, and which seem likely to be contributing to her misery, then oestrogen can be given as an adjunct to the specific psychiatric treatment.

References

1. Gelder MG, Gath D, Mayou R. Oxford textbook of psychiatry, 2nd edn. London: Oxford University Press, 1989.
2. Wing JK, Cooper JE, Sartorius N. The measurement and classification of psychiatric symptoms. London: Cambridge University Press, 1974.
3. Hamilton M. Development of a rating scale for primary depressive illness. Br J Soc Clin Psychol 1967; 6:278–96.
4. Montgomery SA, Asberg M. A new depression scale designed to be sensitive to change. Br J Psychiatry 1979; 131:431–2.
5. Beck AT, Ward CH, Mendelson M, Mock JE, Erbaugh JK. An inventory for measuring depression. Arch Gen Psychiatry 1961; 4:561–71.
6. McKinlay S, Jeffereys M, Thompson P. An investigation of the age at menopause. J Biosoc Sci 1972; 4:161–73.
7. McKinlay SM, Jeffereys M. The menopausal syndrome. Br J Prev Soc Med 1974; 28:108–15.
8. Ballinger B. Psychiatric morbidity and the menopause: survey of a gynaecological out-patient clinic. Br J Psychiatry 1977; 131:83–9.
9. Byrne P. Psychiatric morbidity in a gynaecological clinic. An epidemiological survey. Br J Psychiatry 1984; 144:28–34.
10. Jones MJ, Marshall DH, Nordin BEC. Quantitation of menopausal symptomatology and its response to ethinyl oestradiol and piperazine oestrone sulphate. Curr Med Res Opin 1977; 4, Suppl. 3:12–20.
11. Ballinger B. Psychiatric morbidity and the menopause; screening of a general populative sample. Br Med J 1975; 3:344–6.
12. Hallstrom T, Samuelsson S. Mental health in the climacteric. The longitudinal study of women in Gothenburg. Acta Obstet Gynecol Scand [Suppl] 1985;130:13–18.
13. American Psychiatric Association. Diagnostic and statistical manual of mental disorders, 3rd edn, revised. Washington DC: American Psychiatric Association, 1987.
14. Radloff LS. The CES-D Scale: a self-report depression scale for research in the general population. Appl Psychol Meas 1977; 1:385–401.
15. McKinlay JB, McKinlay SM, Brambila D. The relative contributions of endocrine changes and social circumstances to depression in middle-aged women. J Health Soc Behav 1987; 28:345–63.
16. Kaufert PA, Gilbert P, Hassaret T. Researching the symptoms of menopause: an exercise in methodology. Maturitas 1988; 10:117–31.
17. Goldberg DP. The detection of psychiatric illness by questionnaire. London: Oxford University Press, 1972.
18. Gath D, Cooper P, Bond A, Edmonds G. Hysterectomy and psychiatric disorder II. Demographic and physical factors in relation to psychiatric outcome. Br J Psychiatry 1982; 140:343–50.
19. Cooper P, Gath D, Fieldsend R, Rose N. Psychological and physical outcome after elective tubal sterilisation. J Psychosom Res 1981, 25:357–60.
20. Cooper P, Gath D, Rose N, Fieldsend R. Psychological sequelae to elective sterilisation in women: a prospective study. Br Med J 1981, 82:461–64.
21. Beyene Y. Cultural significance and physiological manifestations of menopause. A biocultural analysis. Cult Med Psychiatry 1986; 10:47–71.
22. George T. Menopause: some interpretations of the results of a study among non-western groups. Maturitas 1988, 10:109–16.
23. Paykel ES, Myers JK, Dienelt MN, Klerman GL, Lindenthal J, Pepper MP. Life events and depression: a controlled study. Arch Gen Psychiatry 1969; 21:753–60.
24. Greene JG, Cooke DJ. Life stress and symptoms at the climacterium. Br J Psychiatry 1980; 136:486–91.
25. Aylward M. Estrogens, plasma tryptophan levels in perimenopausal patients. In: Campbell S, ed. The management of the menopause and post-menopausal years. Lancaster: MTP Press, 1976; 135–47.
26. Coppen A, Bishop M, Beard RJ. Effects of piperazine oestrone sulphate on plasma tryptophan, oestrogen, gonadotrophins and psychological functioning in women following hysterectomy. Curr Med Res Opin 1977; 4, suppl 3:29–36.
27. Cowen PJ. Recent views on the role of 5-hydroxytryptamine in depression. Curr Opin Psychiatry 1988; 1:56–9.

28. Klaiber EL, Broverman DM, Vogel'W, Kobayashi Y. Estrogen therapy for severe persistent depression in women. Arch Gen Psychiatry 1979; 36:550–4.
29. Chalmers JS, Fulli-Lemaire I, Cowen PJ. Effects of the contraceptive pill on sedative responses to clonidine and dapomorphine in normal women. Psychol Med 1985; 15:363–7.
30. Bungay GT, Vessey MP, McPherson CK. Study of symptoms in middle-life with special reference to the menopause. Br Med J 1980, 281:181–3.
31. Gath D, Osborn M, Bungay G, Iles S, Day A, Bond A, Passingham C. Psychiatric disorder and gynaecological symptoms in middle-aged women: a community survey. Br Med J 1987; 294:213–218.
32. Sherwin B, Gelfand M. Sex steroids and affect in the surgical menopause: a double-blind, cross-over study. Psychoneuroendocrinology 1985; 10:325–35.
33. Sherwin B. Affective changes with oestrogen and androgen replacement therapy in surgically menopausal women. J Affeč Dis 1988; 14:177–87.
34. Brincat M, Studd JWW, O'Dowd T, Magos A, Cardozo LD, Wardle PJ. Subcutaneous hormone implants for control of climacteric symptoms. Lancet 1984; i:16–18.
35. Iatrakis G, Haronis N, Sakellaropoulos G, Kourkabas A, Gallos M. Psychosomatic symptoms of postmenopausal women with or without hormonal treatment. Psychother Psychosom 1986; 46:116–21.

Discussion

Baird: It looked initially as though Mr Studd and Dr Gath were in conflict but they have convinced me that they probably have come to the same conclusion.

Fogelman: There is clearly a slight possibility of subjective opinion as to whether somebody has depressive syndrome or just depressive mood. Is this something that requires a psychiatrist to establish the difference, or should any general physician be able to differentiate between the two?

Gath: It is something that is best done by using a standardised measuring instrument, preferably an interview one, and non-psychiatrists can be trained in that. We have non-psychiatrists in our department who have been trained, but the training does require commitment. It takes a daily session for about a week, the use of videos and audiotapes and tests of reliability. One need not be a psychiatrist but one must be trained to use the measure.

Fogelman: Dr Gath said that it was a possibility that there may not be anything more stressful about the menopause compared with, say, child rearing and Mr Studd listed a number of stresses around the time of the menopause. But neither speaker mentioned marital stress, which surprised me. It seems to me that it can be a time of particular problems for women. Their husbands may be becoming successful in their walk of life, for example, and that would seem to be a more obvious source of stress than some of the possibilities that were listed.

Gath: I gave just two examples. These are all what are called loss events and I suppose that the loss of a husband's affections is another example.

Baird: Am I not right in saying that one of the surveys showed that these loss events occurred equally frequently in men of the same age?

Gath: I did not discuss it.

Vessey: Could Dr Gath say more about the importance of symptoms and disease in relation to depression? He mentioned symptoms that are related to meno-pausal syndrome, but I am thinking for instance of his work on hysterectomy and the mood of women who had menstrual bleeding disorders. I am thinking of a paper I heard recently on people who had chronic joint complaints that did not respond too well to treatment and a high proportion of them showed clinical depression. I have no doubt that I could think of other examples.

How important are phenomena of that sort in general in relation to depressive illness and how important might they be specifically to depressive illness at this time and perhaps particularly the exacerbation of gynaecological problems around this time?

Gath: Is the question whether physical illness can induce depressive illness?

Vessey: That is part of the question. There is a clustering of gynaecological illness around this time. How important is that in relation to depression?

Gath: All physical symptoms carry a risk of associated psychical symptoms. That can be shown in general practice. It can be shown in people consulting in the whole range of outpatient clinics. It can be shown in hospital inpatients. There tends to be a gradient of severity going from general practice up to becoming an inpatient, but virtually any physical illness carries the risk of being accompanied by psychiatric symptoms.

Vessey: And the clustering of menstrual symptoms? This is a time at which many hysterectomies take place and I wondered about menorrhagia and irregular menstruation as a physical symptom causing psychical problems. How important might that be in relation to depressive illness?

Gath: In the 550-patient community survey, women who subjectively rated their periods as very heavy had a very high risk for high levels of psychiatric symptoms. Those went together. We do not know whether they were objectively consonant, but subjectively they were.

Baird: Certainly it would make some kind of common sense. Mr Studd has shown that if oestrogen or testosterone implants are imposed on premenopausal women who are having depressive symptoms it makes them better. Similarly if ovarian activity is abolished altogether and they are made artificially meno-pausal many of the psychological difficulties can be abolished using the GnRH agonists. So it may be that it is the actual physical symptoms associated with the menstrual cycle that cause the trouble. Mr Studd's data showed that oestrogen in the postmenopausal woman is no better than the placebo with many of the psychological symptoms.

Anderson: Following on from that, what about the effect of the added pro-gestogen? Is that having any adverse effect?

Studd: That is much more important. We have known for years of the tonic effect of oestrogens and we can suppress cyclic depression in the premenopausal woman [1]. Then we add progestogen to this therapy and the symptoms recur –

that is in the patient with premenstrual depression. The symptoms are often not as bad and not so long but it is quite clear that progestogens do produce these symptoms of depression, anxiety, tiredness, headaches, loss of libido, etc.

It can also happen in the postmenopausal woman, and this is the limiting factor in conventional HRT in women with their uterus. Oestrogens abolish their symptoms and progestogens may cause recurrence of their symptoms. Adam Magos from Oxford showed this in hysterectomised patients. When they were given 10 days of norethisterone or placebo the symptoms were reproduced, which were both dose- and duration-dependent on progestogen [2].

Anderson: How low did he go with dosage?

Studd: 2.5 mg norethisterone.

Anderson: What about 1 mg? Could that be getting down to a level that is not important?

Whitehead: In a recent study [3] one of 67 patients was lost over an 8-month period because of progestogen-mediated side effects with 1 mg/day. It is clearly dose related.

The progestogen dose will depend on the oestrogen dose we are trying to oppose. If the patient is being given oestrogens at a dose that will achieve higher plasma oestradiol levels, she will need to be given higher doses of progestogens.

Selby: Following on from that, our experience of using progestogen alone in postmenopausal women would suggest that they do not get a lot of these adverse side effects. It is probably a phenomenon of giving progestogen to a woman who is oestrogen-primed rather than the progestogen per se. It looks as though it is a combination of the two hormones that is producing the adverse effects.

Whitehead: In 1976, with Stuart Campbell, we did a long placebo-controlled study showing numerous oestrogen benefits as compared to placebo on psychological status [4]. Then at the end of the study when the group was subdivided into those women who complained of vagina dryness and had no flushes and sweats as compared to those who presented initially with vasomotor symptoms, there were still psychological benefits in the non-flushers. Which suggested that oestrogens do have a mood-lifting effect.

I see women who say they are tired, they are listless, they have no drive, no enthusiasm. and they have got adverse social and environmental factors. They will say they would like to try oestrogens for 6 weeks, and they come back and they just feel so much better. It is always a surprise to me. I wonder sometimes if a trial of therapy with oestrogens for six weeks is a grossly undervalued and under-used treatment strategy.

Barlow: Do we have any knowledge from community surveys of the relative influence in menopausal women of depressive mood as compared with the full depressive syndrome? I would suspect that many of the women we see in our clinics who do respond are women with depressive mood. If it turns out that depressive mood is excessively more common than the syndrome, I would suggest that Mr Whitehead's comments are very valid and that it is worth seeing what happens with a short dose of oestrogen. If the woman fails to respond, then maybe that is the time to think of a psychiatrist.

Gath: I am sure depressive mood is much the more common. I tried to stress that at the beginning. In a family of five people only one is likely to have it at some time.

Baird: I am not sure that a therapeutic trial of something for six weeks with symptoms as difficult to define as depressed mood will necessarily tell us very much. There is the dramatic effect of placebo in six weeks.

References

1. Magos AL, Brincat M, Studd JWW. Treatment of the premenstrual syndrome by subcutaneous oestradiol implants and cyclical oral norethisterone: a placebo controlled study. Br Med J 1986; 292:1629–33.
2. Magos AL, Brewster E, Singh R, O'Dowd T, Brincat M, Studd JWW. The effects of norethisterone in post-menopausal women on oestrogen replacement therapy: a model for the premenstrual syndrome. Br J Obster Gynaecol 1986; 12:1290–6.
3. Fraser DI, Parsons A, Whitehead MI, Wordsworth J, Stuart G, Pryse-Davies J. The optimal dose of oral norethindrone acetate for addition to transdermal estradiol: a multicenter study. Fertil Steril (in press).
4. Campbell S, Whitehead M. Oestrogen therapy and the menopausal syndrome. In: Greenblatt R, Studd J. eds. The menopause: clinics in obstetrics and gynaecology IV. Philadelphia: WB Saunders, 1977; 31–47.

Chapter 5

Oestrogen Deficiency and Connective Tissues

M. Brincat, C. Moniz, M. Savvas and J. W. W. Studd

"Their skin is noticeably thin – suggesting that the atrophy is more widespread than just in the bone matrix." Albright et al. (1941) [1]

Introduction

Tissue formed by the cells of the mesoderm is known as mesenchyme and it is from the mesenchyme that the connective tissue of the body develops. Quantitatively some 80% of connective tissue is found in the dermis of the skin and in the bone with the amount of collagen being shared almost equally between them.

Connective tissue is composed of collagen bundles and glycosaminoglycans (GAGs). These are amorphous ground substances, previously known as mucopolysaccharides that are present in between collagen bundles. Both skin and bone share the same types of GAGs. The GAG chains allow rapid diffusion of water-soluble molecules and are responsible for the turgor in the extracellular matrix that resists compressive forces unlike collagen fibrils which resist stretching forces. By weight GAGs amount for less than 5% of the fibrous protein, the rest being composed largely of collagen with some elastin [2]. Skin and bone share a common collagen, type I. Skin contains in addition a further collagen, type III. Type I which constitutes 90% of the total collagen in the body is the most important [2].

After the menopause, profound changes occur in organs containing connective tissue. Evidence suggests that the rapid decline in skin thickness and skin collagen after the menopause, and postmenopausal bone loss shares a common pathology, namely an overall decline in connective tissue that occurs as a result of oestrogen deficiency.

Other sites where connective tissue also plays an important part include blood vessels and the pelvic floor. After the menopause there is an increase in lower urinary tract problems. Likewise there is an increase in easy bruising of the skin which has been related to a higher incidence of osteoporosis [3].

Thus the general atrophy of connective tissues that occurs, although only obvious several years after the onset of the menopause, can be attributable to oestrogen deficiency.

Bone

Bone mass declines rapidly after the menopause reaching rates of 3%–5% per annum in the early postmenopausal years. After 4–10 years this slows down to a rate comparable again to the premenopausal rate of bone loss [4]. This bone loss leads to 50% of the female population sustaining an osteoporotic fracture by the age of 70. The vast morbidity and mortality as a result of osteoporotic fractures leads to a great deal of suffering and huge costs.

Bone is a connective tissue and Albright et al. [1] initially hypothesised that osteoporosis was a connective tissue disorder. This is very often forgotten because the abundance of papers on calcium metabolism gives the impression that the skeleton is composed entirely of chalk [5]. However, dry defatted bone mass is made of roughly one-third organic matrix composed chiefly of collagen and two-thirds mineral [6]. By far the largest proportion of the organic matrix, between 90% and 95%, consists of collagen [7].

Evidence of Bone Collagen Breakdown

An increase in the excretion of urinary hydroxyproline after oophorectomy has been described [8]. This increase is entirely reversible with oestrogens. This has been taken to indicate that an increase in bone resorption occurs with the oestrogen deficiency that occurs after oophorectomy or after the menopause.

Urinary hydroxyproline excretion is a very crude method of assessing collagen breakdown and is only of real use when large changes are occurring such as in Paget's disease. With half the total body collagen content in the skin, it is not possible to use this as an indicator of fine changes in bone metabolism. Furthermore, hydroxyproline excretion is often within the normal range in generalised bone diseases, such as osteoporosis [5]. Due to effective renal reabsorption of free hydroxyproline, even the ingestion of up to 4 g of free hydroxyproline has practically no effect on the total amount of urinary hydroxyproline.

Recently, however, it has been possible to assess the urinary excretion of pyridinium crosslinks. These crosslinks reflect the degradation only of mature collagen and not of any intermediates. These particular crosslinks are not present in the skin, although they might be present in small amounts in tissues. The measurement of urinary pyridinium crosslinks provides sensitive and specific indices of bone resorption [9].

In one study, significantly higher levels of urinary pyridinium were found in a

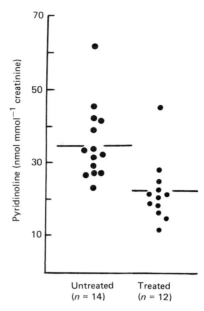

Fig. 5.1. Differences in pyridinoline excretion between age-matched groups of early post menopausal women. The treated group were on oestradiol 50 mg and testosterone 100 mg implants every 6 months. (Untreated: 35.1 ± 10.3 (SD) nmol pyridinoline mmol[1] creatinine; $n = 14$: treated group: 22.9 ± 8.4 (SD) nmol mmol^{-1}; $n = 12$. t test: $t = 3.41$; $F = 1.28$; $P = 0.0023$). (By courtesy of Dr S. Robins, the Rowett Research Institute, Aberdeen.)

population of early postmenopausal women when compared to an age-matched group who were on oestrogen-replacement therapy [9] (Fig. 5.1). This indicated that in the untreated group collagen degradation was occurring at a faster rate. The finding that the excretion of urinary pyridinium was less in oestrogen-treated women is consistent with the finding that bone loss is prevented by oestrogen replacement and occurs as a result of oestrogen deficiency. Such changes were not evident when urinary hydroxyproline alone was measured.

In addition, serum assays of bone specific proteins are being evaluated to overcome problems such as a lack of sensitivity and specificity with alkaline phosphatase (osteoblasts) and acid phosphatase (osteoclasts). Bone specific collagen markers being developed are pro-collagen I peptides (PICP). There are immunoassays using monoclonal antibodies directed towards the carboxy-terminal residues of pro-collagen I and reflect bone collagen synthesis. Pro-collagen III amino-terminal peptide (P III NP) is also being evaluated for collagen turnover but is less specific for bone. Pyridinoline crosslinks, in particular 3-hydroxypyridinium in urine will give an index of bone breakdown and PICP will show bone synthesis.

Thus the turnover of bone connective tissue, as opposed to mineral parameters, is receiving more attention and with increasing sophistication more accurate knowledge of the importance of the organic matrix is being obtained.

The connective tissue matrix of bone contributes to its strength just as the mineral content contributes to its stiffness. Bones therefore become brittle as the connective tissue of the organic matrix is lost. Histological studies have shown that bone biopsies from age-matched groups of osteoporotic population had a lower collagen content than the non-osteoporotic group [10].

Skin

Skin, which constitutes the largest organ in the body, also undergoes changes after the menopause. Many of these changes have formerly been attributed to the ageing process but are in reality due to oestrogen deficiency. The skin of postmenopausal women who are on sex hormone replacement therapy has been shown to contain more collagen than women of the same age who are on no treatment [11].

Skin thickness declines rapidly after the menopause, at a rate very similar to the decline in bone mass. This decline cannot be explained by age alone. Skin collagen declines by some 30% in the first ten years after the menopause, an amount that is comparable to bone loss over the same period [12,13] (Fig. 5.2).

Prospective studies on skin collagen have shown that even though collagen was lost as a result of the duration of oestrogen deficiency after ovarian failure, it was possible to restore collagen to premenopausal levels within six months of initiating hormone replacement therapy [13–16]. If hormone replacement therapy was initiated early, there was no decline in the levels of skin collagen or in skin thickness.

Both oestrogen and androgen receptors have been identified in the fibroblasts of the skin [17]. More recently, oestrogen receptors have been identified on osteoblasts [18], supporting the argument that sex steroids have a direct action

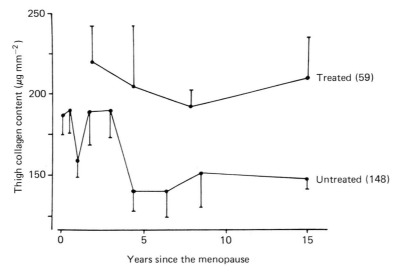

Fig. 5.2. Thigh skin collagen content (mean±SE) with years since menopause in 148 untreated postmenopausal women and in 59 postmenopausal women who had been on sex hormone treatment for between 2 and 10 years.

on osteoblasts. In addition, the possibility of oestrogens working on both fibroblasts and osteoblasts indirectly, through an intermediary hormone such as growth hormone must be considered [19].

Skin Thickness and Postmenopausal Bone Loss

The generalised loss of connective tissue which occurs as a result of oestrogen deficiency after the menopause leads to a postmenopausal decline of skin thickness and postmenopausal bone loss. The loss of organic matrix in bone is followed by a loss of mineral matrix [20]. This hypothesis is supported by highly significant correlations found in postmenopausal women between skin thickness, skin collagen, Metacarpal Index and the mean bone mineral content at 8 cm up the forearm from the styloid processes. Furthermore, all four parameters show a similar decline during the postmenopausal years [13].

The correlation between skin thickness and bone mass has led to the suggestion that skin thickness could be used as a screening test for women who are likely to develop osteoporosis. Further work, however, still needs to be done [20].

The dermis of the skin is a connective tissue composed largely of collagen. McConkey et al. [3] made the observation that elderly women had transparent skin on the backs of their hands which was assumed to be due to a change in the dermis. They showed that the incidence of transparent skin was more common in females over the age of 60. They also found that the prevalence of osteoporosis in women with transparent skin, 83%, significantly exceeded that in women with opaque skin, 12.5%.

McConkey et al. [21] found an association betwen transparent skin and senile purpura, but the likelihood of a patient with senile purpura having osteoporosis depended on whether she also had transparent skin. Purely from anectodal experience, postmenopausal women claim to bruise more easily than they would have in the past. Once on HRT, these same women claim that they are bruising less. The relationship between bruising and connective tissue could be twofold. Either the supporting connective tissue to capillaries, by becoming looser, is more amenable to bruising or vessel wall connective tissue becomes weaker. Whatever the mechanism the process seems to be reversed with oestrogen replacement.

Genitourinary System

The epithelial linings of the vagina and the urethra have the highest concentration of oestrogen receptors in the body and are therefore extremely sensitive to alterations in oestrogen levels. The trigone of the bladder, derived embryologically from the urogenital sinus, appears to undergo atrophic changes after the menopause.

The vagina sustains a decrease in vascularity. Atrophic changes occur and the vaginal epithelium becomes thin, inflamed and ulcerated.

The cervix, instead of protruding into the vagina atrophies, retracts and becomes flush with the apex of the vault. The uterine corpus itself becomes smaller with a return to the 1:2 corpus: cervix ratio of childhood.

Postmenopausal atrophy of the connective tissue and the epithelial linings of the vagina and the urethra have symptomatic sequelae which can continue to be troublesome. These include dyspareunia, apareunia and recurrent bacterial infections. In the urethra, repeated infections may lead to fibrosis which predisposes to frequency, dysuria and urgency referred to as the "urethral syndrome" [22]. The submucosal vascular plexus of the urethra contributes to sphincteric function and is oestrogen dependent [23], as may be the collagen content of the urethral submucosal connective tissue [24]. In this study [24], there were significant correlations between all stress profile variables measured [4] and thigh skin collagen content.

Proximal shortening of the urethra reflects bladder neck incompetence [25] and this was negatively correlated with thigh skin collagen content. This implies that the degree of bladder neck competence is positively correlated with collagen content. Thus this study showed that in all the variables studied, greater sphincteric function was associated with greater collagen content of skin. Once more, this study demonstrates not only the importance of changes in connective tissue after the menopause, but, by identifying correlations between the connective tissue-dependent organs, suggests that generalised connective tissue changes occur as a result of hypo-oestrogenism after the menopause [24].

Oestrogen receptors have been detected in the human female urethra [26] suggesting a direct action of the hormone. It would appear, therefore, that both the genital and lower urinary tract are affected by oestrogens and that at least part of these effects, is due to atrophy of connective tissue brought about by hypo-oestrogenism.

If the assumption that a generalised oestrogen-dependent connective tissue atrophy also affects the urethra is correct then one would expect postmenopausal women to have weaker urethral sphincters than premenopausal women. This has been shown to be the case [25]. It would also be expected that oestrogen therapy would have the opposite effect, and increases in urethral pressure have in fact been reported after oestrogen replacement therapy [27–29].

Since increases in skin collagen with oestrogen replacement therapy have also been noted [14], it is suggested that the beneficial effects of urethral function may be mediated by beneficial effects on collagen content [23].

Discussion

We suggest that oestrogen deficiency leads to an increasing breakdown of connective tissue possibly with a decrease in formation. This action can be direct, as shown by the presence of oestrogen receptors on fibroblasts and osteoblasts, or indirect, through some intermediate hormones. The increase in breakdown in bone connective tissue is due to an increase in osteoclastic activity [30]. The increased breakdown in skin collagen could be due to an increase in macrophage activity [31]. Thus in bone either osteoclasts become more active or osteoblast activity is reduced. Evidence supports both possibilities in bone, but it is not clear which is the more important in the pathogenesis of osteoporosis. It is probably a combination of the two that leads to the overall reduction in connective tissue of the organic matrix of bone [3].

Anecdotal stories abound about postmenopausal women regaining the tone of their tissues, having moister skin, bruising less and looking healthier after being placed on oestrogen replacement. The "urethral syndrome" is likewise vanquished with oestrogen replacement.

We have indicated that there might be substance in these anecdotes. Investigation of postmenopausal bone loss, postmenopausal skin thinning and loss of skin collagen, as well as genitourinary changes, shows the only common pathology is one of a global connective tissue disorder which occurs as a result of oestrogen deficiency after the menopause and which is to some extent reversed with appropriate oestrogen therapy.

Even the moister skin reported after oestrogen therapy can be explained. In addition to an improvement in skin collagen content, work on mice has suggested that glycosaminoglycans in connective tissue also respond to oestrogens. These studies have shown that, the content of hyaluronic acid, one of the major glycosaminoglycans in the skin increases with oestrogens [32,33]. A close linear relationship exists between hyaluronic acid and tissue water and any increase in the former results in an increase in the latter. Likewise the increase in skin collagen, skin thickness and bone mass in postmenopausal women on adequate oestrogen therapy, such as implants, suggests that oestrogen replacement is acting on the common connective tissue matrix [14,16,34]. Hormone implants have been shown to be an effective and safe form of hormone replacement not only in hysterectomised women [35] but also in women with a uterus provided that in addition to the oestrogen contained in the implant, women are also given cyclical oral progestogens so as to prevent endometrial hyperplasia [36,37].

The evidence presented thus shows that postmenopausal oestrogen deficiency leads to a connective tissue disorder, with far-reaching consequences. This being the case it is the only known, potentially preventable and partially reversible connective tissue disorder.

References

1. Albright F, Smith PH, Richardson AM. Postmenopausal osteoporosis – its clinical features. JAMA 1941; 116:2465–74.
2. Alberts B, Bray D, Lewis T et al. Cell–cell adhesion and the extracellular matrix. In: Alberts B, ed. Molecular biology of the cell. New York: Garland Publishing, 1983; 673–715.
3. McConkey B, Fraser GM, Bligh AS, Whitely H. Transparent skin and osteoporosis. Lancet 1963; i:693–5.
4. Lindsay R. Pathogenesis, detection and prevention of postmenopausal osteoporosis. In: Studd JWW, Whitehead MI, eds. The menopause. Oxford, London, Edinburgh: Blackwell Scientific Publications, 1988; 156–67.
5. Smith R. Collagen and disorders of bone. Editorial review. Clin Sci 1980; 59:215–23.
6. Forbes RM, Cooper AR, Mitchell L. The composition of the adult human body as determined by chemical analysis. J. Biol Chem 1953; 203:359–66.
7. Hall DA. Chemical and biochemical changes in ageing connective tissues. In: Hall DA, ed. The ageing of connective tissues. New York: Academic Press, 1976, 79–144.
8. Gallagher JC, Nordin BEC. Oestrogens and calcium metabolism. Front Horm Res 1983; 2:98–117.

9. Robins SP, Duncan A, Reid DM, Paterson CR. Urinary hydroxypyridium crosslinks of collagen as markers of resorption in a range of metabolic bone diseases. Program and abstracts. Tenth international conference on calcium regulating hormones/eleventh annual meeting of the American Society for Bone and Mineral Research. Joint meeting, Montreal. J Bone Min Res 1989; 4:1120.
10. Birkenhager-Frenkel DH. Assessment of porosity in bone specimens, differences in chemical composition between normal bone and bone from patients with senile osteoporosis. In: Gaillard PJ. ed. Fourth European symposium on calcified tissues. Amsterdam: Excerpta Medica, 1966; 8–9.
11. Brincat A, Moniz CJ, Studd JWW, Darby AJ, Magos A, Cooper D. Sex hormones and skin collagen content in postmenopausal women. Br Med J 1983; 287:1337–8.
12. Brincat M, Moniz CJ, Studd JWW, Darby AJ, Magos A, Emburey G, Versi E. Long term effects of the menopause and sex hormones on skin thickness. Br J Obstet Gynaecol 1985; 92:256–9.
13. Brincat M, Moniz CF, Kabalan S et al. Decline in skin collagen content and metacarpal index after the menopause and its prevention with sex hormone replacement. Br J Obstet Gynaecol 1987; 94:126–9.
14. Brincat M, Wong Ten Yuen A, Studd JWW, Montgomery J, Magos A. Savvas M. Response of skin thickness and metacarpal index to estradiol therapy in postmenopausal women. Obstet Gynecol 1987; 70:538–41.
15. Brincat M, Versi E, Moniz CF, Magos A, de Trafford J, Studd JWW. Skin collagen changes in postmenopausal women receiving different regimens of estrogen therapy. Obstet Gynecol 1987; 70:123–7.
16. Brincat M, Versi E, Moniz CF, O'Dowd T, Magos A, Kabalan S, Studd JWW. Skin collagen changes in postmenopausal women treated with oestradiol gel. Maturitas 1987; 9:1–5.
17. Black NM, Shuster S, Bottoms E. Osteoporosis, skin collagen and androgen. Br Med J 1970; 4:773–4.
18. Kaplan JA. Identifications of oestrogen receptors on osteoblast. International Conference on osteoporosis, Aalbourg, 1987. (Unpublished abstract).
19. Vashinav R. Gallagher JA, Beresford NN, Russell RGG. Proliferative effects of oestrogens on bone-derived cells. Calcif Tissue Int 1984; 36:559.
20. Brincat M, Studd JWW. Skin and the menopause. In: Studd JWW, Whitehead MI, eds. The menopause. Oxford, London, Edinburgh: Blackwell Scientific Publications, 1988:85–101.
21. McConkey B, Fraser GM, Bligh AS. Transparent skin and osteoporosis. A study in patients with rheumatoid disease. Ann Rheum Dis 1965; 25:219–23.
22. Smith P. Age change in the female urethra. Br J Urol 1972; 44:667–76.
23. Versi E, Cardozo LD. Urethral vascular pulsations. Proceedings of the International Continence Society, London, 1985; 503–94.
24. Versi E, Cardozo LD, Brincat M, Cooper D, Montgomery JC, Studd JWW. Correlation of urethral physiology and skin collagen in postmenopausal women. Br J Obstet Gynaecol 1988; 95:147–52.
25. Versi E, Cardozo LD, Studd JWW, Brincat M, O'Dowd TM, Cooper D. Internal urinary sphincter in maintenance of female continence. Br Med J 1986; 292:166–7.
26. Josif CS, Batia S, Ed A, Astedt B. Estrogen receptors in the human female lower urinary tract. Am J Obstet Gynecol 1981; 141:817–20.
27. Faber P, Heidenreich J. Treatment of stress incontinence with oestrogen in postmenopausal women. Urol Int 1977; 32:221–3.
28. Walter S, Wolf I, Barlebo H, Jensen HK. Urinary incontinence in postmenopausal women treated with oestrogens. A double blind clinical trial. Urol Int 1978; 33:136–43.
29. Hilton P, Stanton SL. The use of intravaginal oestrogen cream in genuine stress incontinence. Br J Obstet Gynaecol 1983; 90:940–4.
30. Lobo R. Prevention of postmenopausal osteoporosis. In: Mishell DR, ed. Menopause, physiology and pharmacology. Chicago, London: Year Book Medical Publishers 1986; 165–86.
31. Haussler MR, Donaldson CA, Allegretto EA, Marion D, Mangelsdorf J, Kelly MA, Pike JW. New actions of 1,25-dihydroxyvitamin D_3: possible clues to the pathogenesis of postmenopausal osteoporosis. In: Christiansen C, ed. Osteoporosis. Proceedings of the Copenhagen Inter national Symposium on Osteoporosis, Copenhagen, Glostrup Hospital, 1984; 725–36.
32. Grosman N, Hudberg E, Schon J. The effects of oestrogenic treatment of the acid mucopoly saccharide pattern in skin of mice. Acta Pharmacol Toxicol 1971; 30:458–64.
33. Uzuka M, Nakamuza K, Ohta S, Mori Y. The mechanism of oestrogen-induced increase in hyaluronic acid biosynthesis with special reference to oestrogen receptors in the mouse skin. Biochim Biophys Acta 1980; 627: 199–206.

34. Savvas M, Studd JWW, Fogelman I, Dooley M, Montgomery J, Murby B. Skeletal effects of oral oestrogen compared with subcutaneous oestrogen and testosterone in postmenopausal women. Br Med J 1988; 297:331–3.
35. Studd JWW, Cardozo LD, Gibb DMF, Tuck SM, Magos AL, Brincat M, Cooper DJ. Hormone implants in women following hysterectomy and bilateral salpingo-oophorectomy. In: Van Herendael, H, ed. The Climacteric – an update. The Hague: MTP, 1984; 149–55.
36. Studd JWW, Thom MH, Paterson NEL, Wade-Evans T. The prevention and treatment of endometrial pathology in post menopausal women receiving exogenous oestrogens. In: Passeto N, Paoletti R, Ambrus JC, eds. The menopause and postmenopause. Lancaster: MTP, 1980; 127–39.
37. Studd JWW, Thom M. Oestrogens and endometrial cancer. In: Studd JWW, ed. Progress in obstetrics and gynaecology. London: Churchill Livingstone, 1981; 182–98.

Chapter 6

Oestrogen Deficiency and the Bladder

L. D. Cardozo

Introduction

In the female the lower urinary and genital tracts develop in close proximity, both arising embryologically from the primitive urogenital sinus. The urogenital membrane produces the ectodermal covering of the vulva and external urethral meatus. Animal and human studies have shown that the urethra is oestrogen sensitive, and in the human female oestrogen receptors are present in both the urethra and the bladder. Thus it is logical to suppose that changes in oestrogen levels influence the lower urinary tract as well as the genital tract in women.

Epidemiology

Symptoms of lower urinary tract dysfunction, including incontinence, increase with age and are more common in women than men at all ages [1,2]. In cross-sectional epidemiological studies it is difficult to control for single factors that may affect lower urinary tract symptomatology when the aetiology is multi-factorial. It is also difficult to separate the influence of ageing from that of the menopause. Iosif and Bekassy [3] reported that 70% of incontinent elderly women related the onset of their incontinence to their last menstrual period. However, Thomas et al. [1] could not confirm these findings and noted that, although there was a large rise in the prevalence of incontinence at about the age of 35 years, there did not seem to be a further large increase around the time of the menopause. Bungay et al. [4] showed that the symptoms of urgency and frequency of micturition were common in women of all ages, but their incidence was not related to the menopause.

In a study of 228 climacteric women who attended the Dulwich Menopause Clinic, they were designated postmenopausal if more than one year had elapsed since their last menstrual period. Women who had undergone a hysterectomy were regarded as postmenopausal if they had experienced climacteric symptoms for more than one year. All patients had a serum FSH level greater than 40 ng ml^{-1} and an oestradiol level less than 220 pmol ml^{-1}. If only some of these criteria were satisfied, patients were defined as perimenopausal. The normal data on the climacteric women are shown in Table 6.1.

Table 6.1. Normal data on climacteric women from the Dulwich Menopause Clinic

	Years since last menstrual period			
	0	1–2	3–5	6+
Age (years)	47.3	48.9	51.2	56.1
Parity	2.9	3.0	2.3	2.4
Ponderal Index	0.25	0.24	0.26	0.25
n (total = 228)	103	46	35	44

All new patients attending the menopause clinic completed a detailed urological symptom questionnaire under medical supervision and then had full urodynamic investigations.

In climacteric women, not complaining primarily of urological symptoms, who had never been treated for urological disease and who had never received oestrogen therapy, we found that the prevalence of lower urinary tract symptomatology was remarkably high (Table 6.2).

Table 6.2. Prevalence of lower urinary tract symptoms in climacteric women

Symptom (%)	Years since last menstrual period			
	0	1–2	3–5	6+
Diurnal frequency (>7)	28	29	31	33
Nocturia (>1)	22	31	31	29
Stress incontinence	56	54	54	41
Urgency	50	52	63	43
Urge incontinence	20	33	29	23
Poor flow	14	15	17	25
Pain micturition	14	18	9	7

Symptoms tended to be fairly mild although it is notable that one in five climacteric women, regardless of menopausal age, complained of severe urgency and nearly half of them complained of mild stress incontinence.

Diagnosis

Women with lower urinary tract dysfunction usually present with a combination of symptoms. The most common complaints are: stress incontinence, urgency, urge incontinence, frequency (both diurnal and nocturnal), dysuria and voiding difficulties. The correlation between symptoms and urodynamic diagnosis is notoriously poor. Jarvis et al. [5] could confirm the referring gynaecological consultant's clinical diagnosis in only 65% of women, and in 31% the management was significantly altered following urodynamic studies. Bent et al. [6] noted that, although 95% of patients with genuine stress incontinence complained of stress incontinence, 48% also complained of urgency; and only 67% of patients complaining of stress incontinence actually had the diagnosis of genuine stress incontinence. It is, therefore, essential in women who complain of lower urinary tract symptoms to perform adequate investigations prior to treatment.

A full urodynamic assessment was performed on 228 women attending the Dulwich Menopause Clinic for the first time complaining of climacteric symptoms. None of these women was being treated or had previously been treated with oestrogens. They all had a midstream specimen of urine sent for culture and sensitivity, and then underwent uroflowmetry followed by videocystourethrography with pressure and flow studies and urethral pressure profilometry. The prevalence of urodynamic abnormalities did not appear to increase with menopausal age (Table 6.3).

Table 6.3. Prevalence of urodynamic abnormality in climacteric women

Diagnosis (%)	Years since last menstrual period			
	0	1–2	3–5	6+
Normal	55	68	57	61
Genuine stress incontinence	18	13	24	12
Detrusor instability	3	9	5	7
Voiding difficulties	6	6	3	2
Other	18	4	11	19
n (Total = 227)	100	47	37	43

We sought correlations between the urodynamic data and increasing menopausal age in an attempt to identify any specific effect that the menopause may have on the lower urinary tract over and above the effect of ageing. It was found that maximum voiding pressure fell significantly with increasing age and menopausal age, and the height of the isometric detrusor contraction also had a negative correlation with age. Smith [7] proposed that oestrogen deficiency in postmenopausal women may result in distal urethral stenosis and, therefore, voiding difficulties. However, in the majority of women with voiding difficulties, the detrusor is hypotonic or acontractile [8]. It has been found that, at least in part, this may be a consequence of ageing although no age-related fall in the peak flow rate was found.

We sought correlations between age, menopausal age and parameters of the urethral pressure profile. In total 31 different parameters from each urethral pressure profile were measured. Although a number of significant correlations were identified, there was no specific "menopausal" effect on the physiology of the urethra. Rud et al. [9] reported that maximum urethral pressure and urethral length decrease with increasing age. We found that urethral closure pressure declined with increasing age but could not show any difference in urethral length.

The urethra is closely related to the vagina and vulva. Indeed stratified squamous epithelium is commonly seen lining the complete length of the urethra up to the trigone [10]. Oestradiol receptors are present in the urethra in higher concentration than in the bladder (where their greatest concentration is in the trigone) [11]; it is not surprising, therefore, that there is considerable scientific evidence implicating female sex hormones in urethral function.

Continence

For continence to exist, the maximum urethral pressure must exceed the intravesical pressure at all times except during micturition. This positive closure pressure is produced by the four functional layers of the urethra: the epithelium, the connective tissue, the vascular tissue and the muscle. All these layers are affected by oestrogen status.

Epithelium

In animal studies, Zuckerman [12] demonstrated that extragenital tissue derived from the urogenital sinus displayed oestrogen sensitivity. This was shown by maturation of squamous epithelium in response to oestrogen stimulation. Everett [13] postulated that the female urethra could develop "atrophic senile urethritis" similar to senile vaginitis, as a consequence of oestrogen withdrawal.

The close relationship between urethral and vaginal cytology is now well recognised [14,15] and the epithelial linings of both have been shown to change in response to alterations in serum oestrogen levels during the menstrual cycle. Youngblood et al. [16,17] found that the endoscopic and cytological changes of "senile urethritis" returned to normal following oestrogen therapy.

In our own group of patients, symptoms directly attributable to senile urethritis were found in only 1% of perimenopausal and 2% of postmenopausal women, which differs considerably from the experience of Smith [7]. However, he was dealing with a patient population presenting to a urology clinic and our patients were complaining of mixed menopausal symptoms, not of urinary tract dysfunction.

Connective Tissue

Connective tissue is an important component of the female urethra and collagen is its most abundant structural protein. Histological measurements show that collagen fibrils occupy twice the volume of muscle [18] and elastin fibres probably play only a minor role as they are not abundant in the urethra [19]. Collagen is produced by fibroblasts, which have oestrogen receptors [20], and the most common type of collagen is type 1, which accounts for 90% of the total body collagen [21]. Brincat et al. [22,23] have shown that skin collagen declines after the menopause and this decline may be reversed by oestrogen therapy. It is reasonable to assume that the decline in skin collagen may be paralleled by a decline in urethral collagen content; so the relationship between skin collagen content and urethral function was investigated [24].

In a cross-sectional study of normal postmenopausal women, skin collagen content was correlated with various parameters of the urethral pressure profile. For all the parameters studied, a greater collagen content was correlated with improved sphincter function. It is interesting to note that the area under the resting profile in the proximal urethra had a significant positive correlation with collagen content. Yet this did not hold true for the distal part of the urethra. It is our hypothesis, therefore, that the effect of collagen on the urethral closure mechanism is greatest in the proximal part of the urethra.

Vascular Tissue

Submucosal vascular tissue is an important component of the female urethra and contributes about one-third of the urethral closure pressure [9]. There are marked age changes in the vascular tissue [25] with a consequent fall in urethral closure pressure. During urethral pressure profilometry, if the urethral transducer is left at the point of maximum urethral pressure for several minutes, then in some women vascular pulsations, synchronous with the heart beat, can be identified and measured. In normal climacteric women the vascular pulsations decline with increasing menopausal age and this decline may be reversed by oestrogen therapy. Vascular pulsations increase with increasing serum oestradiol levels [26,27].

Muscle

The smooth muscle of the urethra contracts when exposed to alpha agonists [28]. Pretreatment with oestrogen produces a marked increase in the sensitivity of the urethral smooth muscle to alpha agonists [29]. Oestrogen withdrawal following the last menstrual period may result in a reduction in sensitivity of the urethral smooth muscle to sympathetic stimulation and therefore a reduction in muscle tone and closure pressure.

Traditionally, it has been taught that continence in women is maintained at the level of the bladder neck. Thus, opening (beaking) of the bladder neck under stress has been regarded as an indication for incontinence surgery. In a study of 98 women who presented to the Dulwich Menopause Clinic complaining of climacteric symptoms but without a primary complaint of incontinence, it was found by using X-ray screening with contrast medium in the bladder and urethral pressure profilometry, that about 50% of the women had evidence of an open bladder neck in response to stress but were continent as shown by videocysto-urethrography and pad testing [30]. Therefore, opening of the bladder neck under stress in continent climacteric women is common. It is not clear if incompetence of the bladder neck (or internal sphincter) is a consequence of the menopause or if, in fact, it is a common finding in women of all ages.

Lower urinary tract dysfunction is common in peri- and postmenopausal women and forms an integral part of the menopause syndrome. It is still unclear if this is a consequence of ovarian failure and subsequent oestrogen withdrawal or if it is simply age-related.

Treatment

The use of oestrogen therapy for postmenopausal urinary incontinence remains controversial. Early studies were purely subjective, lacked controls and were performed before the advent of urodynamic studies, which enable an accurate diagnosis to be made. However, they did provide evidence of symptomatic improvement. In the first report by Salmon et al. [31], 16 women with dysuria, frequency, urgency and incontinence were treated with intramuscular oestrogen therapy. After four weeks, 12 were symptomatically improved. The authors then discontinued therapy and when symptoms returned, they repeated the course of treatment. They showed that once again there was an improvement in symptoms and concluded that oestrogen must be responsible.

Quinestradol, which is no longer in use, was used by Musiani [32] in the treatment of a series of 110 stress incontinent women. He reported 36 cured and 43 improved. Using oestradiol implants, Schleyer-Saunders [33] showed that of 100 postmenopausal women with mixed urinary incontinence 70 were significantly improved and he felt that this reduced the need for surgery.

With the advent of pressure transducers, the effect of oestrogens on the urethral pressure profile underwent scrutiny. Caine and Raz [34] reported increased maximum urethral pressures together with symptomatic improvement in 26 out of 40 women with stress incontinence who were treated with conjugated equine oestrogens. Also studying stress incontinent women, Faber and Heidenreich [35] showed a significant rise in the urethral pressure profile in 39 of 41 women undergoing treatment with oestriol (a weak oestrogen that is thought to have a specific effect on the urogenital tissues). Interestingly, although they reported clinical improvement, none of the women was cured.

In Norway, Rud [36] treated 24 stress incontinent women with a combination of oral oestradiol and oestriol. He showed a significant increase in transmission of intra-abdominal pressure to the urethra as well as an increase in the maximum urethral pressure and the urethral length at rest. Symptomatic improvement occurred in 70% of his subjects. Similar findings wre reported by Hilton and Stanton [37], who treated 10 women with urodynamically proven genuine stress incontinence with intravaginal oestradiol cream. They showed a significant increase in the stress maximum urethral closure pressure because of improved pressure transmission in the mid-urethra. There was also significant subjective improvement in the symptoms of stress incontinence, urgency and frequency.

More recently, a similar study has shown similar results [38]. In this study 11 postmenopausal women with urodynamically proven genuine stress incontinence were treated with 2 g of conjugated oestrogen vaginal cream daily for a period of 6 weeks. Clinically, six (55%) were cured or significantly improved and a favourable clinical response correlated with urodynamic findings of increased urethral closure pressure and improved abdominal pressure transmission to the proximal urethra. These changes were not found in women who had a poor clinical response. Changes in urethral cytology also correlated well with clinical and urodynamic findings. Those women with a favourable response to oestrogen showed a maturation change from transitional to intermediate squamous epithelium.

Placebo-Controlled Studies

There have been very few properly placebo-controlled studies of oestrogen therapy and the management of urinary incontinence in postmenopausal women. Those which have appeared in the literature are described below.

Twenty years ago, Judge [39] recruited 20 long-stay female geriatric patients into a double-blind placebo-controlled trial of quinestradol. The active preparation significantly reduced the frequency of incontinence during the fifth week of treatment. No placebo effect was noted.

Oestriol is popular in the Scandinavian countries as it is thought to be safe and, as it does not have a major effect on the endometrium, a progestogen is thought to be unnecessary even when it is used for long-term treatment in women with a uterus. In a double-blind placebo-controlled cross-over study [40], 34 women aged 75 years were treated with 3 mg of oral oestriol, or equivalent placebo, daily for 3 months. There was no objective assessment and the women were divided into three groups on the basis of symptoms alone; stress incontinence, urge incontinence or mixed incontinence. The authors noted that oestriol was more effective than placebo in improving women with urge incontinence or mixed incontinence, but there was no difference between oestriol and placebo in those women with stress incontinence. However, only 11 women had stress incontinence alone, all had minimal urogenital atrophy, and the short "washout" period in this study may have obscured potential differences.

A multicentre study comparing the effects of oral oestriol to placebo in women with urgency or urge incontinence has recently been completed (Cardozo et al. unpublished). Patients were assessed symptomatically and urodynamically prior to treatment and at 3 months after receiving either oestriol 3 mg daily or placebo. They also had a subjective improvement check at one month. A total of 56 women completed treatment: 31 received oestriol and 25 received placebo. There was no difference between oestriol and placebo in any of the parameters that were studied, but it is interesting to note that there was a significant improvement in the symptom of urgency at 3 months in all women whether they were taking oestriol or placebo. There were no significant urodynamic changes, but vaginal cytology revealed a significantly increased maturation value in women taking oestriol as compared to placebo. This study underlines the need for some objective form of assessment and for placebo-controlled studies when evaluating treatment of this sort.

Walter et al. [41] also addressed the problem of sensory urge incontinence. A total of 29 postmenopausal women who had urodynamically proven stable bladders received either oestradiol with oestriol, or placebo, for 4 months cyclical therapy. They showed significant improvement in urgency and urge incontinence in seven of 15 women treated with oestrogen, which was significantly more than placebo. However, no improvement was reported in any of the eight women with stress incontinence in either group and no change could be detected in the urethral pressure profile.

A fairly recent placebo-controlled study using subjective and objective parameters has been reported by Wilson et al. [42], in which 36 women with urodynamically proven genuine stress incontinence participated in a double-blind study of cyclical oral piperazine oestrone sulphate for three months. Although there was symptomatic improvement, the authors were unable to find any significant difference in subjective response, urethral pressure profile, or urilos tests (an objective quantification test of urine loss). They concluded that the risk of oestrogen therapy may outweigh the benefit in the management of genuine stress incontinence.

Other/preliminary data have shown similar results. In a study at King's College and Dulwich Hospitals, 46 women, all of whom had urodynamically proven genuine stress incontinence, were randomly allocated to a 50 mg oestradiol implant (24) or a placebo implant (22). All the women completed a medically supervised symptom questionnaire and a visual analogue symptom score. They all underwent urethral pressure profilometry as described by Hilton and Stanton [43] and a pad weighing test [45]. After three months they were reassessed using the same investigations. There was no significant subjective evidence of improvement in either grouping. However, there was significant objective improvement in bladder base descent as seen on the videocystourethrogram. This is noteworthy, as it has long been speculated that oestrogen replacement is beneficial in cases of prolapse, but there has, as yet, been no reported evidence of this.

Side effects

Side effects and complications with oestrogen therapy would appear to be few. In Hilton and Stanton's [37] study one of the 11 women who started treatment with intravaginal cream was withdrawn because of breast tenderness and enlargement. Samsioe et al. [40] reported that four of the 34 elderly women treated with oestriol stopped therapy because of mastodynia or metrorrhagia. In another study [42], two of the 16 women treated with oral oestrone discontinued treatment; one had palpatations and the other suffered a myocardial infarction which was probably unrelated to treatment. There have been no other reported problems despite the use, in some cases, of high doses of oestrogen. However, all the studies reported have been short term: the longest duration of treatment was 4 months.

Fantl et al. [45] have recently assessed the effect of oestrogen supplementation. They studied 72 postmenopausal women, both clinically and urodynamically. Of these women 23 were already taking oestrogen replacement for other indications, and the remaining 49 were not oestrogen supplemented. The only significant difference that these authors reported was a decreased incidence of nocturia in the oestrogen-supplemented group. It was hypothesised that hypo-oestrogenism may affect the sensory threshold of the lower urinary tract.

Combined Therapies

The effect of oestrogen in combination with other drugs has not been widely studied. Ek et al. [46] treated 13 postmenopausal stress incontinent women with oral oestradiol for one month and then with oestradiol plus norephedrine or placebo for another month. They showed that oestradiol alone had no effect on symptoms or the urethral pressure profile, but that oestradiol plus norephedrine significantly improved symptoms and increased the urethral pressure profile. Beisland et al. [47] combined 80 mg of oestriol intramuscularly every four weeks with oral phenylpropanolamine 50 mg twice daily, and found that eight of 13 stress incontinent women became dry; this work was however, uncontrolled. The same authors [48] later performed a controlled cross-over trial of phenyl-propanolamine (50 mg twice daily orally) separately and in combination. Twenty postmenopausal women with genuine stress incontinence were assessed and urodynamic investigations were carried out before and after each period of treatment. Both phenylpropanolamine and oestriol increased maximum urethral closure pressure, but only oestriol increased functional urethral length. Phenyl-propanolamine was clinically more effective than oestriol but did not cause complete continence. However, with the combined treatment eight patients became dry and nine were considerably improved. Two women withdrew because of side effects (vaginal bleeding in one).

Another study has recently been reported [49] in which 36 postmenopausal women with objectively verified stress incontinence were treated with oral oestriol (2 mg daily) and phenylpropanolamine (100 mg daily) alone and in combination. After an initial four week single-blind period with phenylpropanol-amine, either oestriol or oestriol and phenylpropanolamine were given randomly in four-week periods in a cross-over design. Both phenylpropanolamine and oestriol in combination as well as phenylpropanolamine alone raised the intraurethral pressure and significantly reduced the urinary loss by 35% as measured in a standardised test. Most of the women preferred the combined treatment to either drug alone.

A possible application for oestrogen therapy in postmenopausal women with lower urinary tract dysfunction is in the treatment and prophylaxis of urinary tract infection. To date, only preliminary studies and anecdotal experiences have been described in the literature. Privette et al. [50] studied 12 women who experienced frequent urinary tract infections. They were all found to have atrophic vaginitis. They had suffered a mean of four infections per patient per year. Treatment consisted of a combination of short-term douche and antibiotic for one week together with long-term oestrogen therapy. Follow-up was from 2 to 8 years and during that time there were only four infections in the entire group. A large multicentre double-blind placebo-controlled trial is about to commence of oestriol as a prophylactic agent against recurrent urinary tract infection in postmenopausal women. If it proves successful, this type of weak oestrogen therapy could be useful in the prevention of morbidity among both community-dwelling and institutionalised elderly women.

Conclusions

The conclusions which can be drawn from the published data relating to the use of oestrogen therapy in the management of lower urinary tract dysfunction in postmenopausal women are as follows:

1. There have been very few appropriate placebo-controlled studies using subjective and objective parameters for assessment. More are urgently needed.
2. Oestrogen replacement apparently alleviates urgency, urge incontinence, frequency, nocturia and dysuria and possibly recurrent lower urinary tract infection.
3. There is no conclusive evidence that oestrogen alone cures stress incontinence.

However, oestrogen supplementation definitely improves the quality of life of many peri- and postmenopausal women, and therefore makes them better able to cope with their other disabilities. Perhaps the role of oestrogen in the management of postmenopausal urinary incontinence is as an adjunct to other methods of treatment such as surgery, physiotherapy or drugs. This is certainly a hypothesis worth testing and should be included in future research in this field.

References

1. Thomas TM, Plymat KR, Blannin J, Meade TW. Prevalence of urinary incontinence. Br Med J 1980; 281:1243–5.
2. Vetter NJ, Jones DA, Victor CR. Urinary incontinence in the elderly at home. Lancet 1981; ii:1275–7.
3. Iosif CS, Bekassy Z. Prevalence of genito-urinary symptoms in the later menopause. Acta Obstet Gynecol Scand 1984; 63:257–60.
4. Bungay GT, Vessey MP, McPherson CK. Study of symptoms in middle life with special reference to the menopause. Br Med J 1980; 281:181–3.
5. Jarvis GJ, Hall S, Stamp S, Millar DR, Johnson A. An assessment of urodynamic examination in incontinent women. Br J Obstet Gynaecol 1980; 87:893–6.
6. Bent AE, Richardson DA, Ostergaard DC. Diagnosis of lower urinary tract disorders in post-menopausal patients. Am J Obstet Gynecol 1983; 145:218–22.
7. Smith PJB. The effect of oestrogens on bladder function in the female. In: Campbell S, ed. The management of the menopause and post-menopausal years. Lancaster: MTP, 1976; 291–8.
8. Bergman A, Bhatia NW. Urodynamics: effect of urinary tract infection on urethral and bladder function. Obstet Gynecol 1985; 66:366–71.
9. Rud T, Andersson KE, Asmussen M, Hunting A, Ulmsten U. Factors maintaining the intraurethral pressure in women. Invest Urol 1980; 17:343–7.
10. Packham DA. The epithelial lining of the female trigone and urethra. Br J Urol 1971; 43:201–5.
11. Batra SL, Iosif CS. Female urethra: a target for oestrogen action. J Urol 1983; 129:418–20.
12. Zuckerman S. The histogenesis of tissues sensitive to oestrogens. Biol Rev 1940; 15:231–71.
13. Everett HS. Urology in female. Am J Surg 1941; 52:521–659.
14. Del Castillo EB, Argonz J, Mainini CG. Cytological cycle of the urinary sediment and its parallelism with the vaginal cycle. J Clin Endocrinol 1948; 8:76–87.
15. Del Castillo EB, Argonz J, Mainini CG. Smears from the female urethra and their relationship to smears of the urinary sediment. J Clin Endocrinol 1949; 9:1362–71.
16. Youngblood VH, Tomlin EM, Davis JB. Senile urethritis in women. J Urol 1957; 78:150–2.
17. Youngblood VH, Tomlin EM, Williams JO, Kimmelstiel P. Exfoliative cytology of the senile female urethra. J Urol 1958; 79:150–2.

18. Phillips JI, Davies I. A comparative morphometric analysis of the component tissues of the urethra in young and old female C573L/ICRFAt mice. Invest Urol 1981; 18:422–5.
19. Cullen WC, Fletcher TF, Bradley WG. Histology of the canine urethra. I Morphometry of the female urethra Anat Rec 1981; 199:177–86.
20. Stumpf WE, Sar M, Joshi SG. Oestrogen target cells in the skin. Experientia 1974; 30:196–8.
21. Alberts B, Bray D, Lewis J, Raff M, Roberts K, Watson JD. Cell adhesion and the extracellular matrix. In: Alberts B, Bray D, Lewis J, Raff M, Roberts K, Watson JD, eds. Molecular biology of the cell. New York and London: Garland Publishing, 1983; 673–715.
22. Brincat M, Moniz CF, Studd JWW, Darby AJ, Magos A, Cooper D. Sex hormones and skin collagen content in post menopausal women. Br Med J 1983; 287:1337–8.
23. Brincat M, Moniz CF, Studd JWW et al. Long term effects of the menopause and sex hormones on skin thickness. Br J Obstet Gynaecol 1985; 92:256–9.
24. Versi E, Cardozo LD, Brincat M et al. Correlation of urethral physiology and skin collagen in post-menopausal women. Br J Obstet Gynaecol 1988; 95:147–52.
25. Huisman AB. Morphologie van de vrouwelijke urethra. Thesis, Groningen. The Netherlands, 1979.
26. Tapp AJS, Cardozo LD, Versi E. Studd JWW. The prevalence of variation of resting urethral pressure in women and its association with lower urinary tract function. Br J Urol 1988; 61:314–17.
27. Versi E, Cardozo LD. Urethral vascular pulsations. Proceedings of the 15th annual meeting of the International Continence Society, 1985; 503.
28. Ek A, Alm P, Andersson KE, Persson CG. Adrenergic and cholinergic nerves of the human urethra and urinary bladder: a histochemical study. Acta Physiol Scand 1977; 99:345–52.
29. Callahan SM, Greed KE. The effects of oestrogens on spontaneous activity and responses to phenylephrine of the mammalian urethra. J Physiol 1985; 358:35–6.
30. Versi E, Cardozo LD, Studd JWW et al. Internal urinary sphincter in maintenance of female continence. Br Med J 1985, 292:166–7.
31. Salmon UL, Walter RI, Gast SH. The use of estrogens in the treatment of dysuria and incontinence in postmenopausal women. Am J Obstet Gynecol 1941; 42:845–7.
32. Musiani U. A partially successful attempt at medical treatment of urinary stress incontinence in women. Urol Int 1972; 27:405–10.
33. Schleyer-Saunders E. Hormone implants for urinary disorders in postmenopausal women. J Am Geriatr Soc 1976; 24:337–9.
34. Caine M, Raz S. The role of female hormones in stress incontinence. Proceedings of the 16th congress of the International Society of Urology, Amsterdam, 1973.
35. Faber P, Heidenreich J. Treatment of stress incontinence with estrogen in postmenopausal women. Urol Int 1971; 32:221–3.
36. Rud T. The effects of oestrogens and gestagens on the urethral pressure profile in urinary continent and stress incontinent women. Acta Obstet Gynecol Scand 1980; 59:265–70.
37. Hilton P, Stanton SL. The use of intravaginal oestrogen cream in genuine stress incontinence. Br J Obstet Gynaecol 1983; 90:940–4.
38. Bhatia NN, Bergman A, Karram MM. Effects of estrogen on urethral function in women with urinary incontinence. Obstet Gynecol 1989; 160:176–81.
39. Judge TG. The use of quinestradol in elderly incontinent women: a preliminary report. Gerontol Clin 1969; 11:159–64.
40. Samsioe G, Jansson I. Mellstrom D. Svandborg A. Occurrence, nature and treatment of urinary incontinence in a 70 year old female population. Maturitas 1985; 7:335–42.
41. Walter S, Wolf H, Barlebo H, Jensen H. Urinary incontinence in postmenopausal women treated with oestrogens: a double-blind clinical trial. Urol Int 1978; 33:135–43.
42. Wilson PD, Faragher B, Butler B, et al. Treatment with oral piperazine oestrone sulphate for genuine stress incontinence in post menopausal women. Br J Obstet Gynaecol 1987; 94:568–74.
43. Hilton P, Stanton SL. Urethral pressure measurements by microtransducer: the results in symptom-free women and in those with genuine stress incontinence. Br J Obstet Gynaecol 1983; 90:919–33.
44. Versi E. Cardozo LD. Perineal pad weighing versus videographic analysis in genuine stress incontinence. Br J Obstet Gynaecol 1986; 93:364–6.
45. Fantl JA, Wyman JF, Anderson RL, Matt DW, Bump RC. Postmenopausal urinary incontinence: comparison between non-estrogen supplement and estrogen-supplemented women. Obstet Gynecol 1988; 71:823–6.
46. Ek A, Andersson KE, Gallberg B, Ulmsten U. Effects of oestradiol and combined norephedrin and oestradiol treatment on female stress incontinence. Zentralbl Gynakol 1980; 102:839–44.

47. Beisland HO, Fossberg E, Sander S. On incompetent urethral closure mechanism: treatment with estriol and phenylpropanolamine. Scand J Urol Nephrol [Suppl] 1981; 60:67–9.
48. Beisland HO, Fossberg E, Moer A, Sander S. Urethral sphincteric insufficiency in postmenopausal females: treatment with phenylpropanolamine and estriol separately and in combination. Urol Int 1984; 39:211–16.
49. Kinn AC, Lindskog M. Estrogens and phenylpropanolamine in combination for stress urinary incontinence in postmenopausal women. Urology 1988; 32:273–80.
50. Privette M, Cade R, Peterson J. Mars D. Prevention of recurrent urinary tract infections in postmenopausal women. Nephron 1988; 50:24–7.

Discussion

Stevenson: In Fig. 5.2 showing the collagen content of the skin in relation to at time postmenopause, there was no decrease in the skin collagen content until five years after the menopause. Bone density is decreased long before that. We know that the bone is affected by the menopause and the skin is affected by the menopause, but it does not necessarily mean that the two are related together. In fact Dr Brincat's data would suggest that they are not.

Brincat: I would not say that. It was a cross-sectional study. There was a huge individual variation in those particular patients and that is only one of the many figures we have on the subject. That is a problem with all cross-sectional studies I feel, in that because of initial individual variation, one might get a false impression that there is no collagen loss in the first 5 years or in the first 4 years. If we were to consider the loss after 1 year where there is a huge dip in the original figure, we might say that there has been a huge dip after 1 year, it recovers after 3 years, stays up for 5 years and then decreases again. The figure could be interpreted that way, but I would oppose that. It is just one of the problems in interpreting cross-sectional studies and taking a mean out of every cohort that is analysed, or every group that is analysed at 1-year intervals.

Baird: We are here to discuss the role of hormone replacement therapy in osteoporosis in particular and Dr Brincat has made a good case, and Professor Anderson has mentioned it, that the connective tissue is also affected by oestrogen. But I am still totally unsure as to the mode of action of oestrogen either in affecting bone loss or affecting the metabolism of collagen. Dr Brincat has pointed out that there are oestrogen receptors on fibroblasts and there are oestrogen receptors on osteoblasts. But what happens to collagen after the oestrogen reaches the receptors? Is there any information on that?

Brincat: There is only one in vitro study on that. Russell's group in Sheffield did show an increase in the production of pro-collagen in osteoblasts being given oestrogens [1]. They produced similar work on the use of stanozolol and different work on the use of corticosteroids while using the same techniques on their osteoblastic cell lines. That is the only work that I know of showing what actually happens at molecular level.

Stevenson: As far as bone is concerned, it is still rather preliminary evidence that oestradiol receptors are present. They are present on osteoblast-like cells it is thought, but again a really good study in humans is lacking. They are present at very low levels and there is no good evidence that these are functional receptors. So it is still very early days to be talking about those receptors.

Baird: To summarise, we still do not know how oestrogen affects either collagen synthesis or the mineral content of bone.

Brincat: But we are getting more and more evidence. My results indicated a number of mechanisms, not just one, on how oestrogens might possibly affect bone metabolism. There was also a possible mechanism by osteoclasts and possibly by growth hormones.

Lindsay: Professor Baird's statement is probably the appropriate one for our state of knowledge, but Dr Stevenson has made an important comment about the osteoblast-like cells and the fact that those are cells that have been well removed from their in vivo circumstance before one can detect the small number of receptors. It has been very difficult, in fact impossible as yet, to show that osteoblasts in vivo have oestradiol receptors.

These cells differentiate to some degree. There are a number of studies that show that there are changes in the differentiation of these cells on incubation with low doses of oestradiol. It remains to be seen whether those will be physiologically meaningful in the long run with a hormone that clearly inhibits bone resorption in vivo rather than increases bone formation.

Selby: I wanted to pick up on the point that was made about the group looking at stanozolol. I know of the tendency in a number of the studies for giving oestrogen and testosterone. Were Dr Brincat's studies on oestrogen alone or on oestrogen and testosterone?

Brincat: We did comparative studies against oestrogen alone and oestrogen and testosterone and there was no difference between the two groups. We used very low doses of testosterone, 100 mg of testosterone which is relatively low. Although there might be some additive effect we were unable to show it.

Selby: It has been suggested that the changes that might be seen in bone formation may be more related to androgenic changes than oestrogenic changes.

Brincat: The prospective study I showed was oestrogen alone.

Kanis: Our group showed an effect of oestrogens on osteoblast-like cells but I should point out that these effects are rather small compared to the kind of effects that can be demonstrated with PTH or 125. Second, these are mixed cell systems. They are not pure osteoblasts. Third, we have found no evidence of oestrogen receptors, so the question is whether it is mediated by a direct effect on bone cells, or more likely whether it may be affecting other cell populations.

One comment that may be relevant is that it is not necessary to invoke an action of oestrogens on bone cell metabolism. It is clear that oestrogens do affect bone either directly or indirectly, but it is possible (and a lot of morphological evidence would suggest) that oestrogen deficiency has two important effects in osteoporosis. One is to decrease the competence or the numbers of osteoblasts that are attracted to a resorption cavity so that it does not necessarily have to affect the performance of the osteoblasts but only the numbers that are recruited. Second, there is reasonable evidence to suggest that either directly or indirectly oestrogens decelerate bone turnover, which again can be a question of altering the numbers of cells rather than the individual function of those cells.

Whitehead: What does the literature show in terms of the relatively low oestrogen stimulus which is applied with orally administered oestriol, 1 mg or 3 mg daily? Is that really a valid preparation to try to determine whether tissue is or is not oestrogen-dependent? An improvement in genuine stress incontinence (GSI) has been shown using higher dose oestrogen in a placebo controlled fashion and I wondered whether just giving these low doses of oestriol is not almost homeopathic.

Cardozo: From what I glean from the literature, people have been using oestriol on the assumption that because it improves vaginal atrophy it should also improve lower urinary tract (LUT) atrophy. That is obviously a mistaken assumption. Although there are Scandinavian studies that have shown symptomatic improvement [2], in the multicentre study that we have recently finished, placebo showed equal symptomatic improvement and we could show no difference between the two preparations despite a change of vaginal cytology. So oestriol would not seem to be a strong enough oestrogen to use for LUT dysfunction.

The second point is that GSI is not a sensory abnormality; it is an anatomical abnormality. Although many of the studies, including placebo-controlled studies, have shown an improvement in GSI which correlated with changes in the urethral pressure profile, none has affected a cure using oestrogen replacement. This is important and underlines the need for the use of higher doses of oestrogens as an adjunct to therapy, but it is no good sending postmenopausal women with GSI away with the promise of a cure.

Studd: Did any of the patients in the studies report severe recurrent pain on micturition? Clinically if the patient has a number of symptoms and one of them is bladder pain, that is the last one to recover.

Cardozo: In urgency, frequency and dysuria there is definitely an improvement where appropriate oestrogen therapy is used. It may take a long time. The patient needs to use continuous replacement, and oestriol is no good.

Lindsay: A brief comment on hydroxyproline. I should not like anyone to feel that hydroxyproline was a useless measurement. There is a great deal of literature showing that hydroxyproline excretion is reduced with the introduction of oestrogen. The problem is partly that the urinary hydroxyproline has many sources and also that it is a difficult measurement to make. We tend, however, to get wrapped up in the new technologies a lot of the time and fail to examine some of the literature. Evidence for reduced bone turnover biochemically comes from very good measurements of urinary hydroxyproline.

Baird: To sum up, I am somewhat disappointed. I had hoped that a better index of the way oestrogens might affect bone and connective tissue would have been produced, with a view to trying to get a better assessment, albeit indirect, of those people without symptoms who would actually benefit from replacement therapy. If I had to summarise the state of the art, I would say that we probably do not have that information as yet.

References

1. Vaishnav R, Gallagher JA, Beresford JN, Poser J, Russell RGG. Direct effects of stanozolol and estrogens in human bone cell culture. In: Christiansen et al. eds. Osteoporosis. Copenhagen: Glostrup Hospital, 1984; 485–8.
2. Walter S, Wolf H, Barlebo H, Kaalund Jensen H. Urinary incontinence in post-menopausal women treated with estrogens. A double blind clinical trial. Urol Int 1978; 33:135.

Section II
Pathophysiology of Osteoporosis

Chapter 7

Epidemiology of Osteoporosis

R. Lindsay and F. Cosman

Introduction

During the past ten years or so, osteoporosis and its accompanying fractures have been recognised as a major public health problem affecting many countries. In some regions, the problem is epidemic in proportions or is predicted to become so within the next few decades. The consequences, in terms of both cost and the overall impact on the health of the ageing population, are dramatic.

Definition

Osteoporosis is defined as a diffuse skeletal condition in which bone mass is sufficiently reduced that there is an increased risk of skeletal failure, that is fracture even with minimal or no trauma.

Osteoporosis and Fracture Risk

Osteoporosis is only important clinically when fractures occur, but it is self-evident that fractures (usually more traumatic) occur in the absence of significant osteoporosis. The classical distribution of fractures consequent upon osteoporosis mirrors the changes occurring in the skeleton, at least among the adult population. Since in all populations studied thus far, bone mass falls with

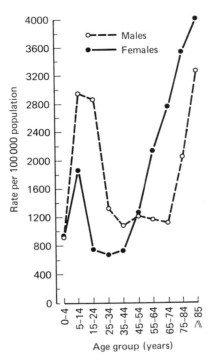

Fig. 7.1. Frequency of limb fractures as a function of age. Note a peak frequency in the very young followed by a continually increasing incidence from age 40 years in women but not until age 70 years in men [1].

age, it is not surprising that the prevalence and incidence of osteoporotic fractures increase with age. Overall this is the pattern that is seen when one examines fracture frequency on a population basis [1], demonstrating the large contribution that is made by osteoporotic fractures to overall fracture frequency (Fig. 7.1).

In addition to the presence of osteoporosis, however, contributions to fracture risk result from a variety of other sources (Table 7.1). In general, these are factors that increase the risk of falls. The relative importance of trauma associated with falling, versus low bone mass *per se* varies according to fracture site but is clearly of importance in two of the three main osteoporotic fractures, those of hip and distal radius. Fractures of the vertebral body are more dependent on the decline in bone mass, and often occur spontaneously with no unusual trauma.

Although falling is common among the elderly, it has been estimated that only 2%–5% of falls result in fracture [2]. Risk factors include the use of sedatives, especially long-acting medications, cognitive impairment, illness or disability, abnormalities of balance and gait, and the presence of foot problems. Individuals who fall are more likely to fall again (for example, patients with Parkinson's disease) and, therefore, identification of recurrent fallers may be a useful strategy for fracture prevention among the elderly [3]. While many of the

Table 7.1. Factors thought to influence fracture risk

Age

Osteoporosis (factors affecting bone mass)

Frequency of falls
Balance
Gait
Sensory capacity
Chronic ill health (frailty)
Cognitive impairment
Drugs (oestrogen, diuretics, antihypertensives, sedatives)
Alcohol
Foot problems
Extrinsic factors (household hazards, weather)

Capacity to resist trauma
Weight (?)
Body composition (?)
Deconditioning (?)
Reflexes (?)

factors thought to affect bone mass (Table 7.2) are commonly discussed and indeed everyone has their own favourite list, the relative importance of all but genetics, gonadal status, and age is probably overrated, at least when considering osteoporosis as a population problem. Thus, the likelihood of prevention of bone loss depends on the judicious use of oestrogen replacement therapy for the postmenopausal population. Further data are required on the control of peak bone mass before simple strategies directed at maximising bone mass among young adults can be introduced on a public health basis.

Table 7.2. Some factors thought to alter skeletal mass

Genetic (gender, race)
Gonadal failure
Age
Physical activity
Nutrition (calcium, caffeine, protein etc.)
Alcohol consumption
Cigarette consumption
Weight (fat mass)
Drugs (oestrogen, thiazides, calcitonin, diphosphonates, steroids, anabolics (androgens), dilantin)
Endocrine disease (thyrotoxicosis, Cushing's syndrome, type I diabetes mellitus)

Epidemiology of Fractures

Throughout life, patterns of fracture frequency change in different ways for different parts of the skeleton (Fig. 7.1) [1]. Fracture occurrence in general tends to be high at the extremes of life, with a secondary peak in young adults [1,4]. Different fractures peak at different ages, and those most common among the aged are thought to be consequent upon osteoporosis. The most common fractures in this category are fractures of the hip, vertebrae (crush fractures) and distal radius (Colles' fractures), although fracture of any bone can probably occur in the presence of osteoporosis. In the USA at present, approximately 1.5 million fractures are thought to occur each year within this category [4]. Of these, there are approximately 500 000 vertebral fractures, although precise data on the incidence of vertebral fractures do not exist, and 250 000 fractures of the hip. Fracture incidence at any age is dependent on both trauma and the capacity of the skeleton to resist the injury. Most fractures of the hip require moderate trauma, usually a fall from a standing height. The increased frequency of hip fracture among the elderly, therefore, depends on low bone mass, falls and reduced capacity to protect the bone from trauma. Vertebral fractures probably occur mostly because of low bone mass [4], and sufficient force to fracture the vertebrae is generated during the normal activities of life. Finally, qualitative changes in the skeleton that accompany reduced bone mass also contribute to the likelihood of fracture, but their contribution in quantitative terms is difficult to evaluate [5,6].

The natural history of osteoporotic fractures is not well understood. It is commonly believed clinically that patients who have one fracture will be at increased risk of other fractures. However, data to substantiate that statement are difficult to find in the literature. Prior fractures of the proximal humerus are twice as common among patients with hip fracture [7], and vertebral fractures may be 2–10 times more common in this population [8]. The converse is also true: there is an increased risk of hip fracture in patients with either radius or vertebral fracture [9]. Melton [4] has suggested that the relationship between fractures is less than would be expected, and this forms one of the bases for the hypothesis that there are two distinct forms of osteoporosis accounting for the difference in fracture relationships.

Fractures of the Proximal Femur

The age-specific increase in hip fracture is exponential in both sexes [10,11] but begins at a much later age among men (Fig. 7.2). The incidence increases from negligible, to more than 3% per year for the very old (>85 years). The fact that 80% of all hip fractures occur among women [4] relates to the greater survival of women to an at risk age. Rates of hip fracture among those at risk, however, are still higher in women than men, with a relative risk ratio of 2:1. This is likely to be due to the increased rate of bone loss which occurs in women after the menopause. In addition, the alterations in skeletal metabolism following ovarian failure, and the documented effects of oestrogen in reducing risk of fracture also support the importance of the menopause in the pathogenesis of hip fracture. The lifetime risk of hip fracture is 15% for the average perimenopausal woman and probably significantly greater for the woman who enters the menopause with low bone mass [12]. The role of other disorders of the skeleton, such as osteomalacia, remains controversial and may vary among populations

Fractures of the hip occur in two types, across the femoral neck itself (transcervical) or between the greater and lesser trochanters (intertrochanteric). Both increase in a similar manner with age, although there appears to be a greater increase in intertrochanteric fractures among the very old. The latter

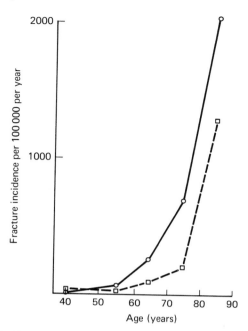

Fig. 7.2 Increasing incidence of fermoral neck fractures with increasing age. Note that in females (○) this incidence increases 10 years earlier than in males (□). (Adapted from Melton and Riggs [43].)

type also appears to have a closer relationship to previous vertebral fractures [7,8]. When a fracture of one type has occurred there is a significantly greater chance of recurrence of the same type of hip fracture on the opposite side [13].

Although most hip fractures are associated with some trauma, usually a fall from standing height, some may be spontaneous, and others associated with local pathology such as malignancy. Factors affecting the frequency of falls are listed in Table 7.1. In addition, women may be at greater risk of falling than men at least up to the age of 75 years [14]. It has been suggested that the increased tendency for the elderly to fracture a hip after a fall is based on the slower gait, and increased tendency to fall to the side or backward, landing directly on the hip. The ability to absorb the trauma without fracturing may relate to fat or muscle mass, good protective reflexes or muscular conditioning. Further investigation is required to elucidate the interrelationship between falls and fracture.

Hip fractures are commoner in all white populations studied, with lower rates in black populations in Africa and America, as well as among Maoris [4,15,16]. The low fracture incidence described in Asian populations may be due to under-reporting and there is some suggestion that the rates of osteoporotic fracture may be higher than previously thought. The risks of fracture among Asian and Mexican populations in the USA, however, may be lower than among the Caucasian population despite their lower bone mass [17,18].

Hip fracture is associated with significant morbidity and mortality. Estimates of post-hip-fracture mortality vary, but the figures suggest a 5%–20% excess mortality (i.e. above that expected for age and sex) [4,19–22] that appears to occur mostly in the first year after fracture, although some excess may continue for several years [23]. The important factors determining mortality appear to be increased age, and frailty (or chronic illness) prior to the fracture. Institutionalised patients are at especially high risk. The complications of urgent surgery, often required to repair the fracture, cause much of the excess mortality, with thromboembolic disease being particularly common after procedures on the hip. Hip fracture is thought to result in some 30 000 deaths each year in the USA.

Of those surviving a hip fracture, half will be unable to walk independently afterward and will experience greater social isolation. For almost one-third of patients, hip fracture precipitates entry to a nursing home, such that almost 10% of nursing home patients have experienced a hip fracture [4].

The financial cost of hip fracture is enormous. About 35% of patients with limb fractures require hospital admission, including all patients with hip fracture, who may require up to 33 days in an acute setting. In 1984 the financial cost to the USA health care system was estimated to be $7 billion. These costs can only be expected to increase as the proportion of elderly increases in the population. By the year 2050 the elderly will account for 22% of the entire population, and those over 85 years old, the fastest growing age group in many societies, will account for 5% of the population [23]. A recent estimate of the costs of hip fracture, based on conservative estimates, indicates that by the year 2040, hip fracture costs will exceed $16 billion per year [24].

These figures may be compounded by increases in the age-specific incidence of hip fracture, as has been noted in a number of European countries including Scandinavia and Great Britain [25–30], although there is some disagreement [31–33]. Data from Canada [34] and some from the USA [35] have also demonstrated an increased incidence, but again not all agree [36]. One major study in the USA found that the age-adjusted incidence of hip fracture increased until the 1950s but has since levelled off. However, our group estimated from hospital discharge data that hip fracture incidence continued to increase through the 1970s (Fig. 7.3) [35] but appeared relatively stable again in the 1980s. Nonetheless, the calculated costs of hip fracture estimated into the next century may well be a considerable underestimate of the real cost.

Vertebral Fractures

The prevalance of vertebral fractures among the ageing population is extremely high and may exceed 75% for very aged women if wedging is included [37]. Vertebral fractures may be painless and gradually progressive, or acute and accompanied by severe back pain. Asymptomatic fractures are detected on radiographs with increasing frequency as age increases. Fractures may be isolated to one vertebra, but most often are multiple and may occur in the thoracic and/or lumbar spine. The suggested higher incidence of acute episodes among younger individuals may be an anomaly caused by the higher activity patterns in that population. True incidence rates have been difficult to determine because of the insidious onset of these fractures [38]. Non-traumatic fractures probably affect about one-third of women by age 65 years. This would represent about 5 million women in the USA currently with radiological evidence of crush fractures. Estimates of incidence based on the prevalence data available show that incidence begins to increase around the time of the

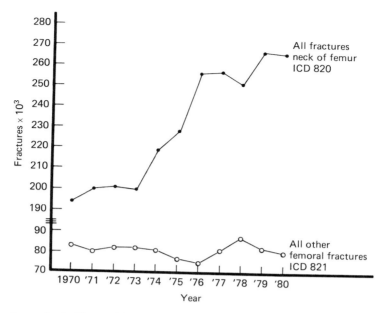

Fig. 7.3. Increasing incidence of femoral neck fractures over the decade 1970 – 1980 [35].

menopause and continues to rise throughout life [38]. Based on these estimates, patients with vertebral fracture outnumber those affected by hip fracture by a factor of three, while the number of vertebral fractures exceeds the number of hip fractures by a considerably greater amount.

Little reliable information is available on the distribution of vertebral fractures in different countries. Most estimates are similar to the USA data, but the difficulty in determining population-based prevalence probably accounts for some data that suggest a lower prevalence in some countries [39]. The influence of race is also poorly documented although clinical experience and one study suggest that black women only rarely have vertebral fractures [40]. Vertebral fracture prevalence among men is probably 8–12 times lower than among women. Why the relative risk of vertebral fracture between men and women is so different from that of hip fracture is unclear, but again this underscores the great importance of ovarian failure in the pathogenesis of vertebral osteoporosis.

As many as 500 000 women, or more, in the USA may suffer vertebral fractures each year, accounting for some 200 000 visits to doctors (since probably over half of these fractures are asymptomatic) and about 5 million restricted activity days each year [41]. This can be added to the 7 million for hip fracture and 6 million for Colles' fracture.

Colles' Fractures

The incidence of Colles' fracture (or fractures of the distal radius) increases among women after menopause but then reaches a plateau, unlike vertebral or hip fractures [42]. The explanation for this phenomenon is unknown. It seems likely that the phenomenon of increased bone loss after menopause accounts for the postmenopausal rise, but the cause of the plateau remains obscure. Explanations based on gradual changes in falling patterns with age seem unsatisfactory although these changes undoubtedly occur. In older women the incidence of Colles' fracture is around 600 per 100 000 person-years, but only 80 per 100 000 person-years among men [43], a relative risk ratio similar to that seen for vertebral fractures. In general, Colles' fractures tend to have a seasonal variation with increased incidence during the winter, presumably related to increased frequency of falling on the ice.

There is little information on the geographical variation in Colles' fracture although in general, regional differences appear somewhat similar to those recorded for hip fracture. This was not found to be the case in certain areas of Yugoslavia associated with a relatively high calcium intake, where hip fractures declined but Colles' fractures remained relatively frequent [44]. The same problem exists for epidemiological studies of Colles' fracture as for vertebral crush fractures. The majority of cases do not require hospital admission and reliable data are, therefore, difficult to obtain.

Other Fractures

Since bone loss after the menopause and with increased age affects all bones to a variable degree, fracture of any bone can occur as part of the osteoporotic syndrome [45]. After the commonest fractures, described above, the most frequent fractures encountered are of the proximal humerus, pelvis and proximal tibia. The age-specific incidence of these fractures follows closely that seen for fractures of the hip, where incidence rates rise with age to a greater extent among women than men, and the rate continues to increase with age.

Consequences of Fracture

It is well accepted that the high prevalence and incidence of osteoporotic fractures result in a major public health problem. Of the 1.5 million new fractures each year in the United States thought to occur consequent upon the development of osteoporosis, estimates of vertebral fracture account for 500 000, hip fracture 250 000, and Colles' fracture 150 000. The remainder include proximal humerus, pelvis and other limb fractures, for which osteoporosis

Table 7.3. Some leading causes of death and morbidity among white postmenopausal women

	Annual mortality per 1000 women	Lifetime risk (%)
Ischaemic heart disease	105	40
Breast cancer	18.8	9
Hip fracture	9.4	16
Endometrial cancer	0.6	2

accounts for one-half of the total fracture incidence in the USA. In 1984 the cost was estimated to be $18 billion for all osteoporotic fractures. These costs can only be expected to increase as the number of elderly in the population continues to grow.

Identifying the "At Risk" Population

Osteoporosis will remain a disorder that is better prevented than treated, and thus identification of those individuals at risk of fracture, prior to fracture occurrence, is a strategy that must be evaluated on a population basis. For a woman entering the menopause the lifetime risk of suffering a hip fracture is of the order of 15% which is equal to the combined risk of breast, uterine, and ovarian cancer (Table 7.3). Applied across the entire population, however, that figure is insufficient to allow recommending preventive therapy for all individuals as they pass the menopause. Nonetheless the menopause, because of its association with acceleration of bone loss, is probably a useful time at which to evaluate women for their risk of osteoporosis and to target for treatment those thought to be at increased risk.

Bone mineral density accounts for 75%–80% of the strength of bone [46]. Therefore, as bone density falls with age so does the strength of bone. Bone strength is, not surprisingly, a major determinant of fracture risk and the likelihood that a fracture will be sustained following an incident of sufficient trauma is determined by bone strength. Recent studies (Fig. 7.4) [45] have demonstrated an increased risk of fracture as bone density falls for the hip, vertebrae, and wrist as well as other limb fractures [38,47–49]. In one study the risk of subsequent fracture was shown to increase with declining bone mass at all ages.

Estimates of bone density can predict the risk of fractures occurring in the

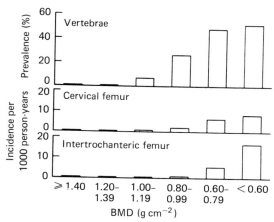

Fig. 7.4. Hip fracture incidence and vertebral fracture prevalence as a function of bone mineral density [45].

future. This is because bone density at one age is fairly predictive of bone density in that individual in later years [50]. Thus, a bone density measurement made at the time of the menopause is a reasonable assessment of what will happen to that woman's skeleton as she ages. A recent model based on these assumptions estimated that the lifetime risk of hip fracture is negligible if a woman has a femoral neck bone density above 1.3 g cm^{-2} at age 40 years, increasing to more than 25% for both intertrochanteric and femoral neck fractures if bone mass is less than 0.6 g cm^{-2} [51]. Thus, bone density at menopause is a useful method of selecting patients for treatment for osteoporosis.

Although bone mass measurements in women with fractures overlap the normal population, their usefulness is to stratify people into groups of varying risks. This is analogous to the use of cholesterol measurement for coronary artery disease, or even blood pressure determination for cerebrovascular risk. Recent data have confirmed the usefulness of bone mass measurements for risk stratification. Measurement of bone mass in the radius or os calcis can predict the risk of fracture [52,53], such that women with the lowest bone mass (in the bottom quintile) had four times the risk of fracture when compared with women in the topmost quintile. Bone mass at one site can predict fracture at another. Measurement of bone mass at the os calcis for example, predicted vertebral fracture risk, as well as risk of radial and os calcis fractures [53]. Measurement in the radius can predict the likelihood of hip fracture.

Clinical data are often used to identify individuals at risk of osteoporosis. Indeed most clinicians have a set of favoured risk factors that are used clinically. However, there are no data which confirm that clinical observations can be used in this way. Risk factors do not allow estimation of bone mass, and patients cannot be stratified into high and low risk using any grouping of clinical facts with the data presently available. Risk factor analysis does have some more general use, since many of those factors that may increase risk for osteoporosis have also been implicated in other disorders of ageing. Evaluation with the patient is a useful way of motivating better general health but to determine risk of future fracture a bone mass measurement is necessary.

Conclusions

Fractures among the elderly are a major public health problem that will continue to enlarge in the years to come. The presence of low bone mass contributes to fracture risk, but other events such as falls, frailty and medication use are clearly important in hip fracture occurrence. Strategies must be developed to identify those individuals in the preclinical phase of the disorder, since early preventive therapy is likely to be more successful than treatment of the already established disorder.

Acknowledgement

This work was supported in part by PHS grant AR 39191–03.

References

1. Garraway WM, Stauffer RN, Kurland LT, O'Fallon WM. Limb fractures in a defined population. Frequency and distribution. Mayo Clinic Proc 1979; 54:701–7.
2. Tinetti ME, Speechley M, Ginter SF. Risk factors for falls among elderly persons living in the community. N Engl J Med 1988; 319:1701–7.
3. Tinetti ME, Speechley M. Prevention of falls among the elderly. N Engl J Med 1989; 320: 1055–9.
4. Melton LJ III, Epidemiology of fractures. In: Riggs BL, Melton LJ III, eds. Osteoporosis: etiology, diagnosis, and management. New York: Raven Press, 1988; 133–54.
5. Dempster DW, Horbert W, Shane E, Lindsay R. A simple method for correlative light and scanning electron microscopy of human iliac crest bone biopsies. J Bone Miner Res, 1986; 1:15–21.
6. Parfitt AM. Trabecular bone architecture in the pathogenesis and prevention of fracture. Am J Med 1987; 82:68–72.
7. Gallagher JC, Melton LJ, Riggs BL. Examination of prevalence rates of possible risk factors in a population with a fracture of the proximal femur. Clin Orthop 1980; 153:158–65.
8. Pogrund H, Makin M, Robin G, Menczel J, Steinberg R. Osteoporosis in patients with fractured femoral neck in Jerusalem. Clin Orthop 1977; 124:165–72.
9. Lewinnek GE, Kelsey J, White AA III, Kreiger NJ. The significance and a comparable analysis of the epidemiology of hip fractures. Clin Orthop 1980; 152:35–43.
10. Melton LJ, Riggs BL. Epidemiology of age-related fractures. In: Avioli LV, ed. The osteoporotic syndrome: detection, prevention, and treatment. New York: Grune and Stratton, 1983; 45–72.
11. Farmer ME, White LR, Brody JA, Bailey KR. Race and sex differences in hip fracture incidence. Am J Public Health 1984; 74:1374–80.
12. Cummings SR, Kelsey JL, Nevitt MC, O'Dowd KJ. Epidemiology of osteoporosis and osteoporotic fractures. Epidemiol Rev 1985; 7:178–208.
13. Dretakis E, Kritsikis N, Economou K, Christodoulou N. Bilateral non-contemporary fractures of the proximal femur. Acta Orthop Scand 1981; 52:227–9.
14. Campbell AJ, Reinken S, Allan BC, Martinez GS. Falls in old age: a study of frequency and related clinical factors. Age Ageing 1981; 10:264–70.
15. Solomon L. Osteoporosis and fracture of the femoral neck in the South African Bantu. J Bone Joint Surg 1968; 50–B:2–13.
16. Stott S, Gray DH. The incidence of femoral neck fractures in New Zealand. N Z Med J 1980; 91:6–9.
17. Bauer RL. Ethnic differences in hip fractures. A reduced incidence in Mexican-Americans. Am J Epidemiol 1988; 127:145–9.
18. Silverman SL, Madison RE. Decreased incidence in hip fracture in Hispanics, Asians and Blacks: California hospital discharge data. Am J Public Health 1988; 78:1482–3.
19. Jensen JS, Tondevold E. Mortality after hip fracture. Acta Orthop Scand 1979; 50:161–7.
20. Mossey JM, Mutran E, Knott K, Craik R. Determinants of recovery after hip fracture: the importance of psychosocial factors. Am J Public Health 1989; 79:279–85.
21. Gallagher JC, Melton LJ, Riggs BL. Examination of prevalence rates of possible risk factors in a population with a fracture of the proximal femur. Clin Orthop 1980; 150:163–71.
22. Weiss NS, Liff JM, Ure CL, Ballard HJH, Abbott GH, Daling JR. Mortality in women following hip fracture. J Chron Dis 1983; 36:879–82.
23. US Bureau or the Census: Current population reports. Series P–25, No. 952. Projections of the populations of the United States by age, sex, and race: 1983 to 2080. Washington, DC: US Government Printing Office; 1984.
24. Cummings SR, Rubin SM, Black D. The future of hip fractures in the United States: numbers, costs, and potential effects of postmenopausal estrogens. Clin Orthop (in press).
25. Baker MR. An investigation into secular trends in the incidence of femoral neck fracture using hospital activity analysis. Public Health (London) 94:368–74.
26. Lewis AF. Fracture of the neck of the femur: changing incidence. Br Med J 1981; 283:1217–20.
27. Wallace WA. The increasing incidence of fractures of the proximal femur: an orthopaedic epidemic. Lancet i: 1413–14.
28. Nilsson, BE, Obrant KJ. Secular tendencies of the incidence of fracture of the upper end of the femur. Acta Orthop Scand 1981; 53:419–26.

29. Zetterberg C, Andersson GBJ. Fractures of the proximal end of the femur in Goteborg, Sweden, 1940–1979. Acta Orthop Scand 1982; 54:681–6.
30. Frandsen PA, Kruse T. Hip fractures in the county of Funen, Denmark. Acta Orthop Scand 1982; 54:681–6.
31. Jensen JS. Incidence of hip fractures. Acta Orthop Scand 1980; 51:511–13.
32. Evans JG, Prudham D, Wandless I. A prospective study of fractured proximal femur: incidence and outcome. Public Health (London) 93:235–41.
33. Engesaeter LB, Soreide O. Incidence of hip fractures based on hospital admission rates. Acta Orthop Scand (abstract) 1984; 55:707.
34. Martin AD, Silverthorn KG, Houston CS. Age-specific increase in hip fractures in Canada. In: Christiansen C, Johansen JS, Riis BJ, eds. Viborg, Denmark: Norhaven A/S, 1987; 111–112.
35. Lindsay R, Dempster DW, Clemens T, Herrington BS, Wilt S. Incidence, cost, and risk factors of fracture of the proximal femur in the USA. In: Christiansen C, Arnaud CD, Nordin BEC, Parfitt AM, Peck WA, Riggs BL, eds. Copenhagen: Aalborg, 1984; 311–15.
36. Melton, LJ, O'Fallon WM, Riggs BL. Secular trends in the incidence of hip fractures. Calcif Tissue Int 1987; 41:57–64.
37. Jensen GF, Christiansen C, Boesen J, Hegedus V, Transbol I. Epidemiology of postmenopausal spinal and long bone fractures; a unifying approach to postmenopausal osteoporosis. Clin Orthop 1982; 166:75–81.
38. Melton LJ III, Kan SH, Frye MA, Wahner HW, O'Fallon WM, Riggs BL. Epidemiology of vertebral fractures in women. Am J Epidemiol 1989; 129:1000–11.
39. Knowelden J, Buhr AJ, Dunbar O. Incidence of fractures in persons over 35 years of age: a report to the MRC working party on fractures in the elderly. Br J Prev Soc Med 1964; 18:130–41.
40. Smith RW Jr, Rizek J. Epidemiologic studies of osteoporosis in women of Puerto Rico and southeastern Michigan with special reference to age, race, national origin and to other related or associated findings. Clin Orthop 1966; 45:31–48.
41. Holbrook TL, Grazier K, Kelsey JL, Stauffer RN. The frequency of occurrence, impact and cost of selected musculoskeletal conditions in the United States. Chicago: American Academy of Orthopedic Surgeons.
42. Owen RA, Melton LJ III, Johnson KA, Ilstrup DM, Riggs BL. Incidence of Colles' fracture in a North American community. Am J Public Health 1982; 72:605–7.
43. Melton LJ, Riggs BL. Epidemiology of age-related fractures. In: Avioli LV, ed. The osteoporotic syndrome: detection prevention and treatment, New York: Grune and Stratton, 1983; 45–72.
44. Matkovic V, Kostial K, Simonovic I, Buzina R, Brodarec A, Nordin BEC. Bone status and fracture rates in two regions of Yugoslavia. Am J Clin Nutr 1979; 32:540–9.
45. Riggs BL, Melton LJ III. Involutional osteoporosis. N Engl J Med 1986; 314:1676–86.
46. Mazess RB. On aging bone loss. Clin Orthop Rel Res 1982; 162:239–52.
47. Melton LJ III, Wahner HW, Richelson LS, O'Fallon WM, Riggs BL. Osteoporosis and the risk of hip fracture. Am J Epidemiol 1986; 124:254–61.
48. Buchanan SR, Myers C, Greer RB, Lloyd T, Varano LA. Assessment of the risk of vertebral fracture in menopausal women. J Bone Joint Surg 1987; 69A:212–17.
49. Eriksson SAV, Widhe TL. Bone mass in women with hip fracture. Acta Orthop Scand 1988; 59:19–23.
50. Hui SL, Wiske P, Norton JA, Johnston CC Jr. Prospective study of change in bone mass with age in postmenopausal women. J Chron Dis 1982; 35:715–25.
51. Johnston CC Jr, Melton LJ III, Lindsay R, Eddy DM. Clinical indications for bone mass measurements: a report from the scientific advisory board of the National Osteoporosis Foundation. J Bone Miner Res 1989; 4(Suppl. 2).
52. Hui SL, Slemenda CW, Johnston CC Jr. Baseline measurement of bone mass predicts fractures in white women. Ann Intern Med 1989; 111:355–61.
53. Wasnich RD, Ross PD, Halbrun LK, Vogel JM. Prediction of postmenopausal fracture risk with use of bone mineral measurements. Am J Obstet Gynecol 1985; 153:745–51.

Chapter 8

Implications of Osteoporotic Fractures in the Elderly

R. M. Francis and A Sutcliffe

Introduction

Osteoporosis is characterised by a reduction in the amount of bone in the skeleton and an increased risk of fracture. Bone is lost with advancing age in both sexes, with women losing 35%–50% of trabecular and 25%–30% of cortical bone, whereas men lose 15%–45% and 5%–15% respectively [1,2]. As the maximum load a bone can withstand without fracture is closely related to its mineral content, this reduction in bone mass with age is associated with an increased risk of fracture. The bone mass at any age and therefore the risk of fracture is determined by the peak bone mass, the age at which bone loss starts and the rate at which it progresses [1,2]. Peak bone mass is influenced by a number of factors including race, sex, heredity, hormonal factors, exercise and diet. The major causes of bone loss with advancing age include the menopause, smoking, excess alcohol consumption, low body weight, reduction in physical activity and the declining efficiency of calcium absorption [1,2].

Falls

Although bone mass and architecture are important determinants of the mechanical properties of bone, the risk of fracture is also influenced by the severity of any trauma applied to the skeleton. Therefore, whilst fractures in young adults usually occur only after extensive injury, as in a road traffic accident, fractures in the elderly may occur after the minimal trauma of a fall. Hence in an elderly population among whom osteoporosis is common, the risk of fracture may be related as much to the frequency of falls as to the severity of osteoporosis. Falls increase with advancing age and are more common in women than men. The prevalence of falls in women is 30% at age 65–69, rising to 40% over the age of 80, whilst in men the corresponding figures are 13% and 34% [3]. The risk of falls may be influenced by intrinsic and extrinsic factors [4]. The intrinsic or host factors include neurological, cerebrovascular and cardiovascular disease and the efects of age on postural stability, visual acuity, co-ordination and gait. Medications such as sedatives, tranquillisers, antidepressants, anti-hypertensives and diuretics, and alcohol, may also contribute to the patho-genesis of falls. Extrinsic or environmental factors include trailing wires, loose carpets, uneven or slippery walking surfaces, steep stairs, poor lighting, ill-fitting clothing or footwear and inappropriate use of walking aids. In many cases, falls are due to both intrinsic and extrinsic factors.

Fracture Incidence

The combination of declining bone mass and increased risk of falls is associated with an escalating incidence of fractures with advancing age [1,5]. The major osteoporotic fractures are those of the forearm, vertebral body, humerus, pelvis and femoral neck [5]. The incidence of each of these fractures increases with advancing age and is considerably higher in women than men, reflecting their lower peak bone mass, the effects of the menopause on bone loss and the higher rate of falls in women [2,3,5]. There are also marked differences in fracture incidence between countries [5], which are probably due to racial differences and to cultural variation in smoking, alcohol consumption and physical activity. The increased fracture incidence with age is also reflected in the cumulative prevalence of fractures. About 7% of women and 3% of men have sustained a fracture of the forearm, vertebral body or femur by the age of 60, rising to 25% and 8% respectively by the age of 80 [6].

Fracture Number

An increasingly elderly population and a rising age-specific incidence of frac-tures have led to an increase in the absolute number of osteoporotic fractures. The proportion of people of pensionable age in the population has increased from 5% in 1901 to 18% in 1981 [7]. If the present mortality rates continue, it has been estimated that the numbers of pensioners will increase from 10.4 million n 1991 to 10.9 million in 2011 and 12.1 million 2021 [7]. Although the numbers of the young elderly will remain reasonably constant, the number of elderly people over the age of 85 will increase considerably. Many of these elderly people will be frail and therefore at particular risk of osteoporotic fractures.

A number of studies show evidence of an increasing age-specific incidence of fractures of the femur, forearm, humerus and vertebral body [8–10], which has been attributed to the survival of more frail individuals and secular changes in smoking, alcohol consumption, diet and physical activity [10]. The data on femoral neck fracture suggest a doubling of the age-specific incidence over the past three decades [8]. If the age-specific incidence continues to rise at the present rate, it has been estimated that the number of femoral fractures in England and Wales will increase from 46 000 in 1985 to 71 000 in 1996, 94 000 in 2006 and 117 000 in 2016 [11]. If, however, the age-specific incidence of femoral fractures remains unchanged, the number of femoral fractures will increase from 46 000 in 1985 to only 54 000 in 1996, 58 000 in 2006 and 60 000 in 2016 [11].

Femoral Fractures

This is the most important of the osteoporotic fractures as it causes greater morbidity, higher mortality and more expenditure than all other fractures combined [5]. The incidence of this fracture rises steeply with age in both sexes. The annual incidence in Oxford in 1983 was 9.3 fractures/10 000 in women aged 55–64, increasing to 322.3/10 000 over the age of 85, whereas in men it was 6.3/10 000 in the age group 55–64 and 131.6/10 000 over the age of 85 [8]. Using current age-specific incidence rates for England and Wales, it has been estimated that 12% of women and 5% of men will have sustained a femoral fracture by the age of 85 [11]. There is a marked geographic diversity in the incidence of femoral fractures [5], which may reflect differences in bone mass due to race and cultural factors as well as variations in the reporting of fractures. The highest rates are seen in the USA, where the incidence is about 60% higher than in the UK [5]. As mentioned above, several studies suggest there has been an increase in the age-specific incidence of this fracture in both sexes in the UK, and Sweden, with a doubling of the rate over the last three decades [8–10]. In contrast, there has been no change in the age-specific incidence of femoral fractures in the USA over the last 35 years, possibly because the incidence was already considerably higher than in the UK or Sweden [12].

Femoral fractures are associated with an appreciable mortality. Early studies showed an in-patient mortality of 12% and a 1 year rate of about 50% [13,14]. Subsequently, Evans reported a reduction in 6 month mortality from 40% in 1975 to 28% in 1985 [15], whereas Greatorex showed a decrease in mortality from 35% in 1968 to 15% in 1982[16]. This reduction in mortality is probably due to improvements in surgical management and rehabilitation following this fracture. These studies did not take into account the expected mortality of subjects in this age group, but recent work shows an excess mortality after femoral fracture of between 12% and 25% at 1 year [17,18]. The mortality is higher in patients who are older and more dependent before the fracture, though premorbid social function appears to be the more important determinant [19,20]. Jensen and colleagues showed that the mortality in individuals who were independent before fracture was 2.7% at 6 months and 12% at 30 months, whereas more dependent patients had a mortality of 27.9% at 6 months and 58% at 30 months [19,20]. In another study, Evans et al. compared the mortality after femoral fracture in two hospitals in Newcastle upon Tyne, and found a 6 month mortality of 53% in one and 28% in the other [21]. The hospital with the higher mortality had significantly more male patients, fewer patients from social classes 1 and 2, a higher proportion with a low mental test score and a greater number of subjects who had sustained their fracture in hospital or a residential home [21].

In addition to the appreciable mortality of femoral fracture, there is also considerable morbidity, with many patients becoming more immobile and dependent after fracture [13,19,20]. In a study from Denmark, Jensen and Bagger [20] showed that 37% of previously independent individuals were more dependent 30 months after fracture. In comparison, 55% of those patients who were already receiving social service and district nurse support were more dependent after fracture. Although 17% of the patients were either living in a nursing home or receiving long-term nursing care at home prior to admission, 39% required continuing nursing care after the fracture. In an earlier British study, Thomas and Stevens [13] demonstrated that 25% of patients were more dependent a year after femoral fracture. Deterioration was more common in women over the age of 75, in those with a poor clinical result and in those who were already dependent to some extent prior to fracture.

The costs of femoral fracture are difficult to measure because of the lack of data on hospital costs and the involvement of other agencies in the after-care of patients. Wallace [22] calculated that in 1966 the hospital cost of femoral fracture in England and Wales was £165 million. This was based on a total number of femoral fractures of 37 500 and a mean hospital stay of 40 days at a cost of £110/day. Although the mean length of stay had been reported as 40 days [9], other data suggest that it may now be between 20 and 30 days [13,23,24]. Nevertheless, the number of femoral fractures now exceeds 46 000/year in England and Wales [11] and the daily bed cost may be a considerable underestimate. The calculation of the financial consequences of femoral fracture examined only the hospital costs and took no account of the expenditure by other agencies. This may include the cost of general practitioner and district nursing services, and the expense incurred by local authority social services departments in providing home helps and places in day centres and residential homes. A considerable burden also falls on the Department of Social Security in providing attendance allowance, invalid care allowance and benefit payments to support private nursing home placement. It is likely that these non-hospital costs exceed the hospital expenditure, so that the total cost of femoral fractures in the UK may be in excess of £500 million/year. The impact of femoral fractures on relatives and informal carers may also generate substantial social and financial costs.

Forearm Fractures

These are the commonest fractures before the age of 75 [5]. The incidence rises steeply at the menopause, but does not alter significantly with age in men [1,25]. The annual incidence for women in Oxford in 1986 increased from 9.8/10 000 between the ages of 35–44 years to 21.1/10 000 at ages 45–54, 60.2/10 000 at ages 55–64 and 62.0/10 000 at ages 65–74, whilst the corresponding figures for men were 10.0, 10.3, 6.5 and 7.3/10 000 [25]. About 5% of women in the UK will have sustained a forearm fracture by the age of 60 rising to 15% in women at the age of 80, compared with 2% and 4% respectively for men [6]. It has been suggested that the increasing incidence with age in women is related to their greater risk of falls [25]. Although this fracture causes pain and inconvenience, there may be few sequelae other than the occasional problem due to mal-alignment, median nerve compression or Sudeck's atrophy. The hospitalisation rate after this fracture is low, and the health service and social service costs are unknown. Nevertheless, a minority of frail elderly people may be incapacitated whilst the fracture is healing, and may require social service input, the support of informal carers or temporary admission to a residential home or hospital.

Vertebral Fractures

The incidence of vertebral fractures is difficult to quantify because most patients with an acute vertebral crush fracture do not present to a hospital or seek medical attention. The precise definition of a vertebral fracture is also debatable as the term may be used to describe biconcavity, anterior wedging in of the vertebral body or a crush fracture, when the height of both the anterior and posterior parts of the vertebral body is reduced. Furthermore, the extent of deformation which constitutes a fracture is uncertain. It has been estimated from a large series of X-rays in Sweden that the annual incidence of vertebral crush fractures in women is 13/10 000 in the seventh decade, 40/10 000 in the eighth decade and 83/10 000 above the age of 80, whereas the incidence in men is 8, 13 and 45/10 000 respectively [10]. A Danish study found radiological evidence of crush fracture in 4.5% of 70-year-old women and wedging a further 18% [26]. Nordin et al. [27], however, suggested that the prevalence of crush fractures in women over the age of 65 was above 5% and that wedging occurred in over 60%. Crush fractures typically produce back pain lasting for six to eight weeks before settling to a more chronic backache, though crush fractures may be asymptomatic on occasions. The occurrence of several crush fractures leads to loss of height, the development of a kyphosis and abdominal protrusion. Although some patients require hospitalisation following an acute crush frac-ture, the proportion is unknown, as are the health and social service costs of this fracture.

Humeral Fractures

The annual incidence of proximal humeral fractures in the USA rises steeply in women over the age of 40, increasing from 4.1/10 000 in the fifth decade to 20/ 10 000 in the seventh and 43.9/10 000 in the ninth decade, with corresponding figures in men of 4.1, 5.2 and 11.2/10 000 respectively [28]. These rates were higher than those reported some 30 years earlier in Oxford and Dundee [29], but comparable with recent data from Sweden [10]. Over 90% of these fractures occurred after modest trauma, which would not normally have been expected to result in fracture [28]. Humeral fractures may result in vascular and neurological problems, and non-union can cause disability. The costs of this fracture are unknown.

Pelvic Fractures

Pelvic fractures occur with increasing frequency with age in both sexes, though the rate is twice as high in women than men. The annual incidence at the Mayo Clinic rises from <5/10 000 at age 45–50 to 45/10 000 over the age of 85 [30]. The rates in the UK 30 years ago were reported to be much lower [29], though they may be more comparable now because of the increasing age-specific incidence of most osteoporotic fractures [10]. Over 50% of pelvic fractures involve the pubic rami, and these fractures mostly occur after only minimal trauma, such as a fall from standing height [30]. The hospitalisation rates are unknown, as is the extent of temporary disability and the costs of this fracture.

Summary

An increase in the number of frail elderly people in the population and the escalating age-specific incidence of osteoporotic fractures will inevitably lead to a steep rise in the total number of fractures. This has implications ranging from devastating personal effects on the individual patient to massive economic impact on health and social service budgets. Although some attempt has been made to quantify the hospital costs of femoral fracture, there is little information on the cost to other agencies of this fracture or on the overall costs of other fractures. This information will be necessary for the future planning of services and for the accurate assessment of the cost-effectiveness of measures to prevent osteoporotic fractures.

References

1. Riggs BL, Melton LJ III. Involutional osteoporosis. N Engl J Med 1986; 314:1676–86.
2. Francis RM. Pathogenesis of osteoporosis. In: Francis RM, ed. Osteoporosis: pathogenesis and management . Dordrecht, Boston, London: Kluwer Academic Pubishers, 1990; 51–80.
3. Prudham D, Evans JG. Factors associated with falls in the elderly: a community study. Age Ageing 1981; 10:141–6.
4. Gibson MJ, Andres RO, Isaacs B, Radebaugh T, Worm-Petersen J. The prevention of falls in later life. Dan Med Bull 1987; 34 [Suppl. 4]:1–24.
5. Cummings SR, Kelsey JL, Nevitt MC, O'Dowd KJ. Epidemiology of osteoporosis and osteoporotic fractures. Epidemiol Rev 1985; 178–208.
6. Nordin BEC, Peacock M, Aaron JE, Crilly RG, Heyburn PJ, Horsman A, Marshall DH. Osteoporosis and osteomalacia. Clin Endocrinol Metab 1980; 9:177–205.

7. Social Trends. No. 17, Central Statistical Office. London: HMSO, 1987.
8. Boyce WJ, Vessey MP, Rising incidence of fracture of the proximal femur. Lancet 1985; i:150–1.
9. Fenton Lewis A. Fracture neck of femur: changing incidence. Br Med J 1981; 283:1217–20.
10. Obrant KJ, Bengner U, Johnell O, Nilsson BE, Sernbo I. Increasing age-adjusted risk of fragility fractures: a sign of increasing osteoporosis in successive generations? Calcif Tissue Int 1989; 44:157–67.
11. Royal College of Physicians. Fractured neck of femur. Royal College of Physicians of London, 1989.
12. Melton LJ III. Ilstrup DM, Riggs BL, Beckenbaugh RD. Fifty-year trend in hip fracture incidence. Clin Orthop 1982; 162:144–9.
13. Thomas TG, Stevens RS. Social effects of fractures of the neck of femur. Br Med J 1974; 3:456–8.
14. Beals RK. Survival following hip fracture – long follow-up of 607 patients. J Chron Dis 1972; 25:235–44.
15. Evans JG. Epidemiology of osteoporosis and fractures of the femoral neck. Int Med 1987 (Suppl. 12): 4–6.
16. Greatorex IF. Femoral neck fractures – improving efficiency in the case of elderly women. Community Med 1986; 8(3):185–90.
17. Melton LJ III, Riggs BL. Epidemiology and cost of osteoporotic fractures. Proceedings of the second international conference on osteoporosis: social and clinical aspects, Athens, Milan: Masson, 1986; 21–31.
18. Aitken JM. Relationship between mortality after femoral neck fracture and osteoporosis. In: Christiansen C, Johansen JS, Riis BJ, eds. Osteoporosis 1987. Denmark: Osteopress ApS 1987; 45–8.
19. Jensen JS, Tendevold E, Sørensen PH. Social rehabilitation following hip fractures. Acta Orthop Scand 1979; 50:777–85.
20. Jensen JS, Bagger J. Long-term social prognosis after hip fractures. Acta Orthop Scand 1982; 53:97–101.
21. Evans JG, Wandless I, Prudham D. A prospective study of fractured proximal femur: hospital differences. Public Health 1980; 94:149–54.
22. Wallace WA. The scale and financial implications of osteoporosis. Int Med 1987 (Suppl. 12):3–4.
23. Jensen JS, Tøndevold E, Sørensen PH. Costs of treatment of hip fractures. Acta Orthop Scand 1980; 51:289–96.
24. Office of Population Censuses and Surveys. Hospital in-patient enquiry. London: HMSO, 1987.
25. Winner SJ, Morgan CA, Evans JG. Perimenopausal risk of falling and incidence of distal forearm fracture. Br Med J 1989; 298:1486–8.
26. Jensen GF, Christiansen C, Boesen J, Hegedus V, Transbøl I. Epidemiology of postmenopausal spinal and long bone fractures. Clin Orthop 1982; 166:75–81.
27. Nordin BEC, Crilly RG, Smith DA. Osteoporosis. In: Nordin BEC, ed. Metabolic bone and stone disease, 2nd edn. Edinburgh, London, Melbourne, New York: Churchill Livingstone, 1984; 1–70.
28. Rose SH, Melton LJ III, Morrey BF, Ilstrup DM, Riggs BL. Epidemiologic features of humeral fractures. Clin Orthop 1982; 168:24–30.
29. Knowelden J, Buhr AJ, Dunbar O. Incidence of fractures in persons over 35 years of age. A report to the M.R.C. working party on fractures in the elderly. Br J Prev Soc Med 1964; 18:130–41.
30. Melton LJ III, Sampson JM, Morrey BF, Ilstrup DM. Epidemiologic features of pelvic fractures. Clin Orthop 1981; 155:43–7.

Discussion

Vessey: Dr Lindsay pointed out, and I agree with him, that the epidemiological studies that take fractures as an end point all suggest a protective effect of HRT. But if we look at those studies we find them very deficient, for instance, in terms of looking at how long the protective effect persists after discontinuation of HRT use. I know about the bone studies on discontinuation of HRT, but nonetheless, I think one needs more satisfactory end-point data than looking at the bone; one really needs fracture data.

The reason I think this is important is that a woman may have 10 years' HRT use from age 45 years to age 54 years or from age 50 years to age 59 years (although many will drop out with bleeding problems and non-compliance), but the great bulk of the femoral neck fractures are in those aged >75 years or >80 years. I do not think one can assume that the protective effect against bone that occurs in those earlier years will necessarily be carried over into a protective effect against femoral fractures 15 or 20 years after discontinuation. Indeed I think there is some evidence to the contrary.

Lindsay: I agree with that comment because most of these studies are very loosely designed. The Weiss [1] study demonstrated that the protective effects were most evident in the women who got oestrogen replacement therapy immediately after the menopause, and they had to have been on treatment for at least five years. But that study did not look at the gap between discontinuing oestrogen and fracture frequency. There is a hole in the data.

There is always the undercurrent in any epidemiological study that there are perhaps biases which we cannot determine simply by reading the studies. Looking at it from a clinical bias, it is entirely possible that epidemiologists are not present in the consulting-room when the doctor prescribes the treatment, and therefore will not be able to determine what sorts of biases are ongoing in that class of physician prescribing that type of treatment.

It would be nice to get those data but I have a suspicion that we would not be able to get them readily. Perhaps the Nurses Study in the United States [2] is one example of a study that will be able to provide some more detailed treatment, particularly now that they have entered the prospective cohort phase.

Anderson: Is there any information on how long women put on to HRT at menopause will continue with it?

Lindsay: That depends on where one looks. The New England data [3] suggest that about one-third of the women who get prescriptions never fill their prescriptions, and that of the other two-thirds, only 10% remain on at the end of 6 months. New Englanders are rather a unique breed, and they are perhaps not related to the rest of the United States, but certainly a large number of people, particularly with the wide variety of prescribing patterns, tend to come off treatment earlier rather than later. Those that do stay on for the first while tend to stay on for a long time in our observations.

Francis: A study in Leeds some years ago [4] showed that at least 50% had stopped HRT after 5 years. This was where a cohort of women was followed through.

Kanis: Even in the prospective studies which have looked at hip fracture, of which there are increasing numbers being published and people are being followed for longer and longer, one omission is the very elderly because they have not been studied for long enough.

It is in fact a very good point that we have no idea of the extent to which oestrogen treatment in the immediate postmenopausal years will affect those fractures which are of the greatest concern to public health, that is the fractures in the very elderly.

Whitehead: We do not know the minimum duration of exposure required either.

Ross: We have been following an elderly population in Southern California. We have been involved in research there for about 15 years and we have established a cohort and have been following a group of about 12 000 residents of a community for about the last 9 or 10 years. About half the women in this community have some history of past oestrogen use and the median duration of use is quite long, somewhere in the neighbourhood of 9–10 years, but almost all of the use is in the distant past. Many of the women used oestrogens for long periods of time beginning around the perimenopausal period, then either discontinued it, or at least discontinued at the time of the endometrial cancer reports in the mid-1970s. The prevalence of current use in the community is now very low, something less than 10% of all women.

We have recently been looking at hip fracture risk in this cohort and we find evidence of protection only among women who have continued to use oestrogen to the present time. We have absolutely no evidence of decrease in risk in women who have discontinued use somewhere in the past.

These are not published data and I am a little reluctant to even talk about them because they have not been peer reviewed. I should certainly like to see some independent evaluation of these data before they become widespread, but it is of interest that the protection we see is limited to women who are on oestrogens.

Anderson: Presumably this is a population of women who still have a relatively low hip fracture risk and who have been on oestrogen. When were they first put on oestrogen?

Ross: It is not a trial. This is an observational study. We collected baseline information on these women in 1981 through a postal survey. We collected detailed oestrogen use information about both their current and past use of oestrogens and we have now been following them forward for various health outcomes. The women were categorised according to oestrogen use or non-use, and among the oestrogen users there were various categorisations of oestrogen use, by duration, dose and so forth. Based on the women who subsequently developed hip fractures during that follow-up, there is no difference in hip fracture risk between lifetime ever-users and between lifetime never-users or between lifetime never-users and women who only used oestrogens in the past. The only reduction in risk we see compared to lifetime never-users is among women who have continued to use them till the present time, or at least till the time of the survey.

Stevenson: If I could speak for the defence, I do not see why giving hormone replacement therapy a number of years ago would not provide any lasting benefit. We know that changes in the so-called peak cancellous bone density seem to reflect the changes in overall risk of osteoporotic fracture, and this has been shown by various studies. Therefore, assuming that stopping oestrogen treatment is no worse than never having had it in the first place, and that any benefit does not instantly evaporate, there is no reason to think that there would not be some lasting benefit which might eventually show up as a reduction in fracture rate. But it may be very difficult with very elderly women to get enough numbers to show a difference in incidence rates.

Ross: I have trouble with the concept too. I reported on what we had observed. I fully expected that 10 years of oestrogen therapy should give some lasting protection, but in fact based on a large number of fractures we do not see any evidence of it.

Studd: It depends so much on the group studied, the dose used and compliance. They may end up with little benefit at all. What do we do when we are confronted with 75-year-old women with fractures? Does oestrogen therapy replace bone? We have to try to give them some sort of therapy that does replace bone and not just maintain it.

Dr Lindsay talked about not being able to build bridges between the discontinuous ends of trabeculi. I am not sure whether I agree with that. I am not sure whether the research has been done using a treatment that works. Using percutaneous oestradiol therapy we can put back 8% of bone density in a year, and proportionately in the older patients who start with a much lower bone density we end up with 10+% per year, and the same thing happens in the second year as well.

Data are presented later of a 10- or 12-year cross-sectional study where women aged 65 end up with a bone density at the 95th centile. Even if therapy is stopped after that sort of bone density level has been achieved, there is bound to be a lasting improvement in fracture rates

Lindsay: It is important for us to understand the physiology of bone remodelling when we are discussing changes that occur when women are given oestrogen replacement, or when they go through menopause and their oestrogen secretion declines. The changes that occur do so in the activation of these remodelling cycles and the first process that happens, whether it be in cortical bone or in trabecular bone, is a change in the rate at which resorption activity occurs. If oestrogens are given and there is a decline in activation frequency, that is, there are fewer new cycles in any unit of time being activated, then there will be an immediate decline in apparent bone resorption. Bone formation (and there are histological data in the literature to support this) continues unabated in those remodelling cycles that are already activated at the time of introducing treatment. As a result, there will be a temporary imbalance between resorption and formation in favour of formation that will be seen in bone mass measurements as a transient increase in density.

Indeed David Hart and I showed this many years ago in our studies on long-term treatment in women who had had no therapy for three years after oophorectomy and then had their treatment introduced at that time. All of the treatment studies in which oestrogen had been introduced after a period of oestrogen deficiency showed a similar transient effect. The magnitude of that transient effect depends on the amount of cancellous bone at the site being measured. It is smaller in sites of cortical bone and it is greater in spine, by as much as 5%–10%. Similar effects are seen with calcitonin.

Studd: But the assumption is that it is a transient, hole-filling effect. We have data for 12 years showing high-normal bone density and nobody has looked at the morphology or histology of those specimens.

Lindsay: There are data from Steiniche et al. [5] that would disagree. And those cross-sectional data unfortunately tell us nothing because these are people whose bone status is not known at the time that they went on to treatment. We need prospective data.

I would agree that prospective long-term data in treatment of established disease are not available, but in younger people they are clearly available and they show transient effects.

Anderson: Is there any evidence as to what the predictive value of uncovering the patients who have had vertebral fractures would be, and about the value of treating them effectively – in other words arresting femoral bone loss in patients with vertebral fractures 10 or 15 years before they are due to get the femoral neck fractures? Are there any data on what the effect of that would be on the incidence of femoral neck fractures? In other words, what percentage of patients with femoral fractures have had vertebral fractures?

Lindsay: I doubt if the data currently available could be used to make any such predictions. Certainly I could not do so as a clinician rather than as a mathematician.

Anderson: Are they totally different populations?

Lindsay: Yes. Everyone talks about the theoretical fracture threshold, which is a mathematical device that we can use to examine populations. But when we get down to looking at the individual patient, the issue of fracture threshold is something that we do not understand. We do not even know if it exists. We do not know, for example, if the patient whose bone mineral density is at the 95th percentile has the same fracture threshold as the person whose bone mineral density is at the 5th percentile. These people may have adequate amounts of peak bone mass for them as individuals, and we have no concept of whether or not their subsequent changes in bone mass will in any way be reflected in fracture frequency that relates to the absolute amount of bone tissue there. We surmise it from population data.

The conclusion we would come to if we looked at the population data is that the people who are in the lowest quintile of peak bone mass would have a five times higher risk of fractures subsequently. Using the data that we generated prospectively, that say that oestrogens would reduce vertebral fractures or vertebral deformity on X-ray by 90%, one could do the sort of calculation, at least for vertebral fractures, that would give an answer. But I know of no way of doing it yet for hip fracture because the data for hip fracture have gaps that do not allow us to determine the real reduction in hip fracture frequency we might see for relatively short-term use of oestrogens.

Francis: The Leeds Group at the First International Meeting in Copenhagen [6] showed that the patients with vertebral crush fractures were at increased risk of femoral fracture, but the increased risk was relatively small and in terms of predictive value was virtually useless.

Kanis: Could I raise the question of morbidity and mortality from hip fracture? A lot of evidence would suggest that patients who have hip fractures are ill, and have other diseases before they fracture their hip. The question is, to what extent is the apparent increase in mortality and morbidity over the normal population in fact increased mortality?

Lindsay: I do not think that it is known. Steve Cummings has coined the term "survival of the frailest" for what we might be doing with the very elderly, and hip fracture might be the last thing that is occurring just prior to their demise. Maybe it is not preventable, or should not be prevented.

Brincat: I remember the Leeds paper at the Copenhagen meeting. These studies are always implicitly flawed as Roger Smith pointed out himself. He said that the problem with these studies that show different treatment modalities in patients who already have fractures is that the other variables change as well once the patient has experienced a fracture. She or he may be more careful, and there are may be other variables. It would be difficult to study individual variables.

Lindsay: It is worth pointing out that the biomechanical forces that are generated on a fall from a standing height are potentially able to break any hip. Those forces do not have to be produced across the hip in vitro; a smaller force can break the hip. We have to be concerned with the protective devices that stop us breaking our hips and that is where a lot of the research has yet to be done.

There are preliminary data from St Louis that I have heard presented but I have not yet seen published that suggest that oestrogen replacement therapy for the older more frail group, changes their cognitive capability and may improve their protective responses to the fall. That may be one reason why we would want to use oestrogen replacement therapy in the very elderly with osteoporosis.

Fogelman: Dr Lindsay mentioned that the single best predictor of later bone density was the starting-off point. Is there any point in trying to identify fast bone losers in that context?

Lindsay: I do not know the answer to that. I would like to see Johnston's data [7] repeated both in terms of identifying fast bone losers and also the usefulness of doing so.

Fogelman: The sting in the tail is that those measurements were based on metacarpal and radius measurements, and we are not certain that spine or femur behave in the same way.

Lindsay: But there is evidence that peripheral bone mass measurements are equally predictive of axial incidence later.

References

1. Weiss NS, Ure CL, Ballard JH, Williams AR, Dalin JR. Decreased risk of fractures of the hip and lower forearm with postmenopausal use of estrogen. N Engl J Med 1980; 303:1195–8.

2. Stempfes MJ, Willett WC, Celditz JA. A prospective study of postmenopausal estrogen therapy and coronary heart disease. N Engl J Med 1985; 313:1044.
3. McKinlay JB, McKinlay SM, Brambilla DJ. Health status and utilization behavior associated with menopause. Am J Epidemiol 1987; 125:110–21.
4. Jones MM, Francis RM, Nordin BEC. Five-year follow-up of oestrogen therapy in 94 women. Maturitas 1982; 4:123–30.
5. Steiniche T, Hasling C, Charles P, Eriksen EF, Mosekilde L, Melsen F. A randomized study on the effects of estrogen/gestagen or high dose oral calcium on trabecular bone remodeling in postmenopausal osteoporosis. Bone 1989; 10:313–20.
6. Marshall DH, Horsman A, Simpson M, Francis RM, Peacock M. Fractures in elderly women: prevalence of wrist, spine and femur fractures and their concurrence. In: Christiansen C, ed. Osteoporosis. Proceedings of the Copenhagen international symposium on osteoporosis. Copenhagen, Glostrup Hospital, 1984; 361–3.
7. Johnston CC Jr, Melton LJ III, Lindsay R, Eddy DM. Clinical indications for bone mass measurement: a report from the Scientific Advisory Board of the National Osteoporosis Foundation (in press).

Chapter 9

Structure of Osteoporotic Bone

A. Boyde

Summary of Professor Boyde's Contribution

Professor Boyde presented illustrations of the structure of bone and discussed methods of obtaining information from images. He began with point-projection radiographs taken in vivo, and compared them with higher resolution images of dead bone. He pointed out that low resolution images can be analysed in the frequency domain rather than the spatial domain, to obtain increased information.

Optical microscope images were illustrated, taken using range-imaging in a confocal microscope, and a new method of three-dimensional image analysis was described.

Older methods of computerised image analysis, using the Quantimet image analysis computer, were also described. Illustrations were shown of the collagen fibril distribution demonstrated by anorganic preparations.

A video demonstration gave a graphic illustration of the thinning and breaking of bone trabeculae that occurs in osteoporosis.

Scanning electron microscope images were shown, and the quantitation of bone using this method was described. The importance of three-dimensional imaging was emphasised. The orientation of collagen fibrils was demonstrated using circularly polarised light. Professor Boyde described how the back-scattered electron imaging process has recently been put on to a fully quantitative basis, using microtomography. This method of calibration gives a measure of bone density that reflects the mineralisation of bone tissue.

Discussion

Anderson: Professor Boyde implied that there was woven bone in there even in the absence of micro-fractures. Is that correct?

Boyde: No. The woven bone was generated in response to the presence in that particular vertebra of a metastasis of carcinoma of pancreas. One of the responses to particular carcinomas may be generation of new bone. That just made a good model showing the difference of scale of woven bone and adult lamellar bone trabeculi, which is not only commonly overlooked in the literature but universally overlooked.

Anderson: Can we be certain that that osteoid never re-mineralises? I was very struck by the statement that the new osteons subsequently pack in a lot of extra mineral, presumably over a number of months.

Boyde: There is no scrap of evidence that old osteoid mineralises, but there is evidence that the new osteoid deposited during the phase in which the vitamin D is administered is probably mineralised. Within the process of give and take in the remodelling, the old osteoid eventually goes, and the reason why eventually no old osteoid can be found is that it has been resorbed and replaced by new osteoid which can mineralise.

Lindsay: I have always been intrigued by those shape changes in the osteoblast population after parathyroid hormone. One of the hypotheses of oestrogen action on bone has always been that oestrogens would increase the resistance of the osteoblast's response to parathyroid hormone. Has anybody ever done the experiment of trying to look at interactions between oestrogens and parathyroid hormone using that as a model?

Boyde: Not that I know of, yet. Both groups of people are working in our laboratories and we may be able to get them to talk to each other!

Kanis: In florid osteomalacia treated with vitamin D there may be islands of osteoid which never mineralise. That is very characteristic, whether it is vitamin D-deficiency or whether it is etidronate induced, and that would very much support Professor Boyde's observations.

In the osteoporotic process many of us tend to think in only two dimensions, and we have difficulties from two dimensions in distinguishing, for example, between plates and rods. In the process of osteoporosis, to what extent do plates of trabecular tissue, particularly in vetebrae, become rods, and to what extent can connectivity on the two-dimensional basis reflect connectivity in a three-dimensional basis?

Boyde: The answer to the latter question has been approached by two-dimensional thinkers but not yet by the three-dimensional thinkers because the strategies for doing so have not yet been widely developed. It is a very interesting question which we would really like to contribute towards, but I do not know the answer.

Rather than "plates", it would be conceptually more correct to describe the bone structure as consisting of a set of interlocking cylinders. It is a honeycomb rather than plates. It is a continuum of sheets of bone that are really wrapped up into cylinders. The normal bone structure is a much more ingenious structure than we realise from calling those things plates. If we call them plates, then they are certainly converted into rods.

Many years ago, it was suggested that osteoporosis in females is more in the nature of removing the total number of rods or plates, whereas in males it may be more of the thinning down of sheets to become rods, so there is a more continuous set of interconnecting rods in the male osteoporotic and less scaffolding to put new bone tissue back on to in the case of the female osteoporotic. This is a very interesting possibility.

Chapter 10

Endocrinology and Osteoporosis

P. L. Selby

Introduction

Although bone is commonly perceived as a metabolically inert tissue it is in fact very active, undergoing continuous renewal of its constituents by resorption of old bone and formation of new. The balance between these two processes is vital to the health of the skeleton, since an apparently small increase of resorption over formation can, over the years, lead to a clinically significant deficit of bone. Because many of the factors that influence these processes are hormonal, it is necessary to have an understanding of the effect of hormones on bone to understand both normal bone physiology and also the deleterious effects on the skeleton of many endocrine disorders.

The hormones that act on bone can be divided into three main groups. The first of these are the classical calcitropic hormones, parathyroid hormone (PTH), calcitriol and calcitonin. The second comprises the ever-growing number of cytokines and related compounds which are increasingly recognised as playing a major role in the control of bone cell behaviour. These two groups of substances fall outside the scope of this review, which is concerned with the role of the third of these groups, the other classical hormones, many of whose members exert profound influences on bone turnover (Table 10.1), and the effect on the skeleton of diseases affecting the concentrations of these hormones.

Table 10.1. Effect of classical hormones on bone metabolism

Hormone	Effect on resorption	Effect on formation
Cortisol	↑	↓ ↓
Thyroxine	↑ ↑	↑
Insulin	?	↑
Growth hormone	?	↑
Oestrogen	↓ ↓	? ↑
Testosterone	? ↓	↑

Corticosteroids

It has been recognised for many years that excessive concentrations of cortico-steroids, either as a result of endogenous overproduction or from exogenous therapy, can have profound effects on bones, leading to osteoporosis and fractures – particularly of the axial skeleton, especially the vertebrae and ribs. Up to 50% of patients with Cushing's syndrome have osteoporosis with evidence of vertebral fractures on radiographs [1,2]. In the case of patients receiving corticosteroid therapy the prevalence of fracture is somewhat lower, at 10%–20% depending on the dose of steroid given and the duration of therapy [3], but corticosteroid therapy is itself so common that this probably represents the most important secondary cause of osteoporosis [4,5].

The marked effects of cortisosteroids on the skeleton result from the fact that they adversely influence both aspects of bone remodelling, not only stimulating bone resorption but also markedly inhibiting the formation of new bone. In addition they have a variety of indirect actions which tend to magnify these actions. The mechanisms underlying the two major effects of glucocorticoids on the skeleton are not clear. Since it is now well established that osteoblasts possess glucocorticoid receptors, it would appear that the action on bone formation may well be a direct receptor-mediated response [5,6]. This is borne out by in vitro studies where corticosteroids directly inhibit the growth and protein synthesis of osteoblast-like cells [7,8]. This action may well be magnified by the tendency of orally administered steroids to suppress adrenal androgen production [9]. Because androgens have an anabolic effect on the skeleton this is likely further to suppress bone formation.

The mechanisms underlying the stimulation of bone resorption are less clear-cut, and indeed some in vitro studies have suggested that corticosteroids actually inhibit the action of osteoclasts [10,11]. In order to try and explain the apparent paradox between these observations and the clinical findings of increased bone resorption, various different indirect mechanisms of action have been postulated. It is known that at high doses corticosteroids inhibit the absorption of calcium from the gut [12]. This is due, in part, to a direct effect on the gastrointestinal transport mechanism and, in part, to an inhibition of the action of calcitriol in promoting calcium absorption. In addition corticosteroids have a tendency to increase urinary calcium losses by a direct action on the renal tubular mech-anisms of calcium reabsorption [13]. As a result of these changes there is an increase in the plasma concentration of PTH [13] and calcitriol [14], both of which tend to increase bone resorption. Furthermore, corticosteroids have been shown to alter the binding of osteoclasts to bone and this may also influence their resorptive efficiency [15]. Once again, exogenously administered steroids tend to exacerbate the increased bone resorption by their suppression of adrenal androgen production. In this instance it is not the androgen lack *per se* that causes problems but the fact that the reduced androgen concentration leads to a decreased peripheral production of oestrogen, which would normally be expected to protect against resorption [9].

A variety of different ways have been proposed to overcome the effects of excess corticosteroids on bone. In the case of Cushing's disease the answer is clearly to treat the underlying condition, although this is frequently less easy than might be expected and drugs which block adrenal steroid production might need to be employed. In the case of corticosteroid therapy it is obviously desirable to limit the treatment to the minimum dose and time possible, but all too often this is still likely to harm the skeleton. Attempts to limit bone loss by concomitant therapy with calcium [16,17] and bisphosphonates [18] are promising but require further investigation. Likewise the steroid deflazacort, which is said to have less severe skeletal effects, is worthy of further study. Once established, corticosteroid-induced osteoporosis is difficult to treat and although calcitonin [19], bisphosphonates [20] and anabolic steroids [3] have all been shown to have some benefit in small studies, large-scale, long-term work is needed before any of these agents can be generally recommended.

Thyroid Hormones

It is well recognised that hyperthyroidism is associated with increased bone resorption and that occasionally this can lead to symptomatic osteoporosis with fracture or hypercalcaemia [21]. Indeed, bone manifestations are occasionally the presenting symptoms of thyrotoxicosis. Although up to 60% of patients with thyroid overactivity can be shown to have disturbed bone metabolism, by using sensitive biochemical markers [22], and 20% to have a bone mass reduced below normal for their age and sex [23], only a small minority develop overt hypercalcaemia or fracture. Thyroid hormones increase the rate of bone turnover but in general the effect on resorption is greater than that on formation, leading to a net loss of mineral from the skeleton [21]. These changes appear to be a result of direct stimulation of bone cell activity. The increased release of calcium from the skeleton causes suppression of plasma concentrations of PTH and calcitriol and consequent reduction of gastrointestinal absorption of calcium [24].

Treatment of thyrotoxicosis leads to a reduction in the rate of bone resorption although bone formation continues at an increased rate for up to a year. This uncoupling of formation and resorption appears to be stimulated by the rise in calcitriol concentration which occurs with treatment, and might be expected to make good some of the deficit in bone mass which had occurred during the toxic phase [24]. Nevertheless the net effect of a period of thyrotoxicosis is frequently a reduction in bone mass which may be additive with other stresses on the skeleton, such as the menopause, in determining overall fracture risk.

In the case of hypothyroidism the picture is a little less clear. It might be expected that the picture would be the opposite of that of thyrotoxicosis, with decreased bone turnover. This has indeed been demonstrated with calcium balance studies [25]. However, one group has demonstrated a reduction in bone mass in patients treated for hypothyroidism following thyroidectomy [26]. The authors suggest that this reflects calcitonin deficiency in these patients compared with goitrous controls, but in all probability this is not the case and it is likely that it results from the slightly higher doses of replacement therapy used in those patients compared with the controls. There is therefore, little evidence that, by itself, hypothyroidism is associated with any increased risk of osteoporosis.

Insulin

Insulin, in addition to its effects on carbohydrate and lipid metabolism, is an important growth factor [27]. Experiments in vitro have shown insulin is important for the growth of bone cells, and observations in animals with diabetes would appear to bear this out. Adolescents with insulin-dependent diabetes (IDDM) tend to have delayed skeletal growth, related to insulin deficiency [28]. More importantly, there is also a deficit of bone mineral associated with IDDM. Unlike the other complications of diabetes this occurs early in the course of the disease, with about 10% of skeletal mass lost over the first five years of diabetes [29]. However, although they are frequently attributed to insulin deficiency it is not clear how much these changes in bone mass might be related to other changes that might be occurring, since hydroxyproline excretion is increased in these patients, suggesting increased bone resorption [30].

In patients with non-insulin dependent diabetes (NIDDM) the picture is a lot less clear [31]. In this condition there is a combination of relative insulin deficiency together with resistance to the action of insulin. Reports of changes in bone mass in NIDDM are contradictory; some authors show quite marked bone loss whereas others demonstrate the opposite. Perhaps the most important marker of skeletal integrity is the fracture rate and this, according to all but one study, is increased in diabetes. The net effect of this is that diabetes has a smiliar effect on fracture incidence to that of oestrogen loss at the time of the menopause, although it is perhaps unlikely that all this increased risk is due to insulin deficiency [31].

Growth Hormone

Deficiency of growth hormone is well known to delay skeletal growth and maturation prior to cessation of linear growth. On the other hand, it is said to have no clinically important effects after growth is complete. Although growth hormone deficiency in the adult has been associated with loss of bone mineral [32] the importance of this in terms of fracture risk has not been estimated, and as yet there is no recommendation that growth hormone deficient adults should receive growth hormone therapy to protect the skeleton. Indeed in many instances there would be associated gonadal steroid deficiencies which are much more likely to have profound effects on the skeleton (see below).

Gonadal Steroids

Perhaps the most important endocrine effects on the skeleton are those exerted by the sex steroid hormones, both male and female. Of these the most important quantitatively is the effect of oestrogen deficiency, since this is inevitable following the menopause. Nevertheless osteoporosis is also an important consequence of hypogonadism in the male.

Oestrogen

The importance of oestrogen for skeletal integrity was first recognised by Albright almost 50 years ago, when he noted that the vast majority of his patients with osteoporosis were postmenopausal women and that he could improve their calcium balance by the administration of oestrogen [33,34]. Although his initial belief was that oestrogen was primarily anabolic for bone, subsequent biochemical, histological and kinetic studies have shown this not to be the case and that its primary action is one of inhibition of bone resorption. In the past there has been considerable controversy as to the mechanism whereby oestrogen brought about these changes, since, until recently, no oestradiol receptors had been detected in bone cells [35–38]. This led to a variety of indirect hypotheses as to the mechanism of action of oestrogen on the skeleton, all of which involved one or other of the calcitropic hormones and all of which have, to a greater or lesser extent, been discredited with the passage of time [reviewed in 39].

The need for such indirect hypotheses was obviated by the recent discovery of oestradiol receptors in osteoblasts [40–42]. Although these receptors are present in low concentration there is no doubt that they are capable of modulating biological activity, in that oestrogen treatment of osteoblasts in vivo leads to the induction of progesterone receptors [40] and activation of the procollagen and transforming growth factor genes [41–43]. However, these actions are either non-specific ones which are common to all oestrogen receptors or are apparently involved with changes that might lead to an increase in bone formation rather than a decrease in resorption. Although no oestradiol receptors have been found on osteoclasts, it must be remembered that many substances that are thought to regulate osteoclastic bone resorption do not act directly on the osteoclast but have their receptors on osteoblasts, which, in turn, modulate osteoclast activity by an as yet ill-defined paracrine mechanism [44–46]. Clearly, oestrogens may exert their effect on bone resorption by precisely such a means but there is some evidence to suggest that it may be a rather more complicated process.

Histological [47] and biochemical [48] studies suggest that oestrogen-induced inhibition of bone resorption takes place over a period of about two to three weeks rather than the hours or days which might be predicted from an inhibitory effect on the action of mature osteoclasts. Furthermore, in tissue culture experiments in vitro it has not yet been possible to replicate the effects of oestrogen on bone resorption in the intact animal. It is possible to do this with other hormones that act on bone, even if they act on osteoclasts through the paracrine influence of the osteoblast. These results suggest that rather than exerting an effect on the mature osteoclast, oestrogens act to decrease the recruitment of oesteoclasts from their precursors. These latter are derived from marrow or circulating cells of the mononuclear series and would not be expected to be present in the sort of tissue culture systems used to look at the effects of oestrogen on bone. Since osteoclast precursors are not yet well defined it remains an open question as to whether they bear oestrogen concentration, or whether they are under paracrine control via osteoblasts, which by themselves are known to influence osteoclast recruitment.

Notwithstanding the precise mechanism whereby oestrogen acts on the skeleton, it is clear that oestrogen deficiency is an important risk factor for the development of osteoporosis and fracture. The major circumstance in which this occurs is after the menopause. This will be dealt with more extensively elsewhere in this volume but suffice it to say that there is a rapid loss of bone from the skeleton at the time of the menopause and that this is associated with a marked increase in fracture risk. Replacement of oestrogen after the menopause halts the loss of bone and reduces the risk of fracture compared to untreated women by about 50% (reviewed elsewhere in this volume and in ref. [39]).

However, the menopause is not the only condition which leads to reduced plasma oestrogen concentrations. For many years it has been recognised that Turner's syndrome and other causes of ovarian dysgenesis are associated with generalised osteoporosis [49]. Although this is based on relatively old radiographic observations and there are no recent data using more modern means of assessing bone mass, the changes were so great as to leave no doubt as to the deleterious effect on the skeleton of the long-term oestrogen deficiency caused by these conditions.

More recently it has been recognised that a variety of conditions which lead to · temporary reduction in plasma oestrogen concentrations lead to a reduction in bone density. Perhaps the most important among these conditions is hyperprolactinaemic amenorrhoea. This is associated with a reduction in bone mass [50–54] which is reversible if the condition is treated and menstruation resumed [54]. That the loss of bone is due to reduced plasma oestrogen is seen from studies which compare the bone mass in women with similar degrees of hyperprolactinaemia but differing oestrogen concentrations: the reduction in bone density is observed only in patients with low oestrogen levels and amenorrhoea [55,56]. Furthermore, patients with amenorrhoea due to other causes in which oestrogen concentrations are preserved do not suffer from increased rates of bone loss. None of these studies has been continued for long enough to determine whether there is a significant increase in fracture risk, but the general inverse relationship between bone density and fracture risk would suggest that this is likely to be the case. In the past it has frequently been standard endocrine practice only to treat patients with hyperprolactinaemic amenorrhoea who wished to conceive. In the light of the adverse effects of this condition on the skeleton, consideration must be given to treating hyperprolactinaemia whether or not infertility is a problem. Since it would appear that correction of amenorrhoea leads to only a partial restoration of bone mass it is particularly important that such treatment be instituted as soon as practicable after diagnosis.

A similar increased rate of bone loss is seen in high-performance female athletes [57,58] and ballet dancers [59] who develop hypothalamic amenorrhoea as a result of intensive training. Since, under other circumstances, exercise is generally of benefit to the skeleton this observation underlines the prime role of oestrogen in the maintenance of bone mass. It is likely that the increased rate of bone loss contributes to the stress fractures suffered by such athletes [60,61] although there is no evidence as yet to implicate it in more serious osteoporotic fractures. However, since ballet dancers in particular often have a late menarche and are involved in intensive training before the attainment of skeletal maturity, they are likely to be left with a low peak bone mass at maturity and hence an increased risk of fracture in later life. Although the reduction in bone mass is, to some extent, reversible by the cessation of training this is frequently unacceptable to the women involved and many doctors caring for such women would suggest the use of a combined oral contraceptive preparation to provide oestrogen to protect the skeleton.

A similar situation arises in anorexia nervosa, where there is hypogonadotrophic amenorrhoea secondary to weight loss [62,63]. Clearly, further nutritional deficiencies secondary to starvation might contribute to bone loss in this condition, although successful treatment of the anorexia with resumption of a normal menstrual cycle is associated with at least partial restoration of bone mass. Once again, consideration should be given to giving oestrogen replacement in the form of the combined oral contraceptive to women with anorexia which is resistant to treatment.

Recently several long-acting gonadotrophin-releasing hormone (GnRH, LHRH) analogues have been introduced into clinical practice. These compounds, after an initial stimulation of gonadotrophin release, result in suppression of gonadotrophin production and hypogonadism. They were initially used for the treatment of endocrine-dependent tumours, particularly carcinoma of the prostate, but have gained increasing acceptance for treatment of benign conditions such as endometriosis, polycystic ovaries, dysfunctional uterine bleeding and fibroids. Treatment with these compounds has been shown to result in rapid loss of bone from the skeleton [64,65]. Although treatment is usually given for only a limited period, following which there is an increase in bone mass, it is possible that the overall effect of such a course of therapy is a net loss of bone. Since many of the indications for this type of treatment might require repeated therapy it is important that the long-term effects of such drugs on the skeleton be clarified.

Androgens

Hypogonadism in males, as in females, is associated with osteoporosis. This is seen both in patients with Klinefelter's syndrome [66] and also in men with hypogonadism from other causes, including hypogonadotrophic hypogonadism [67], tuberculous epididymo-orchitis [67], castration for prostatic cancer (personal observation) and hyperprolactinaemia [68,69].

The mechanisms underlying this bone loss are unclear but bone histomorphometry reveals both increased resorption and decreased formation. In addition there is evidence of malabsorption of calcium due to low plasma concentrations of calcitriol. Administration of testosterone leads to an increase in calcitriol concentration with increased calcium absorption and bone formation [67].

Androgens are less important in women than men. Nevertheless it has been suggested that there may be a reduction in adrenal androgen production ("adrenopause") some years after the menopause and that this might be associated with increased bone loss [70]. This effect is generally believed to be slight and its importance in the genesis of postmenopausal osteoporosis is disputed. It is not clear whether this putative action is mediated by removal of the anabolic effect of the weak adrenal androgens themselves or whether it is due to the reduction of oestrone production which is the result of peripheral aromatisation of androstenedione.

Conclusions

From the foregoing it is clear that many disorders of endocrine function result in altered bone metabolism, with increased risk of osteoporosis and fracture. In considering the appropriate management of patients with these conditions it is important to consider the effects on the skeleton. Even in young patients with no other apparent risk factors for osteoporosis this is important for it must be remembered that anything that reduces the peak bone mass at maturity is likely to increase greatly the risk of osteoporosis and fracture in later life.

References

1. Sprague RG, Randall RV, Scilassa RM et al. Cushing's syndrome. A progressive and often fatal disease. Arch Intern Med 1956; 98:389–98.
2. Howland WJ, Pugh DC, Sprague RG. Roentgenological changes in the skeletal system in Cushing's syndrome. Radiology 1958; 71:69–78.
3. Need AG. Corticosteroids and osteoporosis. Aust NZ J Med 1987; 17:267–72.
4. Francis RM, Peacock M, Marshall DH, Horsman A, Aaron JE. Spinal osteoporosis in men. Bone Mineral 1989; 5:347–57.
5. Chen TL, Aronow L, Feldman D. Glucocorticoid receptors and inhibition of bone cell growth in primary culture. Endocrinology 1977; 100:619–28.
6. Manolagas SC, Anderson DC. Detection of high affinity glucocorticoid binding in rat bone. J Endocrinol 1978; 76:377–80.
7. Peck WA, Brandt J, Miller I. Hydrocortisone-induced inhibition of protein synthesis and uridine incorporation in isolated bone cells in vitro. Proc Natl Acad Sci 1967; 57:1599–606.
8. Choe J, Stern P, Feldman D. Receptor mediated glucocorticoid inhibition of protein synthesis in isolated bone cells in vitro. J Steroid Biochem 1977; 9:265–71.
9. Crilly RG, Marshall DH, Nordin BEC. Metabolic effects of corticosteroid therapy in postmenopausal women. J Steroid Biochem 1979; 11:429–33.
10. Stern PH. Inhibition by steroids of parathyroid induced Ca^{45} release from embryonic rat bone in vitro. J Pharmacol Exp Ther 1969; 168:211–17.
11. Raisz LG, Trummel CL, Wener JA, Simmons H. Effect of glucocorticoids on bone resorption in tissue culture. Endocrinology 1972; 90:961–7.
12. Kimberg DV. Effects of vitamin D and the steroid hormones on the active transport of calcium by the intestine. N Engl J Med 1969; 280:1396–405.
13. Suzuki Y, Ichikawa Y, Saito E, Homma M. Importance of increased calcium excretion in the development of secondary hyperparathyroidism of patients under corticosteroid therapy. Metabolism 1983; 32:151–6.
14. Hahn TJ, Halstead LR, Baron DT. Effects of short term glucocorticoid administration on intestinal calcium absorption and circulating vitamin D metabolite concentrations in man. J Clin Endocrinol Metab 1981; 52:111–15.
15. Bar-Shavit Z, Kahn AJ, Pegg LE, Stone KR, Teitelbaum SL. Glucocorticoids modulate macrophage surface oligosaccharides and their bone binding activity. J Clin Invest 1984; 73:1277–83.

16. Reid IR, Ibbertson HK. Calcium supplementation in the prevention of steroid-induced osteoporosis. Am J Clin Nutr 1986; 44:287–90.
17. Nilsen KH, Jayson MIV, Dixon AStJ. Microcrystalline calcium hydroxyapatite compound in corticosteroid-treated rheumatoid patients: a controlled study. Br Med J 1978; 2:1124.
18. Lindehayn K, Trzenschik K, Buhler G, Wegner G. On the action of prednisolone and ethane-1-hydroxy-1,1-diphosphonate (EDHP) on rabbit bone. Exp Pathol 1982; 21:157–64.
19. Ringe JD, Welzel D, Schmid K. Therapy of corticosteroid induced osteoporosis with salmon calcitonin. In: Christiansen C, Johansen JS, Riis BJ, eds. Osteoporosis 1987. Copenhagen: Osteopress ApS, 1987; 1074–6.
20. Reid IR, King AR, Alexander CJ, Ibbertson HK. Prevention of steroid-induced osteoporosis with (3-amino-1-hydroxypropylidene)-1,1-bisphosphonate (APD). Lancet 1988; i:143–7.
21. Adams PH, Jowsey J, Kelly PJ, Riggs BL, Kinney VR, Jones JD. Effect of hyperthyroidism on bone and mineral metabolism. Q J Med 1967; 36:1–15.
22. Nordin BEC, Crilly RG, Smith DA. Osteoporosis. In: Nordin BEC, ed. Metabolic bone and stone disease. Edinburgh: Churchill Livingstone, 1984; 1–70.
23. Smith DA, Fraser SA, Wilson GM. Hyperthyroidism and calcium metabolism. Clin Endocrinol Metab 1973; 2:333–54.
24. Francis RM, Peacock M. The pathogenesis of osteoporosis in thyrotoxicosis. In: Christiansen C, Johansen HS, Riis BJ, eds. Osteoporosis 1987. Copenhagen: Osteopress ApS, 1987; 166–7.
25. Adams P, Chalmers TM, Riggs BL, Jones JD. Parathyroid function in spontaneous hypothyroidism. J Endocrinol 1968; 40:467–75.
26. McDermott M, Kidd GS, Blue P, Ghaed V, Hofeld FD. Reduced bone mineral content in totally thyroidectomised patients: possible effects of cacitonin deficiency. J Clin Endocrinol Metab 1983; 56:936–9.
27. Zapf, J, Schmidt CH, Froesch ER. Biological and immunological properties of insulin-like growth factors (IGF) I and II. Clin Endocrinol Metab 1984; 13:3–30.
28. Pond H. Some aspects of growth in diabetic children. Postgrad Med J 1970; 46(suppl):616–23.
29. McNair P, Christiansen C, Christensen MS et al. Development of bone mineral loss in insulin treated diabetes; a 12 year follow up study in 60 patients. Eur J Clin Invest 1981; 11:55–9.
30. Selby PL, Marshall SM. Hydroxyproline excretion is increased in diabetes mellitus. Bone (in press) (abstract)
31. Selby PL, Osteopenia and diabetes. Diabetic Med 1988; 5:423–8.
32. Daughaday WH. The anterior pituitary. In: Wilson JD, Foster DW, eds. Williams textbook of endocrinology. Philadelphia: WB Saunders, 1981; 568–613.
33. Albright F, Smith PH, Richelson AM. Postmenopausal osteoporosis: its clinical features. JAMA, 1941; 116:2465–74.
34. Albright F. Hormones and human osteogenesis. Rec Prog Horm Res 1947; 1:293–353.
35. Nutik G, Cruess RL. Estrogen receptors in bone: an evaluation of the uptake of estrogen into bone cells. Proc Soc Exp Biol Med 1974; 146:265–8.
36. Liskova, M. Influence of estrogens on bone resorption in organ culture. Calcif Tissue Res 1976; 22:207–18.
37. Van Paasen HC, Poortman J, Bogart-Creutzburg JHH, Duursma SA. Oestrogen binding proteins in bone cell cytosol. Calcif Tissue Res 1978; 25:249–54.
38. Chen TL, Feldman D. Distinction between alfa-fetoprotein and intracellular oestrogen receptors: evidence against the presence of estradiol receptors in rat bone. Endocrinology 1978; 102:236–44.
39. Selby PL. Oestrogen and bone. In: Francis RM, ed. Osteoporosis pathogenesis and management. Lancaster: Kluwer, 1990; 81–101.
40. Eriksen EF, Colvard DS, Berg NJ, Graham ML, Mann KG, Spelsberg TC, Riggs BL. Evidence of estrogen receptors in normal human osteoblast cells. Science 1988; 241:84–6.
41. Komm BS, Terpening CM, Benz DJ et al. Estrogen binding, receptor mRNA, and biologic response in osteoblast like osteosarcoma cells. Science 1988; 241:81–4.
42. Gray TK, Flynn TC, Gray KM, Nabell LM. 17ß-estradiol acts directly on the clonal osteoblast line UMR 106. Proc Natl Acad Sci 1987; 184:6267–71.
43. Ernst M, Schmid C, Froesch ER. Enhanced osteoblast proliferation and collagen gene expression by estradiol. Proc Natl Acad Sci 1988; 85:2307–10.
44. Rodan GA, Martin TJ. Role of osteoblasts in the hormonal control of bone resorption – a hypothesis. Calcif Tissue Int 1981; 33:349–51.
45. Braidman IP, Anderson DC, Jones CJP, Weiss JB. Separation of two bone cell populations from fetal rat calvaria and a study of their responses to parathyroid hormone and calcitonin. J Endocrinol 1983; 99:387–99.

46. McSheehy PMJ, Chambers TJ. Osteoblastic cells mediate osteclastic responsiveness to parathyroid hormone. Endocrinology 1986; 118:824–8.
47. Frost HM. Bone remodelling and its relationship to metabolic bone diseases. Springfield, Illinois: Charles C Thomas, 1973.
48. Selby PL, Peacock M, Barkworth SA, Brown WB, Taylor GA. Early effects of ethinyloestradiol and norethisterone treatment in post-menopausal women on bone resorption and calcium regulating hormones. Clin Sci 1985; 69:265–71.
49. Preger L, Steinbach HL, Moskovitch P. Roentgenographic abnormalities in phenotypic females with gonadal dysgenesis. AJR 1968; 104:899–910.
50. Klibanski A, Neer RM, Beitins IZ, Ridgway EC, Zervas NT, McArthur JW. Decreased bone density in hyperprolactinaemic women. N Engl J Med 1980; 303:1511–14.
51. Schlecte JA, Sherman B, Martin, R. Bone density in amenorrheic women with and without hyperprolactinaemia. J Clin Endocrinol Metab 1983; 56:1120–3.
52. Koppelman MC, Kurtz DW, Morrish KA, Bou E, Susser JK, Shapiro JR, Loriaux DL. Vertebral body bone mineral content in hyperprolactinaemic women. J Clin Endocrinol Metab 1984; 59:1050–3.
53. Cann CE, Martin WC, Genant HK, Jaffe RB. Decreased spinal mineral content in amenorrheic women. JAMA 1984; 251:626–9.
54. Klibanski A, Greenspan SL. Increase in bone mass after treatment of hyperprolactinemic amenorrhea. N Engl J Med 1986; 315:542–6.
55. Ciccarelli E, Savino L, Carlevetto V, Bertagna A, Isaia GC, Camanni I. Vertebral bone density in non-amenorrhoeic hyperprolactinaemic women. Clin Endocrinol 1988; 28:1–6.
56. Klibanski A, Biller BKM, Rosethal DI, Schoenfeld DA, Saxe V. Effects of prolactin and estrogen deficiency in amenorrheic bone loss. J Clin Endocrinol Metab 1988; 67:124–30.
57. Drinkwater BL, Nilson K, Chesnut CH, Bremner WJ, Shainholtz S, Southworth MB. Bone mineral density of amenorrheic and eumenorrheic athletes. N Engl J Med 1984; 311:277–81.
58. Lindberg JS, Fears WB, Hunt MM, Powell MR, Boll D, Wade CE. Exercise induced amenorrhea and bone density. Ann Intern Med 1984; 101:647–8.
59. Nelson ME, Fisher EC, Catsos PD, Meredith CN, Turksoy RN, Evans WJ. Diet and bone status in amenorrhoeic runners. Am J Clin Nutr 1986; 43:910–16.
60. Heath H. Athletic women, amenorrhea and skeletal integrity. Ann Intern Med 1985; 102:258–60.
61. Riggs BL. Eastell R. Exercise, hypogonadism and osteopenia. JAMA 1986; 256:392–3.
62. Rigotti NA, Nussbaum SR, Herzog DB, Neer RM. Osteoporosis in women with anorexia nervosa. N Engl J Med 1984; 311:1601–6.
63. Szmukler GI, Brown SW, Parsons V, Darby A. Premature loss of bone in chroic anorexia nervosa. Br Med J 1985; 290:26–7.
64. Matta WH, Shaw RW, Hesp R, Katz D. hypogonadism induced by luteinising hormone agonist analogues: effects on bone density in premenopausal women. Br Med J. 1987; 294:1523–4.
65. Johansen JS, Riis BJ, Hassager C, Moen M, Jacobson J, Christiansen C. The effect of a gonadotropin releasing hormone agonist analog (Nafarelin) on bone metabolism. J Clin Endocrinol Metab 1988; 67:701–6.
66. Jackson WU. Osteoporosis of unknown cause in younger people. J Bone Jt Surg 1958; 40B:420–41.
67. Francis RM, Peacock M, Aaron JE et al. Osteoporosis in hypogonadal men: role of decreased plasma 1,25-dihydroxyvitamin D, calcium malabsorption and low bone formation. Bone 1986; 7:261–8.
68. Jackson JA, Kleerekoper M, Parfitt AM. Symptomatic osteoporosis in a man with hyperprolactinaemic hypogonadism. Ann Intern Med 1986; 105:543–5.
69. Greenspan SL, Neer RM, Ridgway EC, Klibanski A. Osteoporosis in men with hyperprolactinaemic hypogonadism. Ann Intern Med 1986; 104:777–82.
70. Crilly RG, Francis RM, Nordin BEC. Steroid hormones, ageing and bone. Clin Endocrinol Metab 1981; 10:115–39.

Discussion

Persson: Patients treated with steroids who develop osteoporosis are a clinical problem. Are there any data to show that the bone loss in these patients, if they are women, can be counteracted by giving them oestrogens?

Selby: There are very few good data on this. The actual use of sex steroids has been very unpromising. More impressive and more interesting data have been generated with the use of either huge dose calcium supplements at the time of steroid administration (the only time that it appears to work) or diphosphonates given at the time of steroid administration. There have been some data to suggest that patients who have been treated with steroids for a long time will benefit from diphosphonate treatment. There are a few data suggesting that calcitonin may reverse these changes and Nordin's group has suggested that anabolic steroids may be of help. But none of these large studies are good data. It is a big clinical problem and one that has not been well addressed.

Studd: Professor Persson is right that it is logical to treat these women with oestrogens. With corticosteroid therapy there is a decrease in androstenedione levels and decreased testosterone in men and decreased oestradiol in women. They are hypogonadal. This may be one very simple cause for corticosteroid osteoporosis.

There is a report about 10 patients who had long-term percutaneous oestrogen therapy on corticosteroids with normal bone density and an increase over a year [1]. It is to me so logical that I cannot understand why the bone physicians do not use it.

Selby: Basically because a lot of people have looked at it in the past, and when patients have end-stage disease, like so many who get sent up to us, it has not been particularly promising.

Studd: Oestrogen is preventive in patients who are having steroids, in asthma for example. Even with end-stage disease bone can still be put back with oestrogens. But they need to be used – not high-dose calcium.

Anderson: Is this in the presence of continuing high levels of glucocorticoid?

Studd: Yes. Twenty years of corticosteroids and 10 and 15 years of oestrogens. Not hole filling, not transient, but permanent.

Anderson: What dose of glucocorticoid? It must be dependent, surely?

Studd: Presumably prednisolone 5–30 mg. Large doses for asthma, and all the patients had asthma.

Stevenson: One point about the effect of gonadotrophin releasing hormone (GnRH) superagonist and hypo-oestrogenism. Not only is there a concern that we may not have put the bone back but it also seems to depend on the site. As we published last year, the decrement seen in proximal femur seems to be greater and certainly does not reverse in the same time period as does that in the spine. Possibly lasting damage is being done, and this is still not known.

Secondly, a point about androgens. There is a very long study undertaken at the Hammersmith by Professor Frank Doyle which found, looking at males with hypogonadotrophic hypogonadism, that by stimulating endogenous testosterone they could show a very nice curvilinear increase in bone density. A plateau was reached at between 3 and 5 years and up to 15 years afterwards there was not really much of an increase. So again, they do not just keep putting bone back all the time; there is a very limited effect.

Selby: We have not followed our Leeds patients as far as that but from what we know about skeletal architecture that is perhaps something we might expect.

To go back to the GnRH agonists, the actual choice of agent was not mentioned. That study was with goserelin, which is probably longer-acting than some of the other agents, and so this may be a factor when we consider what treatment we give. But I would agree that quite a lot of concern needs to be taken over the choice of agent.

Whitehead: In the studies in which androgens were given to hypogonadotrophic males, what was used, what dose, and how often?

Selby: Sustanon 250 mg each fortnight. That took them from below the normal range to well above the normal range of testosterone levels, sometimes as high as 40 for a few days, but mainly kept them within the normal range for plasma testosterone through the fortnight between injections. Some of them were just at the bottom of the normal range by the next time.

Anderson: On average that would be twice the normal male production rate.

On the subject of androgens, does anybody seriously believe that adrenal androgens have anything to do with preventing osteoporosis? It seems to me that they are very low levels of such weak androgens. We are talking about very low levels of androstenedione, which is of dubious biological activity in any event, and DHEA sulphate.

Brincat: Nobody has mentioned the ADFR regimens in use in osteoporotics. I would have expected more comment on these newer regimens. Data are being published referring either to fluoride, to Stromba or whatever, as the active agent, and to calcitonin or diphosphonates for the depressed stage, and they do seem to imply that bone mass is being put on. I do not know of any histological study.

Selby: Although some people have shown some benefit and the first study that showed benefit was a histological study, on the whole they have not been promising. Whatever the regimen chosen for osteoporosis, I do not think we can say at the minute that we have got anything that can lead to sustained increase in bone mass.

I know that Mr Studd will disagree and he will say that oestrogens solve it all, but the general consensus of bone physicians is that in the patients we give oestrogen to we no not see a sustained increase in bone mass. We see the transient increase that we have referred to.

Brincat: Could that be because the treatment is not given for long enough?

Anderson: There is an initial increase, and then a plateau. That it what is suggested.

Studd: One could maintain treatment and try to achieve higher oestradiol levels in the plasma.

Kanis: No prospective studies of the therapeutic modalities that have been mentioned have shown a sustained progressive continuation of a positive increment in bone density which occurs indefinitely. All the inhibitors of bone turnover – anabolic steroids, oestrogens, calcium, diphosphonates – all induce a substantial increment in bone mass which may vary from 1% or 2% at cortical sites to up to 10% or even 15% at trabecular sites with high initial bone turnover, and thereafter bone mass increases no further. Indeed there is some evidence that with some of the treatment modalities (not with oestrogens but with calcium) bone mass will decrease thereafter, albeit at a slower rate of loss than before treatment. The single exception is fluoride. Fluoride acts quite differently and is capable of inducing a progressive, 10% increase in bone mass at least over a period of 10 or 12 years, or perhaps even for ever.

Anderson: But of dubious quality.

Kanis: That is another issue completely

References

1. Studd JWW, Savvas M, Johnson M. Correction of corticosteroid-induced osteoporosis by percutaneous hormone implants (Letter). Lancet 1989; i:339.

Chapter 11

The Measurement of Bone Density

I. Fogelman and A. Rodin

Introduction

The increasing awareness of the problem of osteoporosis has been prompted by
a combination of demographic changes, advances in technology and the realisation that this is an eminently preventable condition. Osteoporosis can be
defined as a reduction in the mass of bone per unit volume throughout the
skeleton leading to risk of fracture following minimal trauma. This condition
predominantly affects older women and is associated with significant morbidity
and mortality. The increasing prevalence of osteoporosis [1,2] imposes a heavy
and growing financial burden on the National Health Service. The average life
expectancy of women in the UK is now 82 years and this has increased
substantially since the 1930s when women could expect to reach 60 years. With
menopausal age remaining static at about 51 years, the woman of the 1990s will
spend a far larger proportion of her lifespan in the postmenopausal era than her
predecessors, and consequently, postmenopausal complications will achieve
more importance to both doctor and patient alike.

The organic matrix of bone is impregnated with mineral salts which confer the
properties of hardness and rigidity. The breaking strength of bone is linearly
related to its mineral content [3] and in osteoporosis there is a significant
reduction in the bone mineral content of the skeleton. Although other factors
such as frequency of falls, are important, the amount of bone present is the
single most important factor determining the likelihood of fracture [4]. The
development of new non-invasive techniques for the measurement of bone
density has led to an improved but still incomplete understanding of the
epidemiology of bone loss. It is now possible to measure bone mass with high

precision and accuracy and therefore critically to evaluate putative regimes for the prevention and treatment of osteoporosis. This chapter reviews recent advances in the measurement of bone density and their application to clinical practice.

Bone Density Measurement

A variety of non-invasive techniques have been developed for the measurement of bone mineral content or bone density. These methods have been reviewed in detail elsewhere [5–7] and this chapter will mainly concentrate on the techniques of photon absorptiometry and quantitative computed tomographic scanning (QCT). In the past radiographic methods were principally used to measure bone mineral but they all lack precision and are now seldom employed. Radiogrammetry relies on morphometric measurement of cortical bone (usually the third metacarpal) and can only be used in the appendicular skeleton. Calliper measurements are taken of the inner and outer diameters of the cortex and an assessment of bone mass can then be calculated from these indices. Although this technique is simple and inexpensive, it is relatively insensitive and gives little indication about bone mass at other, more clinically relevant, skeletal sites. Radiographic photodensitometry involves measurement of the optical density of a radiograph taken at a chosen appendicular site with a density standard such as a calibrated aluminium step wedge included in the exposure for comparison. The precision of this method can be improved by using computer-linked scanning microdensitometry [8]. These radiographic techniques require standardised conditions which are unrealistic in routine clinical practice and they have been largely superseded by photon absorptiometry and QCT.

Single photon absorptiometry was introduced in the 1960s and was originally performed at the midshaft of the radius. However, this site is not prone to osteoporotic fracture and direct measurement at the clinically important sites (distal radius, vertebral bodies and femoral neck) can nowadays be obtained using modern absorptiometry techniques. A single measurement at one site provides limited information about the remainder of the skeleton [9] and may correlate poorly with total body calcium [10]. Trabecular bone is more active metabolically than cortical bone and as the proportions of these two components varies at different sites throughout the skeleton, patterns of bone loss also vary. Mechanical stresses are also different and this may contribute to the inter-site variation in bone density. Direct measurement of bone density at the site of interest is therefore necessary and both QCT and photon absorptiometry facilitate this.

Quantitative Computed Tomography (QCT)

The development of QCT for the quantification of spinal mineral content has been one of the major advances in the field of bone mass measurements. Tomographic imaging techniques allow spatial separation of cortical and the metabolically more active trabecular bone and permit measurement of the amount of calcified tissue within a specific volume of bone.

CT images are derived from measured tissue attenuation values which are themselves dependent on tissue density and composition. Standard CT scanners are, therefore, all potentially capable of making these measurements in the lumbar spine. With QCT, a scout view is used for localisation, and a standard phantom consisting of rods of varying concentrations of K_2HPO_4 or hydroxy-apatite is included in each measurement. The attenuation values are then averaged over regions of interest within the vertebral cortical shell [11]. The slice locations and orientations adopted for these measurements must be accurately reproducible. In this way, a small volume (e.g 5 cm^3) of entirely trabecular bone is sampled. The problems encountered with QCT measurements fall into three categories: problems of precise three-dimensional relocation of the measurement site; problems of changes and differences in the chemical composition of the trabecular bone mixture; and difficulties associated with the physics of the technique.

At the photon energies employed in QCT, the measured attenuation coefficients are dependent on the density of the tissue as well as its elemental composition. Hence the selection of wholly trabecular bone regions results in a much greater influence of the fat content of the trabecular bone on the bone mineral measurement. Corrections may be introduced only for those variations that are, to an extent, predictable, such as age-related change in the red/yellow marrow mixture. Alternatively, scanning consecutively at two different photon energies produces a more accurate, though less precise result [12]. The use of a polychromatic X-ray beam produces inaccuracy due to changes in the photon energy spectrum through a scanned section. The effect of long-term and short-term changes in spectra produced by the scanner can only be corrected by simultaneous scanning and analysis of calibration phantoms. Ultimately, for all these reasons QCT is no more accurate than the photon absorptiometry techniques. Furthermore, it is less precise, more expensive and exposes patients to far higher radiation doses than dual photon absorptiometry. However, it does provide a means of measuring purely trabecular bone in the spine. The accuracy error for QCT in the clinical setting is reported to be between 5%–10% [10,13] and precision in the best hands is 1%–3% [14,15]. The purpose-built isotope CT devices for measurements in the appendicular skeleton, however, although expensive and not widely available, provide measurements of excellent precision at low radiation doses [16]. This makes them ideal for longitudinal therapy monitoring, but they are of limited value in predicting the bone density of the axial skeleton.

Photon Absorptiometry

In this technique, a highly collimated beam of low energy photons is obtained from an isotope source. This is directed at the measurement site and the transmitted beam intensity is monitored with a well-collimated scintillation detection system. The use of beams of known, unique photon energies together with energy-selective detection produces a very stable – hence precise –

measurement system. Synchronous movement of source and detector along a rectilinear path allows data collection from the region of interest.

Single Photon Absorptiometry

Single photon absorptiometry was first described in 1963 [17] and involves measuring the transmission of a monoenergetic photon beam from iodine-125 (28 keV) through bone and soft tissue. Low photon energies are used to produce maximum contrast between bone and soft tissue but attentuation of the beam limits the usefulness of this technique to appendicular body sites. The total thickness of tissue must be constant over the scanning path as varying soft tissue thickness produces transmitted beam intensity variations. This is achieved by surrounding the limb with soft tissue equivalent (water or tissue-equivalent gel). Given that the attenuation of the beam within the bone is exponential, bone mass in the beam can be computed. The forearm is the most convenient measurement site but proportions of cortical and trabecular bone vary markedly along the length of the arm and accurate positioning is vital. Originally, the site (e.g. the distal third of the radius) was determined by measuring along the forearm using the radial styloid and the olecranon as landmarks. Modern instruments incorporate automatic detection of the width of the interosseous space between the radius and ulna and regions of interest are positioned and scanned in relation to some selected value (e.g. 8 mm gap). The non-dominant arm is usually measured and this technique has also been applied to the os calcis [18].

Most authors report accuracy errors of 4%–5% with this technique related to technical factors common to all gamma ray systems and variations in soft tissue [19,20]. Precision of 1%–2% can be achieved in the research setting and 2%–5% in routine use [21]. Radiation exposure is low at <150 μSV (peak skin dose) with negligible whole body dose. In normal subjects, measurements at the distal radius are reasonably well correlated with those in the axial skeleton but this relationship may be poor in osteoporosis [22].

Dual Photon Absorptiometry

Dual photon absorptiometry (DPA) is used mainly to measure bone mineral in the lumbar spine and hip, but it can also be adapted to measure total body calcium. It is similar in principle to single photon absorptiometry but in order to overcome the problem of variable soft tissue thickness, the radiation beam consists of two distinct photon energies. These may be derived from combined radiation sources, but more commonly, a single radionuclide is used which emits at two separate energies. Commercial instruments incorporate gadolinium-153 as the radiation source; its energy spectrum has peaks at 44 keV and 100 keV. Simultaneous transmission measurements are made at the two energies and the thickness of soft tissue and the amount of bone mineral in the beam path can then be computed. This technique does not demand equal soft tissue thickness and permits bone mineral measurement at the clinically important sites where osteoporotic fractures occur. The region of interest is scanned and a point by point determination of bone mineral is made. From this the total bone mineral

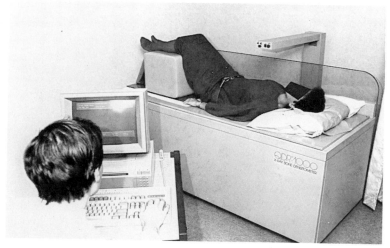

Fig. 11.1. A dual energy X-ray absorptiometry (DEXA) unit with patient positioned for a spinal scan. The legs are elevated to straighten the lumbar lordosis.

value is obtained by summation. Scanner motion and data collection and processing are controlled by a microcomputer. A bone edge detection algorithm is used to define bone and soft tissue. Results are expressed as total bone mineral (grams hydroxyapatite (HA)), bone mineral per unit length of area of interest (grams hydroxyapatite per unit length) and bone mineral per unit area or bone "density" (grams hydroxyapatite per unit area). Most groups now present data as "density", i.e. g HA cm^{-2}.

The accuracy of DPA is about 3%–6% for the spine and 3%–4% for the femoral neck [23]. Short-term precision in our hands is 2% for the spine and femur [24] and reported precision is usually between 1% and 4% [25–27]. Radiation exposure is low with a marrow dose per scan of approximately 20 µSV.

Dual Energy X-ray Absorptiometry (DEXA)

The most recent advance in absorptiometry has been the introduction of DEXA (Fig. 11.1). In this technique, an X-ray source rather than a radionuclide is used to generate a photon flux [28]. Dual energies are obtained by either switching kilovoltage or by filtering X-rays generated from a stable X-ray tube. An X-ray tube produces a much higher photon flux than is possible with a gadolinium-153 source. Thus scan time is considerably less than DPA (approximately 7 min for a spinal measurement compared with 20 min by DPA) and radiation exposure is also reduced [29,30]. Further, the precision of DEXA is excellent and in clinical practice, values in the range 0.5%–1.2% can be achieved [28,30,31]. The stability of the X-ray source eliminates errors related to declining source activity which are sometimes encountered in DPA [30], and there is improved image resolution (Fig. 11.2). These substantial advantages suggest that DPA will soon be superseded by DEXA.

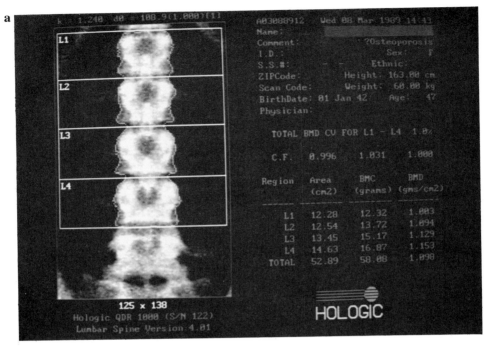

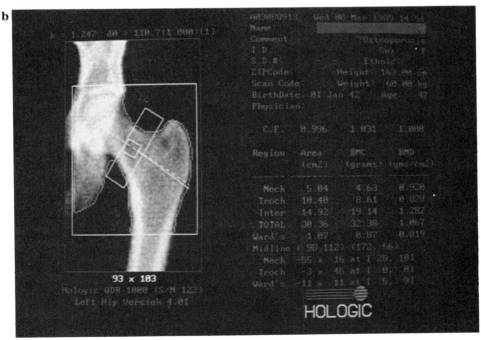

Fig. 11.2. Examples of the analysis of bone mineral density using DEXA in spine (**a**) and femur (**b**). There is improved resolution and counting statistics using an X-ray tube as the radiation source.

The Clinical Application of Bone Mineral Measurements

Age-Related Bone Loss

Ageing is accompanied by a net loss of bone mineral from the skeleton and an increasing likelihood of fracture. However, controversy exists about patterns of bone loss and evidence about the natural history of changes in bone density is incomplete. The majority of studies refer to Caucasian women and there is relatively little information about men. Data are commonly derived from cross-sectional studies which may be biased by secular trends and inadequate sample size [32].

Rickers et al. [33] used single photon absorptiometry to investigate age-related changes in cortical bone density at the mid-radius in 139 normal women (age range 20–88 years). They found that cortical bone in the appendicular skeleton is well maintained until the fifties when slow diminution commences and continues linearly. This diminution in cortical bone mineral is related to the menopause and is in good agreement with other studies [34–36]. Patterns of bone loss from the axial skeleton are more controversial. An early model suggested that bone loss from the vertebrae commenced in young adulthood and was linear [37] but other studies suggest that bone mass increases until the mid-thirties and indeed the bulk of available evidence supports the commencement of bone loss from around the age of 35 [38–40]. In a cross-sectional study of 225 premenopausal Caucasian women spinal bone density was shown to increase to a peak in the mid-thirties and this was followed by a gradual, but significant decrease of 10% of peak bone mass preceding the menopause (Fig. 11.3a) [24]. The femoral neck shows a different pattern with essentially linear loss which commences in the late twenties and proceeds at a slower rate than that seen in the spine (Fig. 11.3b). However, although slower, loss commences earlier and the cumulative premenopausal loss (9%) is similar to that seen in the spine.

The menopause is considered as a watershed for the skeleton and in women it is probably the major determinant of bone loss. Women appear to lose bone at an accelerated rate for several years after the menopause due to a deficiency of oestrogen [41]. The rate of loss decreases as bone density diminishes and a feedback mechanism has been proposed in which diminished density is accompanied by an increasing load on the remaining bone which stimulates bone formation [42]. However, these data have been based almost exclusively on measurements of cortical bone either in the radius or in the metacarpal [42,43]. The situation in the trabecular bone of the axial skeleton is less clear. Riggs et al. in cross-sectional [37] and longitudinal studies [44] found no acceleration in bone loss in the spine around the time of the menopause. However, Krolner and Pors Nielsen [38] found accelerated bone loss after the menopause and recently, a cross-sectional study of 286 women aged between 46 and 55 years showed an acceleration of lumbar bone loss, related to the menopause [45].

Serial studies of spinal bone mass using QCT before and after oophorectomy have shown dramatic rates of bone loss following surgery, thus emphasising the important role of oestrogen [46]. In a longitudinal study, Nilas and Christiansen [47] performed serial bone density measurements in 26 premenopausal women aged 47–49 years by single photon absorptiometry at two forearm sites and by dual photon absorptiometry in the lumbar spine. While confirming accelerated

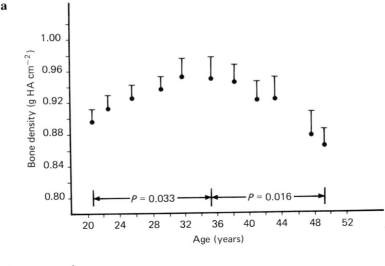

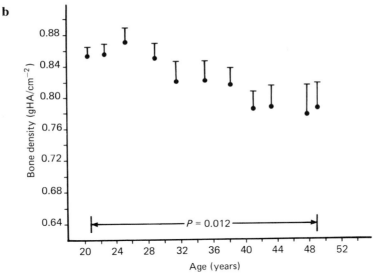

Fig. 11.3. Plots of bone mineral density against age for 225 premenopausal women measured by dual photon absorptiometry. **a** Spinal BMD reaches a peak value in the mid-30s and starts to decline before the onset of the menopause. **b** Femoral neck BMD shows a steady decline with age. In each case the five-year running average ±1SEM is plotted.

bone loss in the forearm they found that the rate of spinal bone loss was identical in late perimenopausal and early postmenopausal women. However, only nine women became postmenopausal during the study and the precision of spinal bone density measurements was 4%, thus the results must be interpreted cautiously. It is difficult to reconcile all the conflicting data in the literature and the debate continues. However, it is probable that the menopause causes accelerated bone loss but this has not always been identified because of the limitations of cross-sectional studies and small sample numbers or poor precision in serial studies.

The mechanism by which oestrogen acts to maintain the integrity of the skeleton remains unclear but it is apparent that oestrogen inhibits bone resorption [47]. Oestradiol receptors have not been detected on osteoblasts [48,49] and it is probable that oestrogen has a direct cellular effect as well as other indirect actions on bone. The menopause is preceded by a transition phase during which the ovaries become increasingly resistant to stimulation by the gonadotrophins and total oestrogen output steadily declines [50,51]. This may be a partial explanation for premenopausal bone loss. An early menopause is widely regarded as a major risk factor for osteoporosis as these individuals are likely to have lower bone density than their peers. However, even such an apparently uncontroversial statement has been challenged and Seeman et al. [52] have recently found that postmenopausal women who had an early menopause do not have lower bone mass than those with normal age at menopause. They suggest that increased fracture risk in these women may be due to prolonged exposure to potential trauma at low bone mass. Nevertheless, the great majority of studies have emphasised the importance of oestrogen exposure to the maintenance of an intact skeleton.

The relative importance of chronological age and menopausal age as determinants of bone density has been discussed extensively [53–56]. In cross-sectional and longitudinal studies Nordin [55] measured forearm bone density by single photon absorptiometry in pre- and postmenopausal women. He found that the menopause is the major determinant of bone loss and there is an additional contribution from ageing. Richelson et al. [53] compared a group of perimenopausal women (mean age 52 years) with a group who had an early menopause (mean years postmenopause 22 years; mean chronological age 54 years) and a group who were on average 22 years postmenopause and had a mean chronological age of 73 years. Bone density was measured in the mid-radius, femoral neck, femoral intertrochanteric region and lumbar spine. The early menopause group and the chronologically older group were of comparable menopausal ages and their patterns of bone loss at all sites was similar. On the basis of these results, it was concluded that oestrogen deficiency and not ageing is the prominent cause of bone loss in the first two decades after the menopause. In old age, when cumulative age-related bone loss has occurred over decades, the menopause becomes less significant. In this situation, chronological age is more important and differences between normal and osteoporotic subjects become less apparent. Indeed, virtually all subjects over 75 years will have values for bone mass that fall into the at-risk range for fracture [37]. Riggs et al. [44] have suggested that if the age of a healthy woman is known then the bone sensity of her lumbar spine or femoral neck can be predicted with a standard deviation of about 10%.

Prediction of Fracture

There is now a considerable body of evidence suggesting that bone mineral measurements provide the single best means of identifying those at risk of fracture [4,18,57–62]. This has also been confirmed in prospective studies, the great majority of which have been carried out using single photon absorptiometry [57,60]. In a prospective study of 699 women of Japanese/American extraction who were followed for a mean duration of 3.6 years (measurements were obtained at four sites – calcaneus, spine, and proximal and distal radius) 39 new spinal fractures occurred (defined as a reduction in vertebral height of >15%) [63]. There was a highly significant correlation between reduction in bone mineral and fracture at all sites. Low bone density in both the calcaneus and radius was a better predictor of spinal fractures than density in the spine itself. Further, the combination of bone mineral measurements at two sites strengthened the relationship with spinal fracture and the best two-site combination was calcaneus and distal radius. In that study, the mean age of women was 63.3 years and as the authors themselves state, the explanation for the apparent discrepancy that spinal measurements are not the best predictors of spinal fracture is likely to arise because of the presence of aortic calcification and degenerative disease in the spine in the study population. This illustrates the difficulty of attempting to answer the question: which sites should be measured with regard to prediction of fracture? The conclusion from the above study may have been very different if women were initially enrolled at a younger age, e.g. the time of the menopause when spinal measurements might have been expected to be the best predictor of subsequent spinal fractures. Of course a follow-up period of around 15 years would have been required to obtain a similar prevalence of fracture. Thus, the age of any study population is important. This is further reinforced by the results of an important recent study from Malmo [57]. There, 1076 women had forearm bone mineral measurements carried out using single photon absorptiometry 10–16 years previously. The subsequent incidence of fragility fractures (defined as distal radius, proximal humerus, hip, vertebra, pelvis or tibial condyle) between 1975 and 1985 were recorded. It was found that for women aged between 50 and 69, those with low bone mass had a significantly increased risk of fracture, but this was not evident for women aged over 70 years. This was due to the high frequency of spinal fractures in that population even when relatively high values for bone mineral were present. It is of interest that in the over 70s those with fracture had significantly lower weight, i.e. weight but not bone mineral content could predict fracture in that population. It was concluded that forearm measurements in those over the age of 70 have no value in predicting fracture. It should be noted that there are no prospective data with femoral neck measurements. This is clearly a glaring deficiency in view of the clinical importance of femoral neck fractures.

With regard to the site of measurement, a correlation of approximately 0.7 has been found between bone mineral measurements in the radius and spine in normal subjects although this may be considerably less good in disease states [22]. Where multiple sites have been measured in the skeleton there is generally a correlation of at least 0.6 between any two sites [4]. Our own experience using dual energy X-ray absorptiometry in 100 normal women aged between 40 and 60 years has shown a correlation of 0.64 between spine and femoral neck. It should be remembered that even at a single site such as the lumber spine the correlation between individual vertebrae is 0.82 [4]. Thus there is no doubt that significant differences in bone mineral content occur between different sites in the skeleton. There is, however, some controversy as to how important this is. In one study measuring three different sites in the forearm, while the ultra-distal radius was the most sensitive indicator of bone loss, each site was equally sensitive with regard to prevalence of fracture [64]. Others have suggested that the particular technique of bone mineral measurement does not matter as much as the site of measurement [4]. This issue is important if screening programmes for the normal population are investigated. A peripheral measurement is likely to be much cheaper and would be particularly suitable for mass screening where many thousands of women are involved. However, in an individual case a peripheral measurement may well be misleading with regard to changes in the spine or hips. Nevertheless, as stated above, there is reasonably good correlation between bone mineral density at various sites throughout the body and this provides supportive evidence that osteoporosis is a systemic disease.

Thus when addressing the question of bone mineral measurements in pre-diction of fracture not only should the age of the study population, the technique and the site of bone mineral measurement in the skeleton be considered, but also, the design of the study. The precision of the technique, the number of study subjects, the number of measurements and the duration of the study should all be considered with regard to statistical significance. Dual energy X-ray absorptiometry provides a major advance with regard to spinal and femoral measurements as precision of 1% can be achieved in clinical practice. As yet, there are no prospective clinical studies using this technique.

The way ahead in the management of osteoporosis is not in treatment of the established disease but in its prevention. It is now generally accepted that oestrogen replacement therapy is the most effective means of preventing postmenopausal osteoporosis [65] and there is recent evidence that subcuta-neous oestrogen implants may even increase bone density [66] presumably due to the high levels of oestradiol achieved by this route of administration. While some advocate a blanket policy of oestrogen replacement therapy for all on reaching the menopause it is more realistic to recognise that a large group of women (and some doctors) remain wary of this form of treatment and will decline it unless given objective reasons to comply. Long-term treatment for all would have to be cost-effective and it would have major implications for the workload of family doctors and gynaecologists. Further, up to 20% of women will discontinue treatment prematurely due to progestogenic side effects such as withdrawal bleeding. In the past, short-term courses of oestrogen therapy have been given to control acute menopausal symptoms, however, there is no evidence to indicate that treatment with oestrogen for less than 5 years provides any real benefit to the skeleton.

A more pragmatic approach is to offer long-term hormone replacement therapy to those who are at particular risk of developing osteoporosis. This implies some form of population screening to identify susceptible women. Traditionally, the fair skinned, the small, the slim, the smoker or the slothful were all considered likely candidates for developing osteoporosis [67]. However, these "risk factors" are a crude means of screening the general population. It has been suggested that a biochemical screen of skeletal metabolism could be of value in identifying fast bone losers [68] but this concept fails to take into account the bone mass on reaching the menopause.

The single best predictor of bone mass in later life is bone mass in earlier life [42]. In the normal population, at any given age, there is a wide range of results for bone density measurement (approximately 30% about the mean) (Fig. 11.4), and in the early years following the menopause an individual's bone density will be largely determined by peak bone mass. In extreme old age this is less relevant

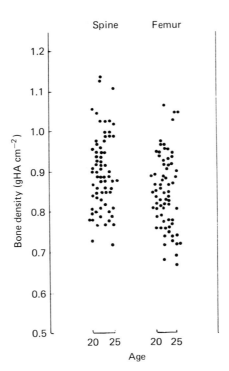

Fig. 11.4. Results for spinal and femoral bone density (measured by DPA) for 100 young normal women. Note the wide range of results obtained.

because of the cumulative effect of age-related bone loss. If an individual's peak adult bone mass is high, then even if a fast bone loser, it may be that bone mass will never be as low as the maximum attained in those commencing with low bone mass. If however, one starts with a low bone mass and is also a fast bone loser, then presumably the likelihood of osteoporosis in later life is greatly increased.

Although some may argue about the feasibility of screening the whole population, in view of the magnitude of the problems related to osteoporosis, some co-ordinated strategy aimed at preventing this insidious condition will have to be instigated.

References

1. Royal College of Physicians Report. Fractured neck of femur–prevention and management. London RCP, 1989.
2. Bengner U, Johnell O, Redlund-Johnell I. Changing incidence and prevalence of vertebral fractures during 30 years. Calcif Tiss Int 1988; 42; 293–6.
3. Bartely MH, Arnold JS, Haslam RK, Webster SSJ. The relationship of bone strength and bone quantity in health, disease and ageing. J Gerontol 1966; 21:517–21.
4. Ross PD, Wasnich RD, Vogel JM. Detection of prefracture spinal osteoporosis using bone mineral absorptiometry. J Bone Miner Res 1988; 3:1–11.

5. Mazess RB, Wahner HM. Nuclear medicine and densitometry In: Riggs BL, Melton III JL, eds. Osteoporosis: etiology, diagnosis and management. New York: Raven Press, 1988; 251–95.
6. Murby B, Fogelman I. Bone mineral measurements in clinical practice. Br J Hosp Med 1987; May:453–8.
7. Mazess RB. Noninvasive bone measurements. In: Kunin A, ed. Skeletal research II. New York: Academic Press, 1983; 277–343.
8. Vogt FB, Meharg LS, Mack PB. Use of a digital computer in the measurement of roentgeno-graphic bone density. AJR 1969; 105:870.
9. Schaadt O, Bohr H. Skeletal metabolism. Lancet 1980; ii:914.
10. Horsman A, Burkinshaw L, Pearson D, Oxby CB, Milner RM. Estimating total body calcium from peripheral bone measurements. Calcif Tiss Int 1983; 35:135–44.
11. Cann CE, Gennant HK. Precise measurement of vertebral mineral content using computed tomography. J Comput Assist Tomogr 1980; 4:493–500.
12. Genant HK, Boyd D. Quantitative bone mineral analysis using dual energy computed tomography. Invest Radiol 1977; 12:545–51.
13. Richardson ML, Genant HK, Cann CE, Ettinger BE. Assessment of metabolic bone diseases by quantitative computerized tomography. Clin Orthop 1985; 185:224–38.
14. Genant HK, Cann CE, Pozzi-Mucelli RS, Kanter AS. Vertebral mineral determination by quantitative CT: clinical and visability and normative data. J Comput Assist Tomogr 1983; 7:554.
15. Graves VB, Wimmer R. Long term reproducibility of quantitative computed tomography for vertebral mineral measurements. J Comput Assist Tomogr 1985; 9:73–6.
16. Ruegsegger P, Dambacher M. Clinical application of peripheral computed tomography. Excerpt Med Int Congr Ser 1983; 617:48–51.
17. Cameron JR, Sorenson J. Measurement of bone mineral in vivo: an improved method. Science 1963; 142:230–2.
18. Wasnich RD, Ross PD, Heilbrun LK, Vogel JM. Prediction of postmenopausal fracture risk with use of bone mineral measurements. Am J Obstet Gynecol 1985; 153:745–51.
19. Sorenson JA, Cameron JR. A reliable in vivo measurment of bone mineral content. J Bone Jt Surg 1967; 49A:481–97.
20. Cameron JR, Mazess RB, Sorenson MS. Precision and accuracy of bone mineral determination by direct photon absorptiometry. Invest Radiol 1986; 3:141–50.
21. Johnston CC Jr. Noninvasive methods of quantifying appendicular bone mass. In: Avioli LV, ed. The osteoporotic syndrome: detection, prevention and treatment. New York: Grune and Stratton, 1983; 73–83.
22. Mezess RB, Peppler WW, Chesney RW, Lange TA, Lindgren U, Smith E. Does bone density on the radius indicate skeletal status? J Nucl Med 1984; 25:281–8.
23. Wilson CR, Matson M. Dichromatic absorptiometry of vertebral bone mineral content. Invest Radiol 1977; 12:188–94.
24. Rodin A, Murby B, Smith MA, Caleffi M, Fentiman I, Chapman MG, Fogelman I. Premeno-pausal bone loss in the lumbar spine and neck of femur: a study of 225 caucasian women. Bone 1990; 11:1–50.
25. Leblanc AD, Evans HJ, Marsh C, Schneider V, Johnson PC, Jhingran SG. Precision of dual photon absorptiometry measurements. J Nucl Med 1986; 27:1362–5.
26. Tothill P, Smith MA, Sutton D. Dual photon absorptiometry of the spine with a low activity source of gadolinium 153. Br J Radiol 1983; 56:829–35.
27. Schaadt O, Bohr H. Bone mineral by dual photon absorptiometry. Accuracy-precision-sites of measurements. In: Dequeker J, Johnston CC, eds. Non-invasive bone measurements. Oxford: IRL Press, 1981; 59–72.
28. Pacifici R, Rupich R, Vered I, Fischer K, Griffin M, Susman N, Avioli LV. Dual energy radiography: a preliminary comparative study. Calcif Tiss Int 1988; 48:189–91.
29. Sartoris DJ, Resnick D. Dual-energy radiographic absorptiometry for bone densitometry: current status and perspective. Am J Radiol 1989; 152:214–16.
30. Kelly TL, Slovik DM, Schoenfeld DA, Neer RM. Quantitative digital radiography versus dual photon absorptiometry of the lumbar spine. J Clin Endocrinol Metab 1988; 67:839–44.
31. Mazess R, Collick B, Trempe J, Barden H, Hanson J. Performance evaluation of a dual-energy X-ray bone densitometer. Calcif Tiss Int 1989; 44:228–32.
32. Sambrook PN, Eisman JA, Furler SM, Pocock NA. Computer modelling and analysis of cross sectional bone density studies with respect to age and the menopause. J Bone Miner Res 1987; 2:109–14.
33. Rickers H, Deding A, Christiansen C, Rodbro P, Naestoft J. Corticosteroid induced osteopenia and vitamin D metabolism. Clin Endocrinol 1982; 16:409–15.

34. Cohn SH, Vaswani A, Zanzi I, Ellis KJ. Effect of aging on bone mass in adult women. Am J Physiol 1976; 230:143.
35. Smith DM, Khairi MRA, Norton J, Johnston CC. Age and activity effects on rate of bone mineral loss. J Clin Invest 1976; 58:716.
36. Aloia JF, Vaswani A, Ellis K, Yuen K, Cohn SH. A model for involutional bone loss. J Lab Clin Med 1985; 106:630–7.
37. Riggs BL, Wahner HW, Dunn WL, Mazess RB, Offord KP. Differential changes in bone mineral density of the appendicular and axial skeleton with aging. J Clin Invest 1981; 67:328–35.
38. Krolner B, Pors-Nielsen S. Bone mineral content of the lumbar spine in normal and osteoporotic women. Clin Sci 1982; 62:329–36.
39. Hansson T, Roos B. Age changes in the bone mineral of the lumbar spine in normal women. Calcif Tiss Int 1986; 38:249–51.
40. Mazess RB, Barden HS, Ettinger M et al. Spine and femur density using dual photon absorptiometry in US white women. Bone Mineral 1987; 2:211–19.
41. Lindsay R, Hart DM, MacLean A, Garwood J, Aitken JM, Clark AC, Coutts JRT. Pathogenesis and prevention of postmenopausal osteoporosis. In: Cooke ID, ed. The role of oestrogen/progestogen in the management of the menopause. Lancaster: MTP, 1978;9–27.
42. Nordin BEC, Polley KJ. Metabolic consequences of the menopause. Calcif Tiss Int 1987; 41s:1–60.
43. Johnston CC Jr, Norton JA Jr, Khairi RA et al. Age-related bone loss. In: Barzel US, ed. Osteoporosis II. Philadelphia: Grune and Stratton, 1979; 91–100.
44. Riggs BL, Wahner HW, Melton JL III, Richelson LS, Judd HL, Offord KP. Rates of bone loss in the appendicular and axial skeletons of women. J Clin Invest 1986; 77:1487–91.
45. Elders PJM, Coen Netelenbos J, Lips P, van Ginkel FC, van der Stelt PF. Accelerated vertebral bone loss in relation to the menopause: a cross sectional study on lumbar bone density in 286 women of 46–55 years of age. Bone Mineral 1988; 5:11–19.
46. Genant HK, Cann CE, Ettinger B, Gordan GS. Quantitative computed tomography of vertebral spongiosa: a sensitive method of detecting early bone loss after oophorectomy. Ann Intern Med 1982; 97:699–705.
47. Nilas L, Christiansen C. The pathophysiology of peri- and postmenopausal bone loss. Br J Obstet Gynaecol 1989; 96:580–7.
48. Komm BS, Sheetz L, Baker M, Gallegos A, O'Malley BW, Haussler MR. J Bone Miner Res 1987; 2:Abstract 237 S1.
49. Eriksen EF, Berg NJ, Graham ML, Mann KG, Spelsberg TC, Riggs BL. J Bone Miner Res 1987; 2:Abstract 238 S1.
50. Sherman BM, West JH, Korenman SG. The menopausal transition: analysis of LH FSH estradiol and progesterone concentrations during menstrual cycles of older women. Clin Endocrinol Metab 1976; 42:629–36.
51. Johnston CC Jr, Hui SL, Witt RM, Appledorn R, Baker RS, Longcope C. Early menopausal changes in bone mass and sex steroids. J Clin Endocrinol Metab 1985; 61:905–11.
52. Seeman E, Cooper ME, Hopper JL, Parkinson E, McKay J, Jerums G. Effect of early menopause on bone mass in normal women and patients with osteoporosis. Am J Med 1988; 85:213–16.
53. Richelson LS, Wahner HW, Melton LJ III et al. Relative contributions of aging and estrogen deficiency to postmenopausal bone loss. N Engl J Med 1943; 11:1273–5.
54. Riggs BL, Melton LJ III. Involutional osteoporosis. N Engl J Med 1986; 314:1676–86.
55. Nordin BEC. The osteoporosis agenda: what we do not know? In: Christiansen C et al., eds. Osteoporosis. Proceedings of the international symposium on osteoporosis. Norhaven A/S Denmark, 1987; 23–30.
56. Nilas L, Christiansen C. Bone mass and its relationship to age and the menopause. J Clin Endocrinol Metab 1987; 65:697–702.
57. Gardsell P, Johnell O, Nilsson BE. Predicting fractures in women using forearm bone densitometry. Calcif Tiss Int 1989; 44:235–42.
58. Wasnich RD, Ross PD, Heilbrun LK, Vogel JM. Selection of the optimal skeletal site for fracture risk prediction. Clin Orthop 1987; 216:262–9.
59. Melton LJ, Wahner HW, Richelson LS, O'Fallon WM, Riggs BL. Osteoporosis and the risk of hip fracture. Am J Epidemiol 1986; 124:254–61.
60. Hui SL, Slemenda CW, Johnston CC Jr. Age and bone mass as predictors of fracture in a prospective study. J Clin Invest 1988; 81:1804–9.
61. Jensen GF, Christiansen C, Boesen J, Hegedus V, Transbol I. Relationship between bone mineral content and frequency of postmenopausal fractures. Acta Med Scand 1983; 213:61–3.

62. Smith DM, Khairi MRA, Johnston CC. The loss of bone mineral with aging and its relationship to risk of fracture. J Clin Invest 1975; 56:311–18.
63. Wasnich RD, Ross PD, Davis JW, Vogel JM. A comparison of single and multi-site BMC measurements for assessment of spine fracture probability. J Nucl Med 1989; 30:1166–71.
64. Price RI, Barnes MP, Gutteridge DH, Baron-Hay M, Prince RL, Retallack RW, Hickling C. Ultradistal and cortical forearm bone density in the assessment of post menopausal bone loss and non-axial fracture risk. J Bone Miner Res 1989; 4:149–55.
65. Lindsay R, Hart DM, Aitken JM, MacDonald EB, Anderson JB, Clarke AC. Long-term prevention of postmenopausal osteoporosis by oestrogen. Lancet 1976; i:1038–41.
66. Savvas M, Studd JWW, Fogelman I, Dooley M, Montgomery J, Murby B. Skeletal effects of oral oestrogen compared with subcutaneous oestrogen and testosterone in postmenopausal women. Br Med J 1988; 297:331–3.
67. Heaney RP, Creighton JA. Risk factors in age-related bone loss and osteoporotic fracture. In: Christiansen et al., eds. Osteoporosis. Proceedings of Copenhagen international symposium on osteoporosis. Aalborg Stiftsbogtrykkeri, Denmark 1984; 245–51.
68. Christiansen C, Riis BJ, Rodbro P. Prediction of rapid bone loss in postmenopausal women. Lancet 1987; i:1105–8.

Chapter 12

Screening Techniques in the Evaluation of Osteoporosis

J. A. Kanis, E. V. McCloskey, K. S. Eyres, D. V. O'Doherty
and J. Aaron

Introduction

Bone disease is now recognised as a major problem of public health. The greatest concern is involutional osteoporosis, which gives rise to fragility fractures, particularly of the spine, wrist and hip. The incidence of vertebral and hip fractures increases exponentially with age. Women are at particular risk from fracture and the incidence in women is twice that of men in this country [1]. The reasons for this relate to the lower bone density of women at the time of maturity (peak bone density) and the accelerated bone loss that occurs after the menopause. Women live significantly longer than men so that the prevalence of osteoporotic fracture among elderly women is six times that of men. The age and sex specific incidence of osteoporotic fracture is rising in all countries and, if the current trends continue, then the prevalence of hip fractures will double over the next 20 years [1].

Awareness of osteoporosis has coincided with the realisation that osteoporosis can be prevented in part, not only with hormone replacement treatment, but also with other interventions which prevent or delay the rate of bone loss. Since the prospects of treatment of the established disorder are significantly less than the ability to prevent skeletal losses [2], much attention has focused on prevention and the use of physical and biochemical techniques which can assess the risk of osteoporotic fracture. This chapter briefly reviews the place of such techniques in the assessment of osteoporosis, and in particular examines the assumptions commonly made and the manner in which these might temper interpretation of the information which the techniques provide. The application of the techniques to screening is reviewed by others in this volume and elsewhere [3].

What is Osteoporosis?

Osteoporosis is a disorder in which there is a diminution of bone mass without detectable changes in the ratio of mineralised to non-mineralised matrix. This definition distinguishes the condition from osteomalacia where the proportion of osteoid to calcified bone is increased. For this reason, measurements of bone mineral content or density provide estimates of skeletal mass in osteoporosis provided that osteomalacia does not coexist. Many techniques have been developed to measure indices of bone mass or loss, often at regional sites (Table 12.1). Since bone mass is one of the major determinants of the compressive and torsional strength of bone, if loss is sufficient, fracture will occur more easily. It has thus become fashionable to consider osteoporosis exclusively in terms of the amount of bone present or in terms of bone mineral content. On this basis, osteoporosis is commonly defined as a decrease in bone density which renders the skeleton more liable to fracture.

Definition of Osteoporosis

Definitions of osteoporosis are somewhat arbitrary, depending on whether it is the clinical end result (fracture) which is described, or the process which gives rise to fracture. From the point of view of a disease process, a decrease in bone

Table 12.1. Some techniques used in the assessment of bone loss

Technique	Site	Reproducibility (CV%)
Metabolic balance		5–15
Serial determination of:		
1. Neutron activation	Hand	2–4
	Spine	2–10
	Whole body	5–10
2. Single photon absorptiometry	Appendicular cortex	1–4
	Appendicular spongy	3–5
	Axial	3–5
	CAT	3–5
3. Dual photon absorptiometry	Appendicular cortex	2–5
	Appendicular spongy	3–5
	Axial cortex	3–5
4. X-ray	DEXA spine	1–2
	Metacarpal width	1–2
	Vertebral morphometry	2–5
	CAT	5–15
5. Bone histology	Ilium	20–30
6. Ultrasound attenuation	Heel	4–6

Table 12.2. Relationship between bone density (BMD) measured by photonabsorptiometry at sites commonly used and estimates of the future probability of fracture in 50-year-old women Computed from Wasnich et al. (10].

SD units	BMD distal radius (g cm^{-2})	BMD proximal radius (g cm^{-2})	BMD lumbar spine (g cm^{-2})	Life-time probability of fracture	% of all fractures	Relative risk
+2	1.17	1.14	1.43	0.6	4	0.28
+1	1.04	1.02	1.29	1.0	6	0.48
0	0.92	0.90	1.15	2.1	14	1.00
−1	0.78	0.78	1.01	3.6	23	1.71
−2	0.65	0.66	0.87	8.2	53	3.90

density is clearly a major factor which gives rise to the increased risk of fracture.

There is a a compelling relationship between the amount of calcium or matrix in bone and the risk of fracture. The lower the bone density, the lower its ability to withstand compressive forces [4], and the greater the risk from fracture [5,6]. Several prospective studies have now shown that measurements of bone mineral content or density at a variety of skeletal sites can provide an estimate of the risk from future fracture [7–9] (*See* Table 12.2). These relationships have markedly influenced the ways in which osteoporosis have been defined.

Thus, osteoporosis has been defined as a decrease in bone density below that of a normal population, either age-matched or the young adult population [11]. An alternative has been to characterise the bone density of an osteoporotic population and to define osteoporosis in terms of bone density below a fracture threshold at which a patient is at risk from fracture [12].

Irrespective of the approach used and the site of measurement there is an overlap between the bone mineral content or density of populations with and without fracture. Indeed, the risk of osteoporotic fracture is stochastic and increases progessively as bone density decreases (Table 12.2). Moreover, factors other than the amount of bone contribute to fracture risk. Thus, bone mineral measurements may give an index of the risk but do not capture all elements of that risk, which vary with the techniques used, age, cause of bone loss and site of interest.

For these reasons osteoporosis might more usefully be defined as a clinical disorder rather than a process. In these terms, osteoporosis represents the occurrence of a fragility fracture and a decrease in bone density (osteopenia) a major risk factor [13]. There are useful analogies to be drawn with other diseases where major risk factors have been identified (Table 12.3). For the purpose of this review, osteoporosis is considered as a disease rather than a process.

Table 12.3. The distinction between risk factors and disease

Disease	Risk/factor measurement	Clinical expression
Coronary artery disease	Hypercholesterolaemia	Myocardial infarction
Cardiovascular accident	Hypertension	Stroke
Osteoporosis	Osteopenia	Fracture
Diabetes	Hyperglycaemia	Retinopathy
Gout	Hyperuricaemia	Arthritis

Diagnosis of Osteoporosis

Can measurements of bone mass be used to provide a diagnostic tool? A number of studies have examined the sensitivity and specificity of bone mass measurements to discriminate osteoporotic patients with fracture from populations without fracture [5,12,14]. In general, both sensitivity and specificity are improved by measuring sites of biological relevance. Thus, measurements of vertebral bone mineral content have a higher predictive value for the detection of spinal osteoporosis than measurements at the wrist. Conversely greater predictability is obtained for the detection of wrist fractures by measurements at this site than by measurements at the spine [15].

The real value of this type of intelligence is, however, limited. The diagnosis of osteoporosis (the detection of fracture) is clinically obvious with a predictive value much greater than can be obtained with density measurements. The strength of such measurements can, in a diagnostic sense, only lie in their ability to provide an estimate of current or life-time fracture risk irrespective of whether an osteoporotic fracture is present or absent. They can also provide information whether a fracture where present was associated with a reduced bone density. Bone types of information are diagnostically useful but do not, and should not be used to assess their value as screening techniques for osteoporotic fracture.

The use of these measurements for screening depends on their ability to measure what they intend (accuracy) and the relationship of a given value to future risk. There have been few critical evaluations of accuracy even though the value of physical measurements depends so critically on their accuracy; for example, the ability of bone mineral content to predict ash weight content of the site examined. The accuracy of the various techniques commonly used for screening varies from 2% to 10% (Table 12.4). These figures have to be considered alongside the variance in measurements of the population to be examined, which ranges from 10% to 50%, depending upon the techniques used for measurement and any normalisation procedures applied [16]. It is evident, therefore, that even techniques with an apparently acceptable accuracy (e.g. 5%–10% for dual photon absorptiometry) cannot define fracture risk with great accuracy where the population variance for photon absorptiometry is in the order of 20% or less (Table 12.4; Fig. 12.1). Notwithstanding, absorptiometric techniques provide the best index currently available and are of greater predictive value than clinical risk factors identified thus far for osteoporotic

Table 12.4. Characteristics of the healthy female population and the accuracy of bone density measured by single and dual photon absorptiometry (SPA, DPA), dual energy X-ray absorptiometry (DEXA) and quantitative computed axial tomography (QCT)

	SPA	DPA	DEXA	QCT
A. Population coefficient of variation (%)	13.3	12.1	14.0	17.9
B. Accuracy (%)	2	4–10	?5	5–10
A/B[a]	6.7	1–3	2.8	1.8–3.6

[a]The ratio A/B provides an index of the relative power of each technique to position correctly a single estimate of bone density within a population reference range.

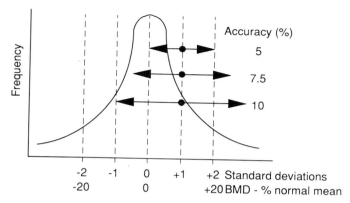

Fig. 12.1. The importance of accuracy of bone density measurements in relation to the variance of a normal population. The curve describes the normal range for density expressed as a percentage of mean values or in standard deviation units. The solid line (arrowed) denotes the confidence estimate for a given bone mineral density measurement assessed as being +1 standard deviation of the healthy population which increases with decreasing accuracy.

fracture (e.g. smoking, body weight, life-style). Nevertheless, the development of techniques with greater accuracy would be of significant value for the diagnostic use of bone mineral measurements.

The Study of Bone Loss and Intervention in Established Osteoporosis

Different considerations apply to the use of bone mass measurements to study patients with established osteoporosis and the effects of treatment. They concern the precision of the methodology and, in particular, the biology of osteoporotic bone loss, which is briefly reviewed below.

The Organisation and Turnover of Bone Tissue

The manner in which osteoporosis arises is, in large part, determined by changes in skeletal metabolism and architecture. The skeleton is composed of compact and cancellous (trabecular) bone. In the healthy adult, bone mass is neither increasing nor decreasing, but there is considerable turnover of bone, and 95% of skeletal turnover in the adult is accounted for by remodelling [17]. The remodelling process comprises a discrete series of cellular events on bone which have been well characterised morphologically. These events occur predominantly on surfaces of bone. The surface of trabecular bone is greater than that of cortical bone, even though trabecular bone may occupy only 25% of total skeletal mass in health and only 10% in an osteoporotic patient. Because of the high surface to volume ratio of trabecular bone tissue, disorders of bone remodelling more commonly affect trabecular sites earlier and more floridly in the disease process.

Remodelling activity is important for skeletal strength in vivo [18]. Clinical and experimental studies both suggest that if the rate of remodelling is decreased substantially, the risk of spontaneous fractures will increase, not due to a decrease in skeletal mass, but due to the inability of the skeleton to undergo self-repair [2].

At the start of the remodelling sequence osteoclasts assemble or differentiate together to excavate a resorption cavity. At the completion of this phase osteoclasts disappear, and several days later bone-forming cells (osteoblasts) are attracted principally to sites of previous resorption and infill the resorption cavity with new bone. This sequence of events permits the self-repair of bone and is one of the mechanisms for preserving both skeletal mass and architecture.

The term "coupling" describes the attraction of osteoblasts to sites of previous resorption, but the basis of this process is ill-understood. Clearly, it allows a moiety of bone to self-repair. The osteoporotic process may involve uncoupling of bone formation to previous resorption (e.g. neoplastic bone disease), but more commonly a decrease in bone mass is due to an imbalance between the amount of mineral and matrix removed and subsequently incorporated into each resorption cavity, so that skeletal mass decreases progressively. In post-menopausal osteoporosis and many other types of osteoporosis, the imbalance between the amount of bone resorbed and that formed at each remodelling site is due to a decrease in the functional capacity of osteoblasts or to a decrease in the number of osteoblasts recruited to resorption sites.

Irrespective of the mechanism, a finite deficit of bone is the end result of each remodelling sequence. If bone turnover is increased, then the number of bone remodelling units extant at any one time also increases. If the imbalance at each site remains constant then the result of increasing bone turnover will be to amplify the rate of bone loss (Fig. 12.2). There is now good evidence that oestrogen deficiency not only induces a focal imbalance at remodelling sites, but also increases the remodelling rate of bone. In this way bone loss is accelerated.

The implications for the measurement of bone loss are that the rate of loss will depend upon the site measured and is clearly greater at trabecular sites than at cortical bone sites. Even within trabecular bone tissue there is a great hetero-

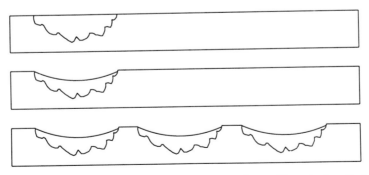

Fig. 12.2. Schematic representation of a trabecular bone surface to illustrate the effect of balance and remodelling on the rate of bone loss. The top panel shows the infilling of a resorption bay with an equal volume of new bone. In osteoporosis less bone is deposited in resorption cavities (centre). If bone turnover is increased without altering this balance (lower panel), the rate of trabecular bone loss will increase in proportion to the increment in bone turnover.

geneity in rates of bone remodelling, so that rates of bone loss similarly differ. As will be reviewed later, the ability to detect a change depends not only on the change but also on the precision of technique. The choice of technique should be determined in part by these biological considerations.

Spatial Organisation of Trabecular Tissue

The continual imbalance between formation and resorption would be expected to result in a progressive decrease in the width of trabecular bone elements. A decrease in trabecular width occurs in many forms of osteoporosis, but it is clear that in postmenopausal osteoporosis there is not only a decrease in trabecular width, but also a marked loss of trabecular elements themselves [19,20]. Indeed, there is little evidence for trabecular thinning in postmenopausal osteoporosis, so that the loss of trabecular elements must be, in part, a result of the generation of resorption cavities which transect or perforate trabecular structures.

The disruption of trabecular architecture characteristic of postmenopausal vertebral osteoporosis has important implications for structural strength. The selective destruction of cross bracing elements leads to failure of the structure out of proportion to the amount of material removed (Fig. 12.3). Even though remaining trabeculae in postmenopausal osteoporosis can thicken, evident even radiographically, this cannot compensate adequately to prevent skeletal failure. Similarly, therapeutic manipulation of the remodelling process might be expected to thicken trabecular structures without necessarily restoring trabecular continuity (Fig. 12.4). The majority of techniques used to measure bone density do not capture information on trabecular continuity. This suggests that changes in bone mass, whether due to natural history or to therapeutic intervention, cannot be

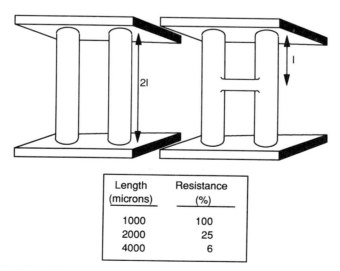

Length (microns)	Resistance (%)
1000	100
2000	25
4000	6

Fig. 12.3. The effect of the loss of cross bracing elements on trabecular strength. A doubling of the length (1) between cross bracing ties decreases the resistance to bending forces fourfold.

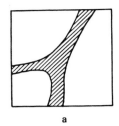 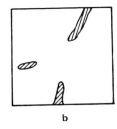 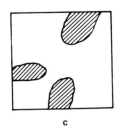

a   b   c

Fig. 12.4. Schematic representation of trabecular bone showing normal trabecular architecture (**a**) and the thinning and discontinuity of trabecular elements during postmenopausal osteoporosis (**b**). The surface deposition of bone by anabolic agents may thicken remnant structures without necessarily restoring trabecular continuity (**c**).

interpreted reliably as changing fracture susceptibility without additional skeletal information.

As in the case of the diagnostic use of density measurements, the site of measurement is important in that changes at one site may not be reflected by parallel changes elsewhere. For example, the therapeutic use of fluoride induces marked increases in trabecular bone volume over several years of treatment, but has less effect on cortical bone [21]. Like all currently used treatments, however, fluoride alters bone mass by affecting bone remodelling and at each remodelling site, the resorption cavity is filled with a greater volume of new bone [22]. Therefore it is to be expected that trabecular width would increase, but its effect on fracture rate in established osteoporosis is likely to be less than would be predicted from the increment in bone density, unless the drug were also to have effects on trabecular continuity.

The less-marked effects of anabolic agents on cortical bone relate in part to bone remodelling. At cortical sites where bone is compact, the resorption cavity is excavated as a cutting cone. The tunnel cannot be overfilled due to the physical constraints of the surrounding compact bone. In contrast, the marrow cavity at trabecular sites does not constrain the overfilling of resorption bays.

Many problems in the interpretation of changes in bone density in established osteoporosis could be overcome by the development of techniques to measure the connectivity of trabecular bone. At present this can be measured reliably only by invasive techniques [20]. X-rays at the hip provide a semiquantitative index in the form of the Singh score [6], which are of value in population studies. It has been suggested that broadband ultrasound attenuation of bone provides an index of skeletal competence [23]. It has recently been shown that this technique discriminates patients with and without osteoporosis at least as well as measurements of bone mineral density [24]. Moreover, it captures some aspects of true bone density not dependent on mineral density (Fig. 12.5; [25]), suggesting the partial dependence of ultrasound attenuation on the intrinsic trabecular architecture of cancellous bone.

Skeletal Versus Extraskeletal Factors

The skeletal abnormalities which increase the risk of osteoporosis are summarised in Table 12.5. Bone density measurements alone do not capture all information

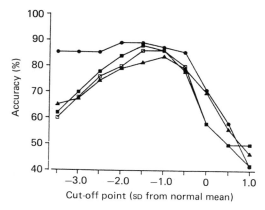

Fig. 12.5. Accuracy of four different techniques to discriminate between normal subjects and patients with axial osteoporosis at various cut-off points expressed as standard deviation units from the normal mean (●, broadband ultrasound attenuation; ■ and □, bone mineral density (BMD) and content (BMC) respectively at the lumber spine measured by dual photon absorptiometry; ▲, single photon absorptiometry at the distal radius). Note that at 2 SDs below the normal mean, ultrasound attenuation had a greater accuracy (89%) than spinal BMD, BMC or forearm BMC (70%, 53% and 50% respectively). (From McCloskey et al. [24].)

Table 12.5. Pathogenesis of osteoporotic fracture

Skeletal
Bone mass
Spatial organisation of bone
Turnover of bone

Extraskeletal
Falls – frequency and severity
Response to trauma – neuromuscular co-ordination

relating to fracture risk. Several studies, including some prospective data, have now shown that age is an independent factor. Thus, for any given bone density, the risk of fracture is greater in the elderly [9,26]. A factor of probable importance is the role of falls which increase with advancing age [27]. The osteopenic skeleton can be likened to a fragile vase. The vase will remain intact forever if left on display, but if it is tipped over it will certainly break. The role of falls differs with different types of fracture as does the importance of protective neuromuscular defences (Table 12.6).

Table 12.6. Relative importance of skeletal and extraskeletal factors in osteoporosis

Type of fracture	Role of falls	Role of bone
Colles	+++	+
Femoral neck	++	++
Vertebral	+	+++

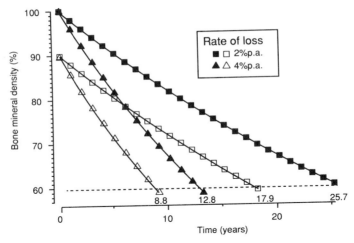

Fig. 12.6. Relationship between peak bone density at maturity and the rate of bone loss. Two rates of bone loss are shown for two different starting values of bone density at the time of the menopause. The graph depicts the time taken in these examples to reach a bone density of 60% of the healthy adult mean value.

Bone Mass and Bone Loss

In the context of postmenopausal osteoporosis, the bone density at any time after the menopause will depend in part on the peak bone mass or density at maturity and the rate of bone loss thereafter. The rate of bone loss after the menopause varies. It has been suggested that there is a bimodal distribution of bone loss [28] but there is very little evidence for this view. It is more probable that the rate of loss is unimodally distributed and that "fast losers" represent the extreme of a normal distribution. Notwithstanding, it is clear that patients who lose bone at the faster rates are more likely to reach a threshold of bone density below which the risk of fracture is unacceptably high (Fig. 12.6).

The question arises as to the relative importance of rates of loss and peak bone density. If rates of loss are important then this implies that the use of biochemical estimates of bone density would improve the assessment of fracture risk. There is some evidence that rates of loss can be reliably predicted from biochemical estimates in the early postmenopausal years [28], but this may bear little relationship to the longer-term outcome unless bone loss continued at the same rate for many years. Indeed, the only study addressing this issue directly suggests that the major determinant of bone density in later life is peak bone density [29].

Technical Considerations

There are several additional biological factors which determine the applicability of bone mass measurements. It is important to be aware of the nature of the measurements made and their physiological significance. For example, measurements of cortical width do not give an indication of bone density, and bone density measurements do not necessarily give an indication of the stress required to fracture a bone. A less dense but larger wrist may be less liable to fracture than a denser, but smaller wrist. Indeed, the techniques used to normalise data are at best arbitrary and are based on assumptions which are difficult to test.

These considerations are at first sight less relevant to the assessment of bone loss or gain where repeated measurements are made in the same individual. However, if bone width alters, if fat distribution changes or extraskeletal calcification occurs due to interventions, apparent changes are liable to misinterpretation. For example, the apparent anabolic effects of oestrogens or decadurabolin on skeletal density is partly artefactual, and the apparent increment observed in bone density is due in part to a significant decrease in fatty tissue surrounding bone [30,31]. Similarly, increases in bone density ascribed to exercise may be due to a decrease in body fat, an increase in lean body fat or both. Conversely, a component, perhaps 50%, of the apparent bone loss after oophorectomy assessed by CT is attributable to an increase in marrow fat.

The precision or reproducibility of the technique used is also a critical factor in determining whether or not a change has occurred. The conditions under which reproducibility is assessed are important. For example, the precision of single photon absorptiometry is less than 1% when bone mineral content of a standard is determined on the same day. But the measurement of greater clinical significance is that derived in real people where the reproducibility is halved (>2%). In osteoporotic patients with a decreased bone mineral content the coefficient of variation exceeds 3% in most laboratories. The importance of determining the coefficient of variation applicable to working conditions in real patients in obvious since the probability of detecting a difference between two measurements (when a difference truly exists) depends on the confidence that can be placed on the single (or repeated) measurement. In the same way individuals must be followed for longer periods with less precise techniques to be sure that a change or lack of change has really occurred (Table 12.7).

Table 12.7. Duration of study necessary to determine significant bone loss ($P<0.05$) in an individual patient

Rate of bone loss (% pa)	Reproducibility (CV %)	Minimum duration of study (years)
1	1	2
	2	4
	5	8
	10	16
2	1	1
	2	2
	5	4
	10	8
5	1	1
	2	1
	5	2
	10	3

From Kanis et al. [16].

Techniques for improving the power of measurements to detect changes in individuals and in populations (reviewed in reference [16]) can considerably enhance the value of density and bone mass measurements.

Conclusions

Bone is a complex tissue. Physical studies of the characteristics of bone have largely been confined to its mechanical properties in vitro, or to the measurement of the amount of bone present. Although the amount of bone present is clearly an important factor which determines structural strength, it is now clear that spatial organisation of bone and its turnover as well as extraskeletal factors are also important for its structural integrity in vivo. Physical measurements of bone density or mineral content do not capture these determinants of skeletal strength and the interpretation of bone mass measurements should take account of these biological considerations as well as statistical and technical factors.

The development of new techniques to assess other determinants of bone strength will form an important component for our further understanding of osteoporosis and the rational use of methodology in the assessment of fracture risk.

Acknowledgements. We are grateful to the Medical Research Council and to Rorer Central Research for their support of our work.

References

1. Hoffenberg R, James OFW, Brocklehurst JC et al. Fractured neck of femur. Prevention and management. J R Coll Physicians Lond 1989; 23:8–12.
2. Kanis JA. Tretment of osteoporotic fracture. Lancet 1984; i:27–33.
3. Johnston CC, Melton LJ, Lindsay RL, Eddy DM. Clinical indications for bone mass measurements. J Bone Miner Res 1990; 4:1–28.
4. Bartley MH, Arnold JS, Haslam RK, Webster SSJ. The relationship of bone strength and bone quantity in health, disease and ageing. J Gerontol 1966; 21:517–21.
5. Jensen GF, Christiansen C, Boesen J, Hegedus V, Transbol I. Epidemiology of postmenopausal spinal and long bone fractures. Clin Orthop 1982; 166:75–81.
6. Cooper C, Barker DJP, Morris J, Briggs RS. Osteoporosis falls and age in fracture of the proximal femur. Br Med J 1987; 295:13–15.
7. Wasnich RD, Ross PD, Heibrun LK, Vogel JM. Selection of the optimal site for fracture risk prediction. Clin Orthop 1987; 216:262–8.
8. Ross PD, Wasnich, RD, Vogel JM. Detection of prefracture spinal osteoporosis using bone mineral absorptiometry. J Bone Miner Res 1988; 3:1–11.
9. Hui SL, Slemenda CS, Johnston CC. Age and bone mass as predictors of fracture in a prospective study. J Clin Invest 1988; 81:1804–9.
10. Wasnich RD, Ross PD, Vogel JM, Davis JW. Osteoporosis. Critique and practicum. Honolulu, Hawaii: Banyan Press; 1989.
11. Nordin BEC. The definition and diagnosis of osteoporosis. Calcif Tissue Int 1987; 40:57–8.
12. Odvina CV, Wergedal JE, Libanati CR, Schulz FE, Baylink DJ. Relationship between trabecular vertebral bone density and fractures: a quantitative definition of spinal osteoporosis. Metabolism 1988; 37:221–8.
13. Kanis JA. Osteoporosis and osteopenia. J Bone Miner Res 1990; 5:209–11.

14. Ott SM, Kileoyne RF, Chesnut CH. Ability of four different techniques of measuring bone mass to diagnose vertebral fractures in postmenopausal women. J Bone Miner Res 1987; 2:201–10.
15. Eastell R, Wahner HW, O'Fallon M, Amadio PC, Melton LJ, Riggs BL. Unequal decrease in bone density of lumbar spine and ultradistal radius in Colles' and vertebral fracture syndromes. J Clin Invest 1989; 83:168–74.
16. Kanis JA, Caulin F, Russell RGG. Problems in the design of clinical trials in osteoporosis. In: Dixon AStJ, Russell RGG, Stamp TCB, eds. Osteoporosis: a multidisciplinary problem. Roy Soc Med Int Cong Symp Series 1983; 55:205–22.
17. Parfitt AM. The physiologic and clinical significance of bone histomorphometric data. In: Recker R, ed. Bone histomorphometry. Techniques and interpretation. Boca Raton: CRC Press, 1982; 143–223.
18. Frost HM. Presence of microscopic cracks in vivo in bone. Henry Ford Hosp Bull 1960; 8:25–35.
19. Parfitt AM, Mathews CH, Villaneuva AR, Kleerekoper M, Frame B, Rao DS. Relationships between surface, volume and thickness of iliac trabecular bone in ageing and in osteoporosis. Implications for the microanatomic and cellular mechanisms of bone loss. J Clin Invest 1983; 72:1396–409.
20. Aaron JE, Makins NB, Sagreiya K. The microanatomy of trabecular bone loss in normal ageing men and women. Clin Orthop 1987; 215:260–71.
21. Kanis JA, Meunier PJ. Should we use fluoride to treat osteoporosis? Q J Med 1984; 53:145–64.
22. Eriksen EF. Normal and pathological remodelling of human trabecular bone: three-dimensional reconstruction of the remodelling sequence in normals and in metabolic bone disease. Endocr Rev 1986; 7:379–408.
23. Langton CM. The measurement of broadband ultrasound attenuation in cancellous bone. University of Hull: PhD thesis, 1984.
24. McCloskey EV, Murray SA, Miller C et al. Broadband ultrasound attenuation in the os calcis: relationship to bone mineral at other skeletal sites. Clin Sci 1990; (in press).
25. McCloskey EV, Murray SA, Charlesworth D et al. Assessment of broadband ultrasound attenuation in the os calcis in vitro. Clin Sci 1990; (in press)
26. Ross PD, Wasnich RD, MacLean CJ, Hagino R, Vogel JM. A model for estimating the potential costs and savings of osteoporosis prevention strategies. Bone 1988; 9:337–47.
27. Cummings SR. Are patients with hip fractures more osteoporotic? Am J Med 1985; 78:487–94.
28. Christiansen C, Riis BJ, Rodbro P. Prediction of rapid bone loss in postmenopausal women. Lancet 1987; i:1105–8.
29. Hui SL, Slemenda CW, Johnston CC. Baseline measurement of bone mass predicts fracture in white women. Ann Intern Med 1989; 111:355–61.
30. Hassager C, Borg J, Christiansen C. Measurement of the subcutaneous fat in the distal forearm by single photon absorptiometry. Metabolism 1989; 35:159–65.
31. Hassager C, Christiansen C. Estrogen/gestagen therapy changes soft-tissue body composition in postmenopausal women. Metabolism 1989; 38:662–5.

Chapter 13

The Patient's View of Osteoporosis

L. Edwards

The National Osteoporosis Society was the brainchild of its present Chairman. Dr Allan Dixon, a rheumatologist; the late Commander Rowe, a charity director; and a gynaecologist, Mr John Studd, the present Vice-Chairman.

It is highly appropriate for the Royal College of Obstetricians and Gynaecologists to devote a Study Group to osteoporosis, as prevention of the disease in women is now considered by the majority in the bone world to be mainly a gynaecological problem.

Of course it is not as simple as that and there are undoubtedly other factors which have a major bearing on the osteoporosis problem. Risk factor lists still include family history, lack of exercise, lack of calcium, smoking, excess alcohol, other medical problems such as thyrotoxicosis; or asthma and arthritis requiring high doses of corticosteroids. But even a lay person asking the question, "Why does osteoporosis apparently affect only 1 in 40 men and yet over 1 in 4 women?" might presume one of the major risk factors for osteoporosis to be – being female. The National Osteoporosis Society see this as a quirk of fate that women should not be prepared to accept, but the Society needs the help of GPs, rheumatologists, endocrinologists, geriatricians, general physicians and, particularly, gynaecologists, to combat the carelessness of Mother Nature.

The National Osteoporosis Society began largely as a registered charity to support sufferers but fortunately the description of the Society's aims for the Charity Commission was very widely written. It became very rapidly obvious that if anything was to be achieved in really helping osteoporosis sufferers and in preventing the disease in the next generation, the Society needed to raise awareness of the whole problem. The National Osteoporosis Society set out with this aim and has been very effective. A major public relations campaign was launched on a general public almost totally unaware of osteoporosis, on media just as oblivious and on a medical profession for whom osteoporosis was really an auntie whom no one wanted to own.

Three years ago a survey by a pharmaceutical company of a representative number of family doctors found that 20% of GPs stated confidently that they had never seen a case of osteoporosis among their patients. Osteoporosis was not only an unwanted auntie, it was largely unrecognised. Women were being fobbed off with painkillers, antidepressants or tranquillisers.

The results of the National Osteoporosis Society's campaign have been very obvious in the media. The Society and osteoporosis have been featured on many major TV programmes: Breakfast Time, TVAM, Tomorrow's World, News At Ten, BBC TV News and a half-hour This Week programme devoted to the National Osteoporosis Society and osteoporosis in September 1988. Radio coverage has been frequent on every local station, and the BBC nationally from the Today programme to You and Yours and Medicine Now. The Press coverage has not been of the "shock/horror" type in the *Sun*, but in-depth articles in the *Guardian*, the *Sunday Times* and all the quality newspapers as well as most of the 3000 local papers in the UK.

Women's magazines often have circulations higher than most national news papers and are very influential and 3 or 4 page in-depth articles in such magazines have been the norm. The National Osteoporosis Society's filing cabinets contain thousands of press cuttings.

Market research surveys by Medical Research Factors Limited show an increased awareness of osteoporosis among the general public as a result of all this coverage. Awareness rose from zero to almost 30% in the eighteen months to 1988. Doctors' awareness has also risen. In 1986 only 10% were aware of the National Osteoporosis Society; two years later 55% knew of the Society's work. The number of GPs in favour of a campaign to prevent or limit the risk of osteoporosis had risen from 78% in 1987 to 91% a year later. At total of 92% of doctors felt that preventive measures should be taken to avert the onset of osteoporosis; this was an increase of 9% on the previous year.

Hormone replacement therapy (HRT) is now seen as the main preventive measure, followed by exercise, and attitudes to both these methods have strengthened. By 1988 80% of GPs believed that HRT could avert the onset of osteoporosis – a 10% increase in 2 years. Incidentally, 67% of GPs thought bone density screening would be useful, a steady increase on 1986, although 68% still did not know where their nearest screening centre was.

It is to be hoped that there have been further and more dramatic increases in all areas of GPs' knowledge since 1988. The National Osteoporosis Society has been working hard in this area and has recently launched a Scientific Section which all medical professionals involved in osteoporosis can join in order to keep up-to-date.

Not all the credit for the increased awareness can be claimed by the National Osteoporosis Society. Womens Health Concern has been working for 15 years or more to improve the lot of menopausal women, as have individuals like Wendy Cooper. Since the National Osteoporosis Society started the Amarant Trust has been launched and many other charities have also begun to do good work on osteoporosis. Many doctors have been tireless in their work on HRT and osteoporosis over many years. They have laid the foundations on which the National Osteoporosis Society was able to launch its publicity campaign and they have given generous support to The National Osteoporosis Society's work.

The NOS also welcomes the largely unsung work of pharmaceutical companies. It is so easy to criticise them but at a time when Government agencies seem reluctant to put money into osteoporosis research and education, it is fortunate that enlightened self-interest spurs pharmaceutical companies into doing so, with perhaps encouragement from the National Osteoporosis Society and others. Nevertheless everyone must be made aware of the independent stance of the NOS and the fact that there is no close alliance to any company or Government agency. The views of the society are the consensus of the Society's Medical Advisory Board and are totally independent and unbiased.

There are three really important aspects with regard to osteoporosis. Is anything really being done:

1. To improve diagnosis
2. To improve treatment; and most important
3. To improve prevention?

The message must be that whatever is being done is **not fast enough**. The authors of this volume are to be congratulated for their work, but they are still lone voices crying in the wilderness.

Part of the job of the National Osteoporosis Society is to reassure medical professionals that the Society does not indulge in destructive criticism. There is no point in blaming those who haven't done enough in the past. A few years ago hardly anyone was aware:

1. Of the seriousness of osteoporosis in terms of cost and numbers
2. Of the possibilities for treatment
3. Of the possibilities for prevention

But that awareness does now exist. Doctors do now know about osteoporosis. A booklet [1] specially designed for GPs has been sent to every family doctor in the UK. Good articles on osteoporosis have appeared in every medical newspaper and magazine over the past two years, so there is now no excuse for ignorance.

However, there is still no room for complacency. Developments are not moving nearly fast enough. The number of prescriptions for HRT is still extremely low. Prescriptions in the USA apparently outnumber those in the UK about tenfold.

Who should be getting HRT? One group who definitely should are oophorectomised women. Mr Nick Siddle (University College Hospital) said recently at public meetings in Sheffield and Newcastle that it is wrong *not* to give oestrogen replacement to women who have their ovaries removed before normal menopause age. He also says he is acutely embarrassed that some of his colleagues will remove ovaries and not consider HRT, thus failing to compensate for the resulting loss of oestrogens.

Recent discussions with bone specialists and gynaecologists indicated that this is no longer a problem. If an oophorectomy is performed the woman is automatically prescribed HRT because otherwise they get osteoporosis [2–4]. They get it severely and often at an early age: 52 or 55 years old is too young to have spinal fractures.

However, the National Osteoporosis Society gets around 1000 letters per day, which show that this assumption is untrue. Of these letters about 19% are enquiring about osteoporosis in general, 5% are enquiring about HRT, and 21% already have real problems with osteoporosis. Most of the questions are answered in free booklets sent in reply.

Some enquirers join us, and the National Osteoporosis Society currently has 10 000 members. About 400 are members of the Scientific Section and 61% have been diagnosed as sufferers of osteoporosis: this is an interesting study group.

At present the National Osteoporosis Society is conducting a research project with its 10 000 members all of whom have been sent a 4-page questionnaire. The response is very good and at least 75% are expected to reply. The responses will be analysed by computer, but an initial analysis has been made of the 1000 responses now on disc.

This is a random sample of 1000 National Osteoporosis Society members throughout the UK, whose names begin with the letters A – E. Although 61% have been diagnosed as sufferers of osteoporosis, the other 39% cannot be taken as a control. For reference in this study they are being labelled "preventers" as opposed to sufferers. However, many of them suspect they have osteoporosis, 10% have actually had fractures without being told by a doctor that they have osteoporosis.

It should be borne in mind that the observations so far are not scientific and cannot necessarily be extrapolated to the general population but some of the information is nonetheless interesting, if not startling.

The average age of suffers is 60 years. This is contrary to the popular image of the typical osteoporosis sufferer as a "little old lady" – 60 years old is not very old. Indeed many GPs and consultants are close to that age. The low average age was no surprise to the Society – many severe sufferers in their 50s have been seen.

Some other interesting figures have emerged. Of the diagnosed osteoporosis sufferers nearly 33% had a family history of osteoporosis, thus indicating that this is a strong risk factor. About 14% had had a hysterectomy and nearly 9% had had an oophorectomy. Nearly 2% had been on high doses of corticosteroids for more than 6 months and almost 4.5% had also suffered thyroid disease. Surprisingly, only 3.9% also have rheumatism or arthritis. About 10% of sufferers had dentures under the age of 30 years. This is an interesting area for further research: perhaps early dental decay is an indicator of bone problems.

None of this particular sample contained any of the special cases on which data are being compiled, which include:

Prolactinoma

Turner's syndrome

Anorexia nervosa

Post-partum osteoporosis

Those given high corticosteroid doses to avoid habitual abortion

Women treated with goserelin and similar drugs to combat endometriosis

This sample also did not contain our youngest sufferer members – a young girl of 17 and a young woman of 22 – or the oldest, a woman of just 100.

Three very striking figures did show up clearly. Only 3.6% of the sufferers had ever been given HRT. Only 1.5% of the sufferers who had had a hysterectomy had ever had HRT. And of our oophorectomised sufferers only 0.6% had ever had HRT.

This situation is far worse than that described by Spector [5] in 1989, in which in a follow-up of over 5000 women around 74% of hysterectomised and oophor-ectomised women had never received HRT. Over 98% of our hysterectomised and oophorectomised osteoporosis sufferers had never received HRT.

And do all women know whether or not their ovaries have been removed? In a recent study of hysterectomy presented to a symposium on risk factors in osteoporosis (organised in Brussels by the European Foundation for Osteoporosis and Bone Disease), operated specimens were inspected to see if ovaries had been removed at the time of hysterectomy. Subsequent questions showed that about half the women were unaware that they had had their ovaries removed. This may be simply because hysterectomy is a term commonly known among women whereas oophorectomy is not.

Furthermore current work at Dulwich [6] shows that women who have only had a hysterectomy should also be on HRT because they lose more bone than comparable age-matched women who have not had a hysterectomy.

A further problem is highlighted by the preliminary findings of the NOS survey. Many women are not remaining on HRT long enough for it to have any significant effect on maintaining their bone mass. The reason for coming off HRT is usually "on doctor's advice".

The National Osteoporosis Society suggests that there are three urgent tasks for gynaecologists who perform oophorectomies and hysterectomies, and for GPs and all consultants who may see these women:

1. Every woman who now has an oophorectomy should be having HRT and this should be monitored to ensure a woman does not come off it for some minor reason. It is important to find the right product to suit the patient. Another booklet for doctors is currently being prepared giving more details on the side effects of HRT, on what to do if a woman comes back after two months with minor problems and on how varying doses and types of HRT can be used to find the right individual prescription.

2. Every woman who has a hysterectomy should be considered for HRT therapy. If she does not have it then she should be closely monitored.

3. All women who have had an oophorectomy in the past should be recalled to consider HRT now before it is too late. The same applies to women who have an early natural menopause [4]. It should be automatic to consider these women for HRT.

Of the sufferers in this initial sample from the National Osteoporosis Society's survey, 14% of women had had an early oophorectomy or hysterectomy, before age 47. The number of osteoporosis sufferers in the UK has been conservatively estimated at 2 million and although it may be speculation and not deduction, 14% of those sufferers could perhaps be saved from their osteoporosis by HRT after a hysterectomy or oophorectomy.

If this is so, gynaecologists have it in their power to save over a quarter of a million women from osteoporosis by following through their work on the operating table. By taking responsibility for compensating a woman for her loss of oestrogens after surgery, enormous savings could be made in human suffering and NHS costs.

In human terms it would mean extending the normal life of hundreds of thousands of women and saving them from terrible pain and deformity and loss of independence. NOS members like:

Mrs D of Wales with five fractures at 55 years after an oophorectomy and no HRT at 37.

Mrs E of Surrey with five fractures at 64 years after a hysterectomy at 43.

Mrs E of Merseyside with three fractures and severe height loss at 70 years after a hysterectomy at 48.

Mrs E of Leicester with a curved spine and height loss at 55 years after an oophorectomy at 40.

Mrs E of Hertfordshire with two fractures at 52 years after a hysterectomy at 41.

Mrs E of Yorkshire with five fractures at 56 years after an oophorectomy at 37.

This is just a small random group from our 1000 sample, all of whom said on their questionnaire that they wish they had had the opportunity of HRT when their hysterectomy or oophorectomy was done.

The NOS suggests that while debate may continue about other risk factors for osteoporosis and about how many of the general population should be considered for HRT, all women who have ever had an early oophorectomy, hysterectomy or early natural menopause should be urgently considered *now*, before the end of 1990, for HRT before thousands more succumb to osteoporosis.

References

1. Paine T, The new approach to osteoporosis, a guide for general practitioners, Bath, National Osteoporosis Society, 1988.
2. Aitken JM, Hart DM, Linday R. Oestrogen replacement therapy for prevention of osteoporosis after oophorectomy. Br Med J 1973; iii: 515–18.
3. Richelson L, Wahner H, Melton L, Riggs B. Relative contributions of ageing and oestrogen deficiency to postmenopausal bone loss. N Engl J Med 1984; 311: 1273–5.
4. Baber R, Abdalla H, Studd J. The premature menopause. In: Studd J. ed. Progress in obstetrics and gynaecology, 1991; in press.
5. Spector TD. Use of oestrogen replacement therapy in high risk groups in the United Kingdom, Br Med J 1989; 299: 1434–5.
6. Edwards L. New research data on hormone replacement therapy. Symposium Newsletter, Issue 9, Bath, National Osteoporosis Society, Sept 1989.

Discussion

Anderson: Dr Kanis said nothing about biochemical indices. Do they not have a place?

Kanis: From a theoretical point of view it is a very attractive area. The difference we observe in patients who are losing bone compared with those who are not losing bone – in other words the degree of change that one sees – is very high compared to the reproducibility of the measurement, so it becomes very attractive. The real questions are: to what extent can we predict bone loss over a period of time and to what extent can we extrapolate that to a time when somebody is liable to get a fracture? Although Klaus Christiansen is one of the greatest advocates of biochemical assessments of bone loss, if we look at his data and look at the relationship between bone density at the beginning of his observation and at the end of his observation, about 90% of the variance is accounted for by initial bone density rather than by rates of bone loss.

So I personally think that this is a fashion that still requires a lot of validation.

Purdie: I would support that, and I would also make the point that Christiansen's data encouraged the concept that women could be partitioned into "fast bone losers" and "slow bone losers" and that there is a biomodality in the population, whereas almost certainly we are dealing with a continuously distributed variable.

Kanis: I do not think that matters particularly.

Anderson: But Dr Kanis implied that the rate of bone loss for a given woman over a number of years was linear (Fig. 12.6). Is there any evidence for that?

Kanis: It was not linear; it was a curved line. It was percentage per annum. We know clearly that after the menopause, rates of bone loss are more rapid than subsequently, but one could develop mathematical models.

One of the issues that I do not think has been well resolved is the question of whether within the individual woman, bone loss is smooth or whether it is an episodic event. There are some interesting data in the literature of repeated measurements to decrease the errors of the measurement, which suggest that bone loss may occur in a stepwise manner, and that there are periods in a person's life where they may have accelerated bone loss for reasons that are not apparent. At other times the reasons may be apparent) e.g. when somebody goes to bed or is immobilised. But all these kinds of events would suggest that an estimation at one point is most unlikely to predict what may happen 20 years in the future.

Brincat: For a number of patients repeatedly, and postmenopausally, there were periods of rapid bone loss, followed by a resting phase with no apparent bone loss, followed by variable rates of bone loss. Had they been measured over a 6-month period they might have been thought of as being "fast bone losers", if such a concept exists, yet had they been looked at in the following six months they would have been thought of as being "slow bone losers". I would agree with the idea that fast and slow bone losers do not really exist.

Vessey: The early studies that looked at elderly women who had femoral neck fractures, and then measured bone mineral density in the contralateral femur or perhaps in the spine, and which also made comparisons with age-matched controls, tended to produce variable findings in regard to bone mineral density. Some of them found remarkably little difference. This was regarded as evidence against the notion that osteoporosis and fracture are linked, and perhaps pointed to the greater importance of falling over or something of that sort. Then it was argued that there could be some analogy with cholesterol and coronary heart disease (CHD): we are all very far over the threshold with regard to CHD risk, and we are talking about small variations.

But the follow-up studies discussed here suggest a rather clear relationship between bone mineral density and fracture rates.

I am one of those who remains confused about this area.

Kanis: With modern technology there is clearly a difference in the bone mineral density between those who have a hip fracture and those who do not, but like all fractures there is an enormous overlap between the two populations. But that is not to say that bone density measurements cannot be used to obtain a gradient of risk, and we have had examples of that being applied with a relatively low specificity and sensitivity of about 60% or 70%.

We have good prospective data in relatively young people, in cohorts that we have followed up for 10, 15, getting on for 20 years. However, we do not have reliable information in the very elderly, which again is the economic problem. We shall have to wait for a time to see if these kind of risk ratios can be applied to the elderly population.

Fogelman: There is also the problem with regard to fracture diagnosis as compared to fracture risk. Any woman aged ›75 years who has not had HRT will have relatively low values, perhaps those which one would consider below a fracture threshold. And if we are talking of an elderly population with a fracture, what is an appropriate control group for them? It may be that a control may go out and fracture a hip the next day.

Vessey: I have heard that as an argument for not screening for osteoporosis but that everyone should be treated.

Studd: It is worth discussing this question of screening further. We should remember that we are looking at women and not skeletons. We know that oestrogen therapy has considerable benefits as regards the cardiovascular system, the bones and depression, and it may be that the logic is to offer it to all women rather than to screen and encourage putting a bone density machine in every regional hospital at vast expense. It costs as much to screen somebody once as to treat for a couple of years and it is clearly more logical to treat the whole age group. If there are worries about breast cancer, then the funds should be transferred to mammography. To me that makes more sense.

There is a group who will not have hormone therapy and may need it on clinical grounds, and perhaps they are the patients who need the skills and technology and expense of screening. But I may be a lone voice.

Vessey: I do not think so.

Persson: I have doubts about giving HRT to all women from an ethical standpoint. We aim not to harm people and this is preventive treatment of something that might appear. I think we are obliged to select those women who are at increased risk of having the disease that the treatment prevents.

Anderson: I would agree with Mr Studd that generally speaking, all women should be offered HRT. If a woman comes in and asks for HRT then we need to have a good reason not to give it to her.

Persson: She should be fully informed about all the aspects.

Anderson: Yes. The danger is with increasing practice of defensive medicine, do we have to cover ourselves for every eventuality, if the balance of evidence comes out in favour of the woman feeling better and being more healthy? Has there been a study examining, in large numbers of hysterectomised women, whether apparently asymptomatic postmenopausal hysterectomised women feel better, even though they are not complaining, on HRT?

Hart: Certainly Mr Studd is not a lone voice. What I think we should perhaps pay a little more attention to is distinction between people who can get unopposed oestrogen and people who have either cyclical or combined oestrogen/progestogen. I have no doubt that more lives would be saved and more women would have more years of high-quality life if every woman who has had a hysterectomy is offered unopposed oestrogen, because that is what has been shown to have a cardioprotective effect.

Where I am in some doubt is on giving all women with an intact uterus oestrogen/progestogen, particularly the continuous combined oestrogen/progestogen. What is the effect of long-term combined oestrogen/progestogen? There is no doubt that the cyclical or continuous combined treatment will protect against osteoporosis. It may have no effect one way or the other on the cardiovascular system, in which case we are doing good. But we have to be cautious about very long-term oestrogen/progestogen because we do not have very long-term data on its effects on the cardiovascular system.

Then of course there is the worry about whether very long-term therapy is likely to increase breast cancer, although the answer to that is that if there is a slight increase in breast cancer and a considerable decrease in fractures and cardiovascular disease, more lives will be saved in the long term. We must not ignore the possibility of an increase in breast cancer with very long-term therapy, but the people who have been frightened too much about breast cancer are perhaps forgetting that we may, at the expense of producing one or two more breast cancers, be saving many more people from other conditions.

Selby: The use of ultrasonic techniques of assessing bone, has not been discussed.

Kanis: This is being validated in vitro and in vivo. This is a measurement made at the heel, on the face of it a very unlikely site, but the sensitivity and specificity to distinguish an osteoporotic population from a young healthy control group are as good as bone mineral density measured at the lumbar spine and if we take the cut-off point at two or three standard deviations below the normal it is in fact better.

That is the kind of argument that people would use to say we should be doing lateral DPA or lateral Dpx. I am not convinced by those arguments because I think these techniques assessed in those ways give an index of the reliability of that technique to measure fracture, and in a screening sense we are not interested in detecting fracture because we can do that much better clinically or on an X-ray. The important question is what is their specificity and sensitivity, say in a perimenopausal population, to predict fracture in the future? We have absolutely no idea with ultrasound attenuation.

Hip fracture can certainly be diagnosed by ultrasound – but not nearly as well as by looking at the patient. And I do not think that has much relationship to the problems of its application for screening.

Baird: If I might broaden the issue. I noticed that Ms Edwards was very careful to say it was her view that among the patients who should be considered are those who have been hysterectomised and I think that is wise. We are discussing this prematurely before we have had a formal assessment of risk/benefit. If we were to go to the other extreme and offer HRT to every woman whose ovaries had failed but whose uterus remained intact – and we should not forget that this is the vast majority of the population – then one of the major constraints, one that is a determinant of whether or not the woman continued with the therapy, would be the problems of menstruation.

Women are prepared to go to gynaecologists and ask to have their uterus removed because of the inconvenience and the morbidity associated with having monthly periods, and we should not forget that this is incontinence of blood and mucus for up to a week once a month. It is then difficult at the menopause to try to persuade them to go back to that to counter the prospect that perhaps 30% of them might fracture their neck of the femur when they get to age 85 years. A lot of women for that reason will start off with HRT on their gynaecologist's advice because of flushes, or because they are not feeling very well, and they will then give up because the symptoms that have replaced those for which they have been prescribed the treatment are worse.

I say this not in the mode of not offering women HRT. I am merely saying that we have not yet discussed the risk/benefit ratio in an intelligent way to be able to make this sort of statement.

Anderson: It is an interesting paradox that a great deal of our discussion has concerned hip fractures, which we are told is where the real cost to the Health Service and to the country lies, although there seems to have been some doubt as to whether these patients with a high morbidity and a high mortality are expensive to keep alive whether or not they fracture their hips, and that some of the costs might not relate to hip fractures but to other diseases. Yet the National Osteoporosis Society is clearly seeing the kind of patient I get referred to my metabolic clinic with osteoporosis – the woman in her late 50s or early 60s with multiple vertebral fractures. Clearly they are the majority of the members with an average age of 60 years.

Perhaps we are not discussing quite the same thing. We are discussing HRT for women starting at 50, with or without screening, with a view to preventing femoral neck fractures, for which I do not think there is any good evidence. Are we discussing two different diseases, and should we be concentrating more on the late middle-aged or elderly patient with established osteoporosis, even if she does not cost a lot?

Edwards: That is where it costs a lot in human suffering. A hip fracture is a horrible way to go and it is expensive to the Health Service. But for a woman it is probably more significant to have spinal fractures in her fifties. She may live for another 20 years with those spinal fractures getting progressively worse and worse.

Kanis: One of the difficulties is that we have very little idea of the size of the problem. For hip fracture we have reasonably good statistics, though there are problems with the statistics, some of which have been mentioned. But we have no idea of the prevalence of vertebral osteoporosis in the UK. We are setting up a survey at the moment to try and find out. Estimates vary from about 10% of the population aged ›50 years to as high – if we are to believe the Mayo Clinic data – as 30%, 40% or 50% of the population. The truth is that we do not know.

Given that, we have no idea to what extent vertebral osteoporosis is a clinical disorder as defined earlier; is it 1% or is it 50% of the population? Ms Edwards knows of those with pain and those who join the Society, but we have no idea what the reference base is and in an economic sense we have no way of gauging this at the moment.

Lindsay: I agree. Epidemiological data on vertebral fracture are virtually impossible to get without good community examination. The problems with that are the end point that we decide to look at. If we look at those who complain we will get a very much smaller proportion than if we X-ray everybody in the community and look at radiographic abnormalities. That explains some of the disparity in the data that are available from, for example, the Kaiser Permanent Health Maintenance Organisation where the X-rays were looked at every year and somebody decided that 40% had vertebral osteoporosis as related to structural abnormalities on the X-ray. We do not even understand what the relationship is between those structural abnormalities and any process of bone loss, never mind any disease process or symptoms. Most of those are asymptomatic.

Nonetheless, Ms Edwards makes a very valid point. The biggest priority for the younger female population is the avoidance of kyphosis, avoidance of loss of height, and the severe upset of body image that the patient with vertebral osteoporosis ends up having. They do not want to avoid hip fracture; frankly they do not care about hip fracture. They want to avoid the deterioration that they see in themselves, the fact that they cannot get clothes to fit any more, that their abdomens protrude, that they are constipated and so on. They see mother or grandmother like that and that is what they want to avoid, yet we tend to ignore it because it is not the business end of the health care system.

Anderson: Is Ms Edwards's suggestion that for the early 1990s this group of women who have been hysterectomised with or without any knowledge of what has happened to their ovaries should be singled out? I understood that the suggestion is that hysterectomised women go through the menopause five or six years before control women, although that might be biased because many of them might have their hysterectomy because of problems related to the perimenopausal state. Is that a thesis that we can accept, and if so are we in danger (or is the National Osteoporosis Society in danger) of raising expectations too high before we have put the actual systems in place and before the Department of Health has found the funding to support them?

Are there the experts or enthusiasts around in sufficient numbers to do this? Should there be more organisation before this is advocated?

Baird: Ms Edwards suggested that these women should be considered for HRT.

Edwards: No one can make them take it. But it should be offered.

Baird: It should be considered. But would it be right to give HRT to a woman aged 48 years whose three sisters have died of breast cancer?

Edwards: That is not my decision. It is a decision for the woman and her own doctor – I would hope he is well enough informed. We never say as a Society that all women should go on HRT.

Persson: What is the rationale for removing the ovaries in the premenopausal woman? I was surprised to hear of it. It is said to prevent ovarian carcinoma but what is the lifetime risk of getting ovarian carcinoma?

Studd: One in 100.

Persson: Is that reason enough to remove the ovaries?

Purdie: No, it is not. I would be interested to know about London practice, but the practice in the provinces of England and in Scotland as I understand it is that if a woman is having a hysterectomy for a non-malignant indication at the age of 45 years or over, it is general practice to remove the ovaries at the same time.

Persson: I think that is bad.

Studd: A questionnaire to the Members and Fellows of the Royal College of Obstetricians and Gynaecologists showed that 79% of gynaecologists would take out the ovaries after the menopause and about 45% after age 49 years. I would support the concept that prophylactic oophorectomy is a good thing at 45 years for many reasons; and there would be an obligation to give hormone therapy afterwards.
  It is a complex argument, but I think the balance lies in favour of oophorectomy and HRT. The problem is that if all these arguments are correct then there is the question of availability and compliance. It is no good removing the ovaries at age 40 years if the patient will not have hormone therapy or there is no doctor available to prescribe it.

Anderson: Are there perceived to be problems for example with patients having a hysterectomy or an oophorectomy for endometriosis?

Studd: No. In most cases they would get oestrogens straight away.

Baird: There can be problems. I have seen women with kidney stones having oestradiol implants with residual endometriosis and blocked ureter.

Studd: In our experience of 109 patients with endometriosis who had hysterectomy, there was one patient who had a ureter blockage. However, she had had nine previous operations.
  Someone asked if there are people available to give this therapy. Menopause is normally a simple diagnosis and hysterectomy is an even simpler diagnosis and the treatment is cheap and straightforward. It does not need anyone with great skill to prescribe HRT and it is a straightforward and safe therapy with a lot of benefits, and we await the long-term work on the breasts. It does not take great skill or great expense to prescribe hormone therapy.

Anderson: I was thinking more of the logistics in tracing these women. If we follow it to its logical conclusion, the responsibility should fall on the people who have done the hysterectomies and oophorectomies, at least to initiate it. Some thought perhaps needs to be given to the logistics.

There will no doubt be different views about the preferred forms of HRT, and maybe some clearer guidelines, particularly for some of the newer forms of therapy (when to give patches, etc.) ought to be given before this blanket recommendation is made.

Boyde: Dr Fogelman and Dr Kanis used various terms for what they were screening for, i.e. "mass", "density", "bone mineral content", and "bone mineral density". Dr Fogelman talked about one method which can be used to derive a reasonable estimate of density. But these methods do not measure density at all. Most of these methods measure optical density and for the record we should use the correct terms.

"Density" is mass per unit volume. The data that I am querying could be translated into measurements of mass per unit volume and what we have found (on a limited dataset which is not yet ready for publication) is that the density in osteoporotic bone increases. The density of osteoporotic bone fabric increases and what matters is that there is less of it. More densely mineralised bone is more brittle.

Fogelman: Professor Boyde is absolutely right, but the problem is that it is universally accepted with this technology to call it "bone density", which is $g\ cm^{-2}$, which is bone mineral which is corrected for area. It is not a volume correction.

Boyde: It is physically incorrect to use the term "density" for that.

Anderson: With regard to that true increase in density – is that because there is proportionately less matrix than mineral?

Boyde: No. Because proportionately more of the potential mineral fillable space, which is in the proteoglycan component of the bone matrix, is filled up so that there are more packets of bone which have reached a higher degree of mineralisation. And all of that is complicated by whether those more highly mineralised packets are connected together by less densely mineralised bone. It is a very complicated story. To take a global measurement of how much calcium is present in the path of a photon beam is not exactly measuring density.

Fogelman: Which is why Dr Kanis and I both suggested that it is better to do it earlier. We agree that in the osteoporotic subjects there are problems. We are talking about perhaps screening a woman at age 50 years.

Kanis: To pick up on what Professor Boyde was saying. I tried to say we should not make too many assumptions: we should think about what we are doing and what it means. This is another area where we glibly talk about density. We do not measure density, as Professor Boyde correctly says, and the idea of trying to correct for density or for shape or area is quite arbitrary. Intellectually we do not know what are the proper things to adjust to normalise somebody within a population. We pick area because we can measure it. Other people might pick lean body mass because we can measure it, or height, and these are quite arbitrary. None of them gives measures of density, all of them are quite arbitrary.

Section III

Risks and Benefits of HRT

Chapter 14

Hormone Replacement Therapy and the Risk of Cancer in the Breast and Reproductive Organs: A Review of Epidemiological Data

I. Persson, H. O. Adami and L. Bergkvist

HRT and Prevention of Osteoporosis

Hormone replacement therapy (HRT), by means of oestrogens (and cyclic progestogens), has become recognised as the only well-established prophylactic measure against postmenopausal bone loss [1,2]. Numerous clinical studies have reported a bone-mass preserving effect during study periods extending from 2 to 8 years [3]. Furthermore, the results of several epidemiological studies, of both retrospective and prospective designs, indicate that such treatment can also reduce the risk of fragility fractures in the vertebrae, distal radius and hip [3]. As postmenopausal bone loss, with ensuing bone fragility (osteoporosis), is a major cause of fractures, it has, according to a consensus development conference in 1987 [1], been considered justified to give HRT to women identified to be at increased risk of developing osteoporosis.

Treatment Principles

The principles of HRT in order to achieve efficient fracture prevention were specified by the consensus conference as follows [1,3]:

1. The minimum effective doses of oral oestrogens are 0.625 mg for conjugated oestrogens, 2 mg for 17 ß-oestradiol and 25 µg for ethinyloestradiol;

2. HRT should be commenced in the early peri- or postmenopausal phase;
3. HRT should be continued long term, probably for at least 10 years;
4. HRT should include the regular addition of cyclic progestogens in order to control the bleeding pattern and to prevent endometrial hyperplasia and neoplasia.

Risk-Benefit Evaluation

If HRT is to be implemented for osteoporosis prevention, a major problem would be identification in the perimenopausal years of women who would be at increased risk of having fractures at an old age, most importantly hip fractures. No methods of adequate sensitivity or specificity exist today for identification of patients at risk [4]. Therefore, such a programme would have to include a substantial proportion of all postmenopausal women to have an effect on the population.

Before introducing HRT along such principles, other effects, notably harmful ones, need a full assessment. Of particular importance is the risk of malignancies.

This chapter summarises the epidemiological data on HRT and cancer risk in the main target organs of oestrogens and progestogens, i.e. the breast, the uterus (endometrium and cervix), and the ovaries.

Breast Cancer

Public Health Importance

From a public health point of view, the influence of HRT on breast cancer risk may be important. Breast cancer is by far the most frequent malignant tumour in women. In Sweden the age-standardised incidence is four times higher [5] and the cumulative rate of developing breast cancer to the age of 75 years is 4 to 5 times greater [6] than for endometrial cancer. Furthermore, the excess mortality among breast cancer patients is considerable, amounting to 30%–40% after 15-20 years [7]. Therefore, if a large proportion of the population receives long-term HRT, even a moderate true increase of the risk after HRT would cause a substantial number of new cases of breast cancer.

Conflicting Epidemiological Data

The association between HRT and breast cancer risk has been studied extensively ever since oestrogens were introduced for replacement therapy. An early cohort study published in 1976 showed a twofold increase in relative risk after 15 years of observation [8]. A large number of subsequent studies, 21 of case-control and four of cohort designs, have produced conflicting results (Fig. 14.1), [8-33]. Twenty-one did not report a significant alteration of the overall risk,

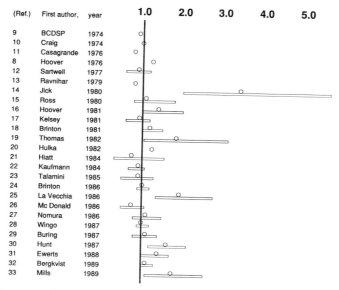

Fig. 14.1. Summary of results from 26 epidemiological studies of breast cancer risk after HRT. Relative risk estiamtes (represented by circles) and 95% confidence intervals (lines).

whereas five found a significant increase in the risk of developing breast cancer, mainly after exposure to conjugated oestrogens [14,19,25,30,33]. For a proper interpretation of these overall results, a careful evaluation of methodological issues in each study is necessary. Furthermore, the interpretation is complicated by the observations that the risk differed among various subgroups of women, i.e. with regard to type of menopause, natural or surgical (hysterectomy, with or without oophorectomy), and presence of previous "benign breast disease", indicating that the effects of exogenous exposure are modified by characteristics of the treated women. However, the type and magnitude of interaction by such factors differ among the studies [24].

Detailed Analysis of Risk Relationships

Sixteen studies reported risks in association with protracted intake, classified in different ways (Fig. 14.2). In all but three, the relative risk estimates (RR) were greater than unity, ranging from 1.5 to 5.3. Seven of them reported significantly elevated estimates [8,16,21,27,30–32], three borderline values [15,25,29] and two showed a significant trend with increasing duration [24,33].

Some of the recently published studies provide further details on risk relationships. A large multicentre case-control study was based on 1960 post-menopausal breast cancer cases recruited within a mammography screening programme and 2258 control subjects from the underlying population [24]. A significant overall trend of increasing risk with increasing duration of use of HRT (both for conjugated and synthetic oestrogens) was found. The RR reached 1.5 (95% confidence limits = 0.9, 2.3) after 20 years of treatment.

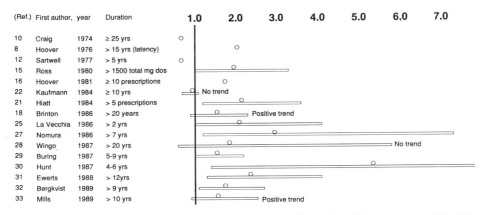

Fig. 14.2. Summary of results from 16 studies reporting relationship of breast cancer risk with protracted use of HRT, according to various types of classification.

Elevations associated with such long-term use were apparent in all menopausal subgroups (natural; surgical with ovaries retained; surgical with ovaries removed). Adverse effects seemd to be the strongest following long-term treatment that was initiated subsequent to a diagnosis of "benign breast disease" (RR = 3.0, 1.6, 5.5). The pattern of a duration-risk increase was most prominent for women with in situ or small (≤ 1 cm) tumours; RR = 1.9 and 1.5 after 10+ years of treatment, respectively, whereas for those with larger tumours the risk was the lowest; RR = 1.3.

Results from a cohort study in Sweden [32], based on an average follow-up of 5.7 years among over 23 000 women, showed a slightly elevated overall risk of breast cancer (RR = 1.1; 1.0, 1.3). Exposure to any oestrogenic compound was associated with a duration-dependent risk increase, from RR = 0.7 after ≤ 6 months to RR = 1.7 after more than 9 years of treatment, the trend being statistically significant (P = 0.002). A similar duration-risk gradient also appeared in the subgroups of women, who took oestrogens alone and who took oestrogens combined with progestogens (mainly levonorgestrel 250 μg for 10 days of each cycle), during the whole or part of the treatment period. For those exposed to oestradiol compounds (oestradiol valerate 1–2 mg) the risk became higher with increasing length of treatment, being increased twofold after 6–9 years (RR = 2.3, 1.2, 4.3). No such pattern was evident for conjugated oestrogens. These results indicated that added progestogens may not prevent the risk increase associated with long-term oestrogen exposure.

Another cohort study [30] among over 4500 women in the UK who used various types of oestrogens, in 43% combined with progestogens, also reported an increased incidence of breast cancer; overall RR = 1.6 (1.2, 2.1) and after more than six years of intake, RR = 3.6 (0.9, 15.0).

A population-based case-control study in Denmark [31], based on 1386 women with breast cancer and 1336 controls, provided evidence of an association with long-term exposure, the risk increasing from RR = 0.9 after less than three years of exposure to 2.3 (1.3, 4.1) after more than 12 years. Furthermore, an elevated overall risk was found among users of oestrogen–progestogen (RR = 1.4) and oestrogen–androgen combined regimens (RR = 2.3).

Finally, the large cohort study among some 20 000 Seventh Day Adventist women in California [33] found a 70% increased risk among current users of conjugated oestrogens (RR = 1.7; 1.1, 2.6) and a significant trend with length of HRT, reaching an almost 3-fold increase after 6–10 years (RR = 2.8; 1.6, 4.6).

Interpretation of Epidemiological Data

Although to some extent contradictory, these epidemiological studies, especially those published in recent years [24,30–33], have provided evidence that extended use of potent oestrogens entails a moderately increased risk of breast cancer, maybe with the greatest risk of early stage tumours [24]. Certain subgroups of women might be particularly sensitive, e.g. those with a history of benign breast disease [15,18,24] or with a history of maternal breast cancer [16,18]. A few studies provide tentative evidence that added cyclic progestogens might not alter the risk increase after long-term oestrogen exposure [30,32].

Especially important issues for further research concern the duration of risk increase after cessation of therapy; the effect of adding progestogens; and case fatality rates for cancers associated with HRT. In addition, the combined effect of long-term exposure to combined oral contraceptives and HRT on breast cancer risk needs to be evaluated in future studies.

Endometrial Cancer

Consistent Epidemiological Data

Since 1975 a large number of retrospective and two prospective epidemiological studies have reported a 2–12 times increased risk of endometrial cancer after postmenopausal HRT (Table 14.1) [30,34–44]. The validity of the results from

Table 14.1 Postmenopausal oestrogen treatment and the risk of endometrial cancer, overall risk estimates (95% confidence limits)

Reference	Author	Year	Relative risk (95% confidence limits)
34	Smith	1975	7.5 (4.4, 14.4)
35	Ziel	1975	7.6 (4.3, 13.3)
36	Mack	1976	8.0 (3.5, 18.1)
37	McDonald	1976	2.0 (1.1, 3.3)
38	Gray	1977	2.1 (1.2, 3.5)
39	Antunes	1978	6.0 (3.7, 9.7)
40	Horwitz	1978	12.0 (4.0, 47.7)
41	Weiss	1979	6.0
42	Hulka	1980	4.1 (1.8, 9.6)
30	Hunt	1987	2.8 (1.5, 5.0)
43	Paganini-Hill	1989	10.0 ($P<0.0001$)
44	Persson	1989	1.7 (1.4, 2.2)

case-control studies has been debated on account of methodological short-comings, but consensus is that the data reflect a true and causal association [45,46]. The wide variation in the magnitude of risk estimates can be explained by differences in study designs and in the definition of exposure [46].

Risk Patterns

Aggregated data from these studies have clarified how various patterns of exposure influence the risk. The strongest determinant of risk is the duration of oestrogen treatment. The risk becomes significantly elevated after 2–4 years of treatment and rises thereafter, in either a linear or an exponential fashion, to about a 10-fold increase after 10 years' duration (Fig. 14.3). The risk level appears in most studies to return to baseline 2 years after the discontinuation of the treatment [46], though in one study some excessive risk seemed to remain [43]. The dose of the administered hormone also affects the risk. Conjugated oestrogens in a daily dose exceeding 1 mg were associated with a twofold higher risk as compared with a lower dose [38]. The selection of patients for treatment may be of importance, since the presence of other risk factors for endometrial cancer, e.g. obesity and late menopause, may potentiate the risk associated with the oestrogen exposure [47]. Endometrial cancers developing after oestrogen exposure seem to have less aggressive biological characteristics, since in these instances an early clinical stage, a low histopathological grade of differentiation with no or little invasiveness into the myometrium [46] and excellent 5-year survival rate (around 95%) [48] have been consistently reported.

These findings, short latency period, rapid decline of risk after discontinuation of treatment and development of biologically less-aggressive tumours, indicate that oestroens act as carcinogens mainly by promotion (stimulation of the growth of pre-existing premalignant cell clones) rather than by initiation [49].

Most of these epidemiological data reflect the consequences of the particular

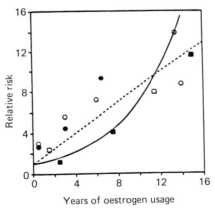

Fig. 14.3. Dose–response between relative risk for endometrial cancer and length of oestrogen usage: linear fit (interrupted line) versus exponential fit (continuous line). ○, Mack et al. [36]; ●, Ziel and Finkle [35]; □, Gray et al. [38]; ■, McDonald et al. [37]. (Reprinted with permission from the Editor and the authors.)

practice regarding HRT that was predominant in the USA at the time when the study materials were generated, i.e. in the 1960s and 70s [45]. Features of that practice were liberal treatment indications, the use of high doses of potent oestrogens (mainly conjugated oestrogens, given in daily doses above 1 mg), and no addition of progestogens (unopposed exposure). Combination with added progestogens for 10 to 12 days in each treatment can, according to data from clinical trials, prevent the occurrence of endometrial hyperplasia [50].

Effect of Added Progestogens on Endometrial Cancer Risk

The cohort study among over 23 000 postmenopausal women in Sweden [44], provides data on the risk of endometrial neoplasia after exposure to various oestrogenic compounds, both opposed and unopposed by cyclically added progestogens. After approximately 6 years of observation, exposure to any unopposed oestrogen compound for more than 6 years yielded about a three times increased risk of endometrial neoplasia including premalignant lesions (RR = 2.7; 1.8, 4.2). Among women exposed to potent oestrogenic compounds for more than 3 years without added progestogens, the risk of endometrial neoplasia was 2 to 3 times elevated; RR = 2.7 (1.5, 5.0) and RR = 3.0 (1.7, 5.3) for oestradiol compounds (1–2 mg) and conjugated oestrogens (0.625–1.25 mg), respectively. When the treatment had been combined with progestogens (predominantly levonorgestrel 250 µg) for 7–10 days of each treatment cycle, no significant risk increase was observed. These data give the first evidence that cyclically added progestogens can prevent the excess risk of developing endometrial neoplasia after long-term oestrogen exposure.

Ovarian Cancer

Long-term use of combined oral contraceptives (COCs) among young women has consistently been reported to reduce the risk of ovarian cancer by 20%–60% [51,52]. The underlying mechanisms of this protective action are believed to be the inhibition of ovulation and the suppression of gonadotrophin levels [51]. Epidemiological data concerning HRT and ovarian cancer risk are more conflicting. One study reported an increased risk of ovarian cancer after exposure to diethylstilboestrol (DES) and conjugated oestrogens [53], whereas in other studies a slightly protective effect or no alteration of the risk was found [54–56]. In the Swedish cohort [56] the relative risk of ovarian cancer was 1.0 (0.7, 1.2), and the risk was seemingly unrelated to the type and duration of HRT. In a recent case-control study [57], a 20%–50% reduced risk of epithelial ovarian cancer after exposure to mainly conjugated oestrogens was found. The magnitude of the risk reduction became greater with increasing treatment duration and decreased after discontinuation of the treatment. The authors interpreted their finding as a possible true protective effect, possibly mediated by reduced pituitary gonadotrophin stimulation due to negative feed-back by the oestrogen exposure.

Due to contradictory results in available studies, definite conclusions can not be made at present. Ovarian cancer risk is, due to the seriousness of this disease, an extremely important issue that needs to be addressed in additional studies.

Cervical Cancer

Epidemiological data on HRT and cervical cancer risk have not been reported. Among women in reproductive age groups hormone exposure in the form of combined oral contraceptives has been linked to an increased risk of cervical neoplasia (carcinoma in situ and invasive carcinoma) [57]. However, the difficulty of adequately accounting for a large number of confounding variables and the impact of cytological screening in such studies preclude firm conclusions on the effects of the hormones *per se*. Moreover, results based on a younger population and a different type and amount of hormonal exposure, i.e. oral contraceptives containing comparatively higher doses of combined oestrogens and progestogens, cannot be extrapolated to postmenopausal women.

With regard to invasive cervical cancer, data from the Swedish cohort [56] indicated that women below the age of 60 at the time of recruitment into the cohort had a rather lower risk than expected (RR = 0.6; 0.4, 1.0), supposedly due to a higher degree of cytological screening among these women.

General Summary and Conclusions

HRT in the postmenopausal period is associated with a broad panorama of potential effects, both beneficial and harmful. In the context of preventing postmenopausal bone loss and subsequent fragility fractures, an effective HRT regimen would need to involve long-term exposure (10–15 years) to potent and high-dose oestrogens that are cyclically combined with progestogens and started in the early postmenopausal period. On introducing such preventive treatment among a substantial proportion of healthy women in a population, a full assessment of risks and benefits is necessary. It is then of importance to consider the risk of malignancies, chiefly in the target organs of sex hormones – the uterus, ovaries and breast.

A review of epidemiological data allows the following conclusions:

1. Long-term HRT (exceeding 10–15 years) with potent oestrogens is associated with a moderate increase in the risk of postmenopausal breast cancer, of the order of 1.5–3 times, supposedly with the highest risk among specific subgroups of women and for small tumours. Data from recent studies are consistent in showing such a risk pattern, and tentative evidence is provided that the addition of progestogens may not prevent the risk increase.

2. Exposure to potent oestrogens, like oestradiol compounds and conjugated oestrogens, without added progestogens gives rise to a duration-dependent increase in risk of endometrial cancer, reaching about a tenfold level after 10–15 years. Added progestogens for at least 10 days of each treatment cycle may prevent the risk increase. Tumours developing after HRT are characterised by low biological aggressiveness and excellent 5-year survival.

3. There is no consistent evidence of HRT effects on the risk of developing ovarian cancer.

4. No documentation of an increased risk of invasive cervical cancer after HRT has been presented.

References

1. Consensus development conference. Prophylaxis and treatment of osteoporosis. Br Med J 1987; 295:914–16.
2. Editorial. Osteoporosis. Lancet 1987; ii:833–5.
3. Cummings SR, Kelsey JL, Nevitt MC, O'Dowd KJ. Epidemiology of osteoporosis and osteoporotic fractures. Epidemiol Rev 1985; 7:178–208.
3. Peck WA, Riggs BL, Bell NH et al. Scientific workshop: research directions in osteoporosis. Am J Med 1988; 84:275–82.
5. National Board of Health and Welfare. The Cancer Registry. Cancer Incidence in Sweden 1983. Stockholm 1986.
6. Waterhouse J, Muir C, Shanmugaratnam K et al., eds. Cancer incidence in five continents, vol IV. IARC, Lyon, 1982.
7. Adami H-O, Holmberg L, Persson I, Stone B. The relation between survival and age at diagnosis in breast cancer. N Engl J Med 1986; 315:559–63.
8. Hoover, R, Gray LA, Cole P et al. Menopausal estrogens and breast cancer. N Engl J Med 1976; 295:401–5.
9. The Boston Collaborative Drug Surveillance Program. Surgically confirmed gallbladder disease, venous thromboembolism, and breast tumours in relation to postmenopausal estrogen therapy. N Engl J Med 1974; 15–18.
10. Craig TJ, Comstock GW, Geiser PB. Epidemiologic comparison of breast cancer patients with early and late onset of malignancies and general population controls. J Natl Cancer Inst 1974; 53:1577–81.
11. Casagrande J. Gerkins V, Henderson BE et al. Brief communication: exogenous estrogens and breast cancer in women with natural menopause. J Natl Cancer Inst 1976; 56:839–41.
12. Sartwell PE, Arthes FG, Tanascia JA. Exogenous estrogens, reproductive history, and breast cancer. J Natl Cancer Inst 1977; 59:1589–92.
13, Ravnihar B, Seigel DG, Lindtner J. An epidemiological study of breast cancer and benign breast neoplasias in relation to oral contraceptive and estrogen use. Eur J Cancer 1979; 15:395–405.
14. Jick H, Walker AM, Watkins RN et al. Replacement estrogens and breast cancer. Am J Epidemiol 1980; 112:586–94.
15. Ross RK, Paganini-Hill A, Gerkins VR et al. A case-control study of menopausal estrogen therapy and breast cancer. JAMA 1980; 243: 1635–9.
16. Hoover R, Glass A, Finkle WD et al. Conjugated estrogens and breast cancer risk in women. J Natl Cancer Inst 1981; 67:815–20.
17. Kelsey JL, Fischer DB, Holford TR et al. Exogenous estrogens and other factors in the epidemiology of breast cancer. J Natl Cancer Inst 1981; 67:327–33.
18. Brinton LA, Hoover R, Szklo M, Fraumeni JF. Menopausal estrogen use and risk of breast cancer. Cancer 1981; 47:2517–22.
19. Thomas DB, Pershing JP, Hutchinem WB. Exogenous estrogens and other risk factors for breast cancer in women with benign breast disease. J Natl Cancer Inst 1982; 69:1017–25.
20. Hulka BS, Chambless LE, Deubner DC, Wilkinson WE. Breast cancer and estrogen replacement therapy. Am J Obstet Gynecol 1982; 638–44.
21. Hiatt RA, Bawol R, Friedman GD, Hoover R. Exogenous estrogen and breast cancer after bilateral oophorectomy. Cancer 1984; 54:139–44.
22. Kaufmann DW, Miller DR, Rosenberg L. et al. Noncontraceptive estrogen use and the risk of breast cancer. JAMA 1984; 252:63–7.
23. Talamini R, La Vecchia C, Franceschi S et al. Reproductive and hormonal factors and breast cancer in a northern Italian population. Int J Epidemiol 1985; 14:70–4.
24. Brinton LA, Hoover R, Fraumeni JF. Menopausal oestrogens and breast cancer risk: an expanded case-control study. Br J Cancer 1986; 54:825–32.
25. La Vecchia C, Decarli A, Parazzini F, Gentile A, Liberati C, Franceschi S. Non-contraceptive oestrogens and the risk of breast cancer in women. Int J Cancer 1986; 38:853–58.

26. McDonald I, Weiss N, Daling J, Francis A, Pollisar L. Menopausal estrogen use and the risk of breast cancer. Breast Cancer Res Treat 1986; 7:193–9.
27. Nomura AMY, Kolonel LN, Hirohata T et al. The association of replacement estrogens with breast cancer. Int J Cancer 1986; 37:49–53.
28. Wingo PA, Layde PM, Lee NC, Rubin G, Ory HN. The risk of breast cancer in postmenopausal women who have used estrogen replacement therapy. JAMA 1987; 257:209–15.
29. Buring JE, Hennekens CH, Lipnick RJ et al. A prospective cohort study of postmenopausal hormone use and risk of breast cancer in US women. Am J Epidemiol 1987; 125:939–47.
30. Hunt K, Vessey M, McPherson K, Coleman M. Long-term surveillance of mortality and cancer incidence in women receiving hormone replacement therapy. Br J Obstet Gynaecol 1987; 94:620–35.
31. Ewerts M. Influence of non-contraceptive exogenous and endogenous sex hormones on breast cancer risk in Denmark. Int J Cancer 1988; 42:832–8.
32. Bergkvist L, Adami HO, Persson I, Hoover R, Schairer C. The risk of breast cancer after estrogen and estrogen–progestin replacement. N Engl J Med 1989; 321:293–7.
33. Mills PK, Beeson WL, Phillips RL, Fraser GE, Prospective study of exogenous hormone use and breast cancer in Seventh Day Adventists. Cancer 1989; 64:591–7.
34. Smith DC, Prentice R, Thompson DJ, Herrman WL. Association of exogenous estrogen and endometrial carcinoma. N Engl J Med 1975; 293:1164–7.
35. Ziel HK, Finkle WD. Increased risk of endometrial carcinoma among users of conjugated estrogens. N Engl J Med 1975; 293:1167–70.
36. Mack TM, Pike MC, Henderson BE et al. Estrogens and endometrial cancer in a retirement community. N Engl J Med 1976; 294:1262–7.
37. McDonald TW, Annegers JF, O'Fallon WM, Dockerty MB, Malkasin GD, Kurland LT. Exogenous estrogen and endometrial carcinoma: case-control and incidence study. Am J Obstet Gynecol 1977; 127:572–80.
38. Gray LA, Christophersen WM, Hoover RN. Estrogens and endometrial carcinoma. Obstet Gynecol 1977; 49:385–9.
39. Antunes CMF, Stolley PD, Rosenshein NB et al. Endometrial cancer and estrogen use. Report of a large case-control study. N Engl J Med 1979; 300:9–13.
40. Horwitz RI, Feinstein AR. Alternative analytical methods for case-control studies of estrogens and endometrial cancer. N Engl J Med 1978; 299:1089–94.
41. Weiss NS, Szekely DR, English DR, Schweid AI. Endometrial cancer in relation to patterns of menopausal estrogen use. JAMA 1979; 242:261–4.
42. Hulka BS, Fowler WC, Kaufman DG et al. Estrogen and endometrial cancer: cases and two control groups from North Carolina. Am J Obstet Gynecol 1980; 137:92–101.
43. Paganini-Hill A, Ross RK, Henderson BE. Endometrial cancer and patterns of use of estrogen replacement therapy: a cohort study. Br J Cancer 1989; 59:445–7.
44. Persson I, Adami HO, Bergkvist L et al. Risk of endometrial cancer after treatment with oestrogens alone or in conjunction with progestogens: results of a prospective study. Br Med J 1989; 298:147–51.
45. Ziel HK. Estrogen's role in endometrial cancer. Obstet Gynecol 1982; 60:509–15.
46. Hulka BS. Effect of exogenous estrogen on postmenopausal women: the epidemiologic evidence. Obstet Gynecol Surv 1980; 35:389–99.
47. Davies JL, Rosenshein NB, Antunes CMF, Stolley PD. A review of the risk factors for endometrial carcinoma. Obstet Gynecol Surv 1981; 36:107–16.
48. Collins J, Donner A, Allen LH, Adams O. Oestrogen use and survival in endometrial cancer. Lancet 1980; ii:961–4.
49. Fox H. Endometrial carcinogenesis and its relation to oestrogens. Pathol Res Pract 1984; 179:13–19.
50. Whitehead MI, Townsend PT, Pryse-Davies J et al. Effects of estrogens and progestins on the biochemistry and morphology of the postmenopausal endometrium. N Engl J Med 1981; 305:1599–605.
51. Ory HW, Layde PM, Webster LA, Wingo PA. Oral contraceptive use and the risk of ovarian cancer. JAMA 1983; 249:1596–9.
52. Weiss NS, Lyon JL, Liff JM et al. Incidence of ovarian cancer in relation to use of oral contraceptives. Int J Cancer 1981; 28:669–71.
53. Weiss NS, Lyon JL, Krishnamurthy S et al. Non-contraceptive estrogen use and the occurrence of ovarian cancer. J Natl Cancer Inst 1982; 68:95–8.
54. Smith EM, Sowers MF, Burns TL. Effects of smoking on the developing of female reproductive cancers. J Natl Cancer Inst 1984; 73:371–6.

55. Kaufman DW, Kelly JP, Welch WR et al. Noncontraceptive estrogen use and epithelial ovarian cancer. Am J Epidemiol 1989; 130:1142–51.
56. Adami HO, Persson I, Hoover R, Schairer C, Bergkvist, L. The risk of cancer in women receiving hormone replacement therapy. Int J Cancer 1989; 44:833–9.
57. Hartge P, Hoover R, McGowan. et al. Menopause and ovarian cancer. Am J Epidemiol 1988; 127:990–8.
58. Vessey MP, Lawless M, McPherson K, Yeates D. Neoplasia of the cervix uteri and contraception: a possible adverse effect of the pill. Lancet 1983; ii:930.

Chapter 15

Oestrogens and Cancer

M. P. Cust, K. F. Gangar and M. I. Whitehead

Introduction

The fear that hormone replacement therapy (HRT) may provoke cancer currently prevents many women from seeking such treatment and many physicians from prescribing it. Although the evidence linking oestrogens and cancer is reassuring for most tumours, there are still uncertainties. This chapter discusses the current evidence for an association of HRT with genital cancers, cancers of the large bowel and melanomas.

Endometrial Carcinoma

Cyclical Oestrogen Therapy

Until the mid-1970s, oestrogen was usually prescribed on a cyclical basis, for 3 weeks out of each 4-week cycle, without a progestogen. By 1975–1976, the first retrospective studies were published [1–3] linking endometrial adenocarcinoma with cyclical oestrogen administration. These early studies were criticised for various methodological flaws, but subequent work confirmed the findings of an increase in risk. From an overall background or untreated risk of approximately one case per 1000 women per year, the risk rises to approximately four to five per 1000 oestrogen users per year. Thus, although the annual increase in risk is small in absolute terms, the increase in risk is cumulative. In the fifth year of oestrogen exposure, endometrial cancer would be expected to develop in 20–25 cases per 1000 women and in the tenth year in aproximately 40–50 per 1000 women.

The prognosis with most oestrogen-related cancers is favourable [4], but some oestrogen users who have developed this malignancy have died [5]. The survival rates for users (92.4%) are greater than for non-users (81.3%). However, unopposed cyclic oestrogens also cause irregular bleeding and endometrial hyperplasia, and when added to carcinoma, this triad contributed to an increased prevalence of hysterectomy among cyclic oestrogen users. Ettinger et al. [6] reported that 28.2% of oestrogen users had a hysterectomy, compared to 5.3% of non-users. Thus, unopposed cyclical oestrogen therapy has both medical and financial implications.

A recent study [7] has identified an increased risk of developing endometrial cancer among women who took cyclical oestrogen therapy in the past, but who have now ceased. Even for women who stopped this unopposed therapy more than 15 years previously there was still an almost sixfold increase in risk compared to women who had never received HRT. No strategy has yet been proposed to monitor women after ceasing cyclical oestrogen therapy.

Combined Therapy: Oestrogen and Progestogen

Various approaches have been suggested to reduce the risk of endometrial hyperstimulation. It is logical that by reducing the dose of oestrogen, the risk can also be reduced. However, as the dose is lowered, so the beneficial effects of therapy are reduced. For doses of oestrogen that may be expected to provide symptom relief and prevent bone loss, only progestogen addition has been shown to reduce the incidence of hyperplasia [8]. A seven-day course of progestogen reduces the incidence to 3%–4% [8]; extending the duration to ten days reduces the incidence further to 2% [9] and the incidence is 0 if a progestogen is added for 12–13 days [9,10].

Until recently, only large-scale cross-sectional studies were available on the results of combined therapy as compared to oestrogen alone on cancer risk. These studies reported that combined therapy reduced the incidence to below that in an untreated population [11]. A recent prospective Swedish study [12] has observed that the incidence is increased with unopposed cyclical oestrogen therapy, but not with combined oestrogen–progestogen therapy. The relative risk was 1.8 (95% confidence intervals 1.2–4.4) for women who took oestrogen for more than 6 years, whereas the risk was 0.9 (95% confidence intervals 0.4–2.0) for women who added a progestogen.

Cigarette smoking reduces the risk of endometrial cancer in both users and non-users of HRT [13]. Any increased risk of endometrial carcinoma among women taking unopposed cyclical oestrogen is negated by cigarette smoking. However, the morbidity and mortality from cigarette smoking is substantial.

Risks of Progestogens

Progestogens can give rise to unwanted physical effects such as mastalgia, headaches, nausea, bloatedness and backache. These symptoms are similar to those observed in premenstrual syndrome. Progestogens have also been shown to have potentially adverse effects on lipid metabolism [14]. Both C_{19} and C_{21}

steroid derivatives cause reductions in HDL-cholesterol [15,16]. However, the clinical consequences of these metabolic changes are as yet uncertain.

Because the physical and metabolic side effects of progestogen are dose-dependent, it is important to prescribe the lowest effective dose. From studies carried out at King's College Hospital, histological and biochemical changes were assessed for five commonly used progestogens (norethisterone, dl-norgestrel, oral progesterone, dydrogesterone and medroxyprogesterone acetate). Progestogen potency was measured in endometrial samples from women receiving continuous oestrogen and cyclical progestogen therapy [17–19]. Biopsies were taken on day 6 of progestogen addition when endometrial responses are maximal. Part of the tissue was examined histologically for proliferative, secretory or hyperplastic changes. Secretory histological features (subnuclear glycogen, giant mitochondria, nucleolar channel systems) were scored using transmission electron microscopy. Homogenised samples were assessed for enzyme activity (isocitrate dehydrogenase and 17ß-oestradiol dehydrogenase), DNA synthesis and concentration of nuclear oestradiol receptor. From these studies, the minimum effective dose of progestogen was calculated (Table 15.1).

Table 15.1. Daily dosage of various oral progestogens required to prevent endometrial abnormalities when given for 12 days each cycle (with continuous oestrogen)

Progestogen	Daily dose
Norethisterone	0.7–1.0 mg
dl-Norgestrel	150 µg
Medroxyprogesterone acetate	10 mg
Dydrogesterone	10–20 mg
Oral progesterone	200–300 mg

Pattern of Bleeding

When a progestogen is given for 12 days each cycle with continuous or cyclical oestrogen, approximately 90% of patients will experience a regular withdrawal bleed. It has been argued that the re-establishment of vaginal bleeding will reduce patient compliance. However, in our studies of symptomatic women, only 2%–4% of patients refused therapy because of this.

Clinically the bleeding pattern can be used to advantage. It is well recognised that there is a large interpatient variation of response to added progestogen [20]. For reasons stated previously, the minimum effective dose should be administered. With the doses stated above, the majority of patients will exhibit progestational changes within the endometrium, but some may not. Padwick et al. [21] demonstrated that the day of commencement of withdrawal bleeding is a reliable guide as to whether adequate progestational effects have been achieved or not. In these studies, patients who had been on oral combined therapy for at least 3 months were asked to record the day of onset of their bleeding for a further 3 months and the mean was calculated. Bleeding which commenced on or after day 11 of progestogen addition was associated with secretory transformation within the endometrium. In patients who bled earlier, the endometrium tended to be proliferative (devoid of progestational activity) or of a mixed pattern (part secretory and part proliferative). In clinical practice, the dose of progestogen can be increased until bleeding occurs at an appropriate time in the cycle (day 11 of progestogen addition or later), thus obviating the need for regular endometrial biopsy. The pattern of bleeding appears to be slightly different with transdermal oestradiol therapy [20], occurring earlier in the cycle despite adequate endometrial protection.

Continuous Oestrogen/Progestogen Therapy

Some patients, especially those starting therapy some years after the menopause, do not relish the continuation of their periods. To overcome this problem, and to minimise the daily dose of progestogen administered, various authors have tried a "continuous combined" oestrogen/progestogen regimen whereby both oestrogen and progestogen are taken every day throughout the cycle. The continuous progestogen should induce an atrophic endometrium and the patients will not bleed. Various groups have attempted to find an ideal combination [22–24]. In the majority of patients, amenorrhoea is eventually achieved. However, the early months are characterised by many patients experiencing chronic irregular spotting [23,24] which leads to a significant proportion of withdrawals. Because there are no data on the long-term endometrial safety of such regimens, it is recommended that endometrial biopsies be repeated regularly.

Ovarian Carcinoma

Ovarian carcinoma is more common than endometrial carcinoma and has a much greater mortality. Certain risk factors are shared by both (e.g. nulliparity) and once the increased risk of endometrial carcinoma with unopposed oestrogen therapy was established, it was suggested that there may be a similar increase in risk of ovarian carcinoma. Others argued that oestrogens may exert a protective effect on the ovary, because the oral contraceptive pill is known to reduce the risk.

There is agreement between epidemiological studies that there is no significant overall increase in risk of ovarian carcinoma among oestrogen users. Cancer screening programmes in the USA have shown no increase in ovarian carcinoma risk in recent years, where an increase might have been expected because of the more widespread use of oestrogen therapy [25]. The Third National Cancer Survey (TNCS), undertaken between 1969 and 1971, a time before the widespread use of oestrogen therapy, was compared with the Surveillance, Epidemiology and End Results (SEER) programme, performed between 1975 and 1977, when there had been a substantial increase in oestrogen use. Although there was no significant overall increase in incidence between the two studies, there appeared to be an increase in certain histological types, namely the endometrioid and clear-cell tumours. These epithelial carcinomas are similar histologically to endometrial carcinoma. Three further studies have investigated the incidence of endometrioid carcinoma in more detail [26–28]. A small increase in risk was reported, but this was not statistically significant and the increases could be due to chance. Another explanation of this apparent increase for certain histological types with no overall increase in incidence may be underreporting of these types prior to 1975. Further work is needed to clarify the exact relationship between postmenopausal oestrogen use and these types of ovarian malignancy.

Cervical Carcinoma

The peak incidence of cervical intraepithelial neoplasia (CIN) and cervical carcinoma both occur premenopausally. A causal relationship between post-menopausal oestrogen therapy and cervical carcinoma is therefore unlikely. However, few epidemiological studies have specifically evaluated such a risk. Hunt et al. [29] observed only two cases of invasive cervical cancer among their cohort recruited from menopause clinics in the UK (relative risk 0.47, 95% confidence intervals 0.05–1.70). Our current understanding is that HRT may be used safely in patients treated for cervical carcinoma.

Breast Carcinoma

This is perhaps the most controversial issue concerning the risks of oestrogen therapy at present. The breast is a target tissue for gonadal hormones and it is assumed that they influence breast cancer risk. It is well recognised that an early menarche [30] and a late menopause [32] are both associated with an increased risk of breast carcinoma. It has been estimated that a woman whose menopause occurred at the age of 55 years or later has twice the risk of developing breast carcinoma compared to a women who had a natural menopause before the age of 45 [31]. Therefore, it is not unreasonable to assume that "delaying the menopause" with oestrogen therapy may also increase this risk.

Many epidemiological studies have investigated the association between postmenopausal oestrogens and breast cancer. Unfortunately, many of the early studies were carried out on small numbers of patients and drew different conclusions. Some of these studies were methodologically flawed and failed to control adequately for factors known to influence the risk of breast cancer such as family history, age at menarche, menopause, and first live birth and also to control for surveillance bias. Thus the results may be of only limited value. However, even the results of recent well-cotrolled studies are inconsistent.

Most of the recent epidemiological studies of breast cancer were performed in the USA and the vast majority of women were taking unopposed conjugated equine oestrogens. Four case-controlled studies [32–35] reported an increase in relative risk (1.3–1.9) with long-term oestrogen use, and three of these reported a dose-dependent association [32–34]. In contrast, three other studies found no evidence to suggest that breast cancer risk was increased overall or with long-term use [36–38]. Two of these studies [36,37] were criticised for the use of hospital-based controls as a comparison group as these women may have had an excess of disease compared to the general population. However, the third study [38] used population-based controls.

Many of these studies have tried to establish whether there is a particular group most at risk. A recent large-scale study from the American National Cancer Institute [39] found no significant overall increase in risk of breast cancer with postmenopausal oestrogen use. The data were analysed in terms of duration of oestrogen use. With 5 years of use, the relative risk was 0.89 for oestrogen users whereas for 20+ years of use, the risk was 1.47. A trend test of increasing risk for increasing duration of use was significant ($P<0.01$).

It is unclear whether women with previous benign breast disease are more at risk of breast cancer with subsequent HRT use than those with no preceding history. The National Cancer Institute study [39] suggested that women with biopsy proven "benign breast disease" were at increased risk if the diagnosis preceded oestrogen therapy. Interestingly, those women developing benign breast disease after commencing HRT did not in the long-term, have an increased risk of breast cancer. Thomas et al. [40] suggested that women with breast biopsies showing epithelial hyperplasia and microcalcification were most at risk of developing malignancy with later HRT use. However, a recent study [41] failed to confirm this association. It is also far from clear whether women with a strong family history of breast carcinoma, although already at increased risk of developing the disease, are at any further increased risk because of postmenopausal oestrogen use.

The type of menopause does not appear to be relevant; some studies have reported that the greatest increase in risk occurs following oophorectomy [33,34] whereas others have reported the greatest risk following natural menopause [32]. The data from the National Cancer Institute [39] indicate an increased risk for all menopausal subgroups (natural; hysterectomised with ovarian conservation; bilateral oophorectomy).

Combination Oestrogen/Progestogen Therapy

The most recent controversy is whether progestogen addition modifies the risk of breast cancer. A prospective Swedish study [42] suggested that the risk of breast cancer was highest among women who took combination oestrogen/progestogen therapy for extended periods. The relative risk was 4.4 (95% confidence intervals 0.9–2.2) in women who used combination therapy for more than 6 years. The wide confidence intervals are accounted for by the small number of cases (10 cases). A study from Denmark [43] also found an increased risk among combination oestrogen/progestogen users (relative risk 1.6; 95% confidence intervals 0.98–1.87). Conversely, Gambrell [44] found a protective effect of long-term oestrogen/progestogen use on breast tissue. Between 1975 and 1983, the incidence rates for oestrogen/progestogen users was 66.8 per 100 000, for oestrogen only users was 142.3 per 100 000 and for non-users was 343.5 per 100 000. However, these data have been criticised for possible bias in selection of patients to receive treatment.

Breast and endometrial tissue may respond differently to the effects of progestogen. Whilst progestogens have a clear antimitotic effect on the endometrium by reducing DNA synthesis and the level of oestradiol receptor, it is unclear whether they have similar actions in the breast. Anderson et al. [45] studied breast tissue in perimenopausal women and found that DNA synthesis in breast epithelium does not appear to be suppressed by endogenous progesterone. The recent International Consensus Conference on Progestogens [46] concluded that there were insufficient data on breast protection to recommend the routine prescribing of progestogens to hysterectomised women taking oestrogens.

Oestrogen Therapy in Women with Breast Carcinoma

Clinicians are divided over the advisability of prescribing HRT to women with a history of breast carcinoma. The majority counsel against its use because of the potential for stimulating growth in metastatic carcinoma cells. Progestogen therapy alone has a role in the treatment of breast cancer and may also have some effect in relieving climacteric symptoms and protecting against postmenopausal bone loss [47]. These effects have been utilised to treat symptoms in postmenopausal women with breast cancer.

There are reports of women who, after removal of a malignant breast tumour, have been treated with either a combined oral contraceptive [48] or HRT [49]. In these short-term studies, the patients noted a reduction in their menopausal symptoms with no evidence of tumour reactivation. Larger studies with longer follow-up are needed to establish the safety of such regimens. On our present knowledge, it would seem safest to assume that oestrogen therapy in women with a preceding history of breast carcinoma may influence the growth of tumour cells, and should therefore be avoided. However, for certain patients, the quality of life may be so poor without oestrogen therapy that any possible risk is worth taking.

Colorectal Cancer

Among women diagnosed as having endometrial cancer, the subsequent incidence of colorectal cancer is more than twice that expected in the female population [50,51]. One explanation for this observation would be that these tumours share

Table 15.2. Risk ratios from studies of colorectal cancer in women receiving oestrogen therapy

Author	Year	Site of cancer	Oestrogen therapy	Risk ratio	95% CI
Weiss [51]	1981	Colon and rectum	None	1.0	
			≤5 years	1.1	0.7–1.9
			≥5 years	1.0	0.6–1.6
Potter [52]	1983	Colon	Never	1.0	Referent
			Ever	0.8	0.5–1.5
		Rectum	Never	1.0	Referent
			Ever	1.5	0.8–3.0
Davis [53]	1989	Colon and rectum	Current	1.5	0.8–2.7
			Past	1.1	0.7–1.9

a common aetiology. The association between postmenopausal oestrogen therapy and endometrial cancer has been discussed above. Various authors [51–53] have evaluated a possible relationship between such therapy and the subsequent finding of colorectal cancer (Table 15.2). Their conclusions were that, within the groups studied, there was no evidence to suggest an overall increase in risk of colonic or rectal carcinomas among postmenopausal oestrogen users.

Malignant Melanomas

Several lines of evidence suggest a relationship between sex hormones and the behaviour of malignant melanomas. A cytoplasmic "oestrogen receptor" has been discovered among various melanoma tumour cell lines [54,55]. Animal studies have produced conflicting results as to the effect of oestradiol on tumour growth in vivo. Both enhancement [56] and inhibition [57] of tumour growth have been reported.

In epidemiological studies, the overall prognosis is better for women than for men [58], but the prognosis is worse for postmenopausal than for premenopausal women [58]. Pregnancy has been reported to either worsen or have no effect on melanoma [59,60]. Worryingly, there are anecdotal reports of rapidly worsening disease soon after starting treatment with oestrogens [61,62]. There are no studies relating postmenopausal oestrogen therapy and disease prognosis, but Shaw et al. [58] found no significant difference in 5-year survival between oral contraceptive users and non-users. Without any relevant data, it is difficult to advise the postmenopausal woman who has had a melanoma removed whether HRT is safe or not. However, the possibility of tumour reactivation must be considered.

Conclusions

Other chapters have dealt with the undoubted and well-defined benefits of HRT. In common with almost any drug therapy, the use of oestrogen and progestogen in postmenopausal women is not without risk. There is an increased incidence of endometrial carcinoma with unopposed oestrogen therapy, although the addition of a progestogen for 12 days each cycle at an adequate dose appears to abolish this increase. Although the data on breast cancer are confusing, there may be a small increase in risk with long-term oestrogen use. There is no overall increase in risk of ovarian cancer but there may be an excess of clear cell and endometrioid tumours. The data on cervical cancer and oestrogen/progestogen therapy are sparse but reassuring. From the published studies, large bowel cancer is unaffected by HRT. Anecdotal reports suggest that the behaviour of malignant melanoma may be altered by postmenopausal hormone therapy, but there are no epidemiological studies to indicate risk.

Work still needs to be done to quantify these risks. New well-designed studies are required and those already reporting results should be continued long term. Until these results are available, our advice to patients on the risks of cancer must of necessity be incomplete.

References

1. Smith DC, Prentice R, Thompson DJ et al. Association of exogenous estrogens and endometrial cancer. N Engl J Med 1975; 293:1164–7.
2. Ziel H, Finkle W. Increased risk of endometrial carcinoma among users of conjugated estrogens. N Engl J Med 1975; 293:1167–70.
3. Mack TM, Pike MC, Henderson BE et al. Estrogens and endometrial cancer in a retirement community. N Engl J Med 1976; 294:1262–7.
4. Chu J, Schweid AI, Weiss NS. Survival among women with endometrial cancer: a comparison of estrogen users and non-users. Am J Obstet Gynecol 1982; 143:569–75.
5. Elwood JM, Boyes DA. Clinical and pathological features and survival of cancer patients in relation to prior use of estrogens. Gynecol Oncol 1980; 10:173–80.
6. Ettinger B, Golditch IM, Friedman G. Gynecologic consequences of long-term unopposed estrogen replacement therapy. Maturitas 1988; 10:271–82.
7. Paganini-Hill A, Ross RK, Henderson BE. Endometrial cancer and patterns of use of oestrogen replacement therapy: a cohort study. Br J Cancer 1989; 59:445–7.
8. Whitehead MI, King RJB, McQueen J, Campbell S. Endometrial histology and biochemistry in climacteric women during oestrogen and oestrogen/progestin therapy. J R Soc Med 1979; 72:322–7.
9. Studd JWW, Thom MH, Paterson MEL, Wade-Evans T. The prevention and treatment of endometrial pathology in postmenopausal women receiving exogenous oestrogens. In: Pasetto N, Paoletti R, Ambrus JL, eds. The menopause and postmenopause. Lancaster: MTP, 1980; 127–39.
10. Whitehead MI, Townsend PT, Pryse-Davies J et al. Effects of various types and dosages of progestogens on the postmenopausal endometrium. J Reprod Med 1982; 27:539–48.
11. Gambrell RD. Prevention of endometrial cancer with progestogens. Maturitas 1986; 8:159–68.
12. Persson I, Adami H-O, Bergkvist L et al. Risk of endometrial cancer after treatment with oestrogens alone or in conjunction with progestogens: results of a prospective study. Br Med J 1989; 298:147–51.
13. Franks AL, Kendrick JS, Tyler CW, Postmenopausal smoking, estrogen replacement therapy, and the risk of endometrial cancer. Am J Obstet Gynecol 1987; 156:20–3.
14. Crook D, Godsland IF, Wynn V. Ovarian hormones and plasma lipoproteins. In: Studd JWW, Whitehead MI, eds. The menopause. Oxford: Blackwell Scientific Publications, 1988; 168–80.
15. Silverstolpe G, Gustafson A, Samsioe G, Svanborg A. Lipid metabolic studies in oophorectomised women: effects of three different progestogens. Acta Obstet Gynecol Scand 1979; 88:89–95.
16. Ottoson UB, Johansson BG, von Schoultz B. Subfractions of high-density lipoprotein cholesterol during estrogen replacement therapy. A comparison between progestogens and natural progesterone. Am J Obstet Gynecol 1985; 151:746–50.
17. Whitehead MI, Townsend PT, Pryse-Davies J, Ryder TA, King RJB. Effects of estrogens and progestins on the biochemistry and morphology of the postmenopausal endometrium. N Engl J Med 1981; 305:1599–604.
18. Lane G, Siddle NC, Ryder TA, Pryse-Davies J, King RJB, Whitehead MI. Effect of dydrogesterone on the oestrogenised postmenopausal endometrium. Br J Obstet Gynaecol 1986; 93:55–62.
19. Lane G, Siddle NC, Ryder TA, Pryse-Davies J, King RJB, Whitehead MI. Is Provera the ideal progestogen for addition to postmenopausal estrogen therapy? Fertil Steril 1986; 45:345–52.
20. Fraser DI, Parsons A, Whitehead MI, Wordsworth J, Stuart G, Pryse-Davis J. The optimal dose of oral norethindrone for addition to transdermal estradiol; a multicenter study. Fertil Steril 1990 (in press).
21. Padwick ML, Pryse-Davies J, Whitehead MI. A simple method for determining the optimal dose of progestin in postmenopausal women receiving estrogens. N Engl J Med 1986; 315:19.
22. Staland B. Continuous treatment with natural oestrogens and progestogens: a method to avoid endometrial hyperstimulation. Maturitas 1981; 3:145–56.
23. Magos AL, Brincat M, Studd JWW, Wardle P, Schlesinger P, O'Dowd T. Amenorrhoea and endometrial atrophy with continuous oral estrogen and progestogen therapy in postmenopausal women. Obstet Gynecol 1985; 65:496–9.
24. Whitehead MI. Prevention of endometrial abnormalities. In: Greenblatt RB, ed. A modern approach to the perimenopausal years. Berlin: de Gruyter, 1986; 189–206.
25. Cramer DW, Devasa SS, Welch WR. Trends in the incidence in endometrioid and clear-cell cancers of the ovary in the United States. Am J Epidemiol 1981; 114:201–8.

26. Weiss NS, Lyon JL, Krishnamurthy S, Ditert SE, Liff JM, Daling JR. Noncontraceptive estrogen use and the occurrence of ovarian cancer. J Natl Cancer Inst 1982; 68:95–8.
27. La Vecchia C, Liberati A, Franceschi S. Noncontraceptive estrogen use and the occurrence of ovarian cancer. J Natl Cancer Inst 1982; 69:1207.
28. Cramer DW, Hutchison GB, Welch WR, Scully RE, Ryan KJ. Determinants of ovarian cancer risk. Reproductive experiences and family history. J Natl Cancer Inst 1983; 71:711–16.
29. Hunt K, Vessey M, McPherson K, Coleman M. Long-term surveillance of mortality and cancer incidence in women receiving hormone replacement therapy. Br J Obstet Gynaecol 1987; 94:620–35.
30. Pike MC, Henderson BE, Casagrande JT, Rosario I, Gray GE. Oral contraceptive use and early abortion as risk factors for breast cancer in young women. Br J Cancer 1981; 43:72–8.
31. Trichopolous D, Macmahon B, Cole P. The menopause and breast cancer risk. J Natl Cancer Inst 1972; 48:605–13.
32. Ross RK, Paganini-Hill A, Gerkins VR. A case-control study of menopausal estrogen therapy and breast cancer. JAMA 1980; 243:1635–40.
33. Brinton LA, Hoover RN, Szklo M, Fraumeni JF. Menopausal estrogen use and risk of breast cancer. Cancer 1981; 47:2517–22.
34. Hoover R, Glass A, Finkle WD et al. Conjugated estrogens and breast cancer risk. J Natl Cancer Inst 1981; 67:815–20.
35. Hiatt RA, Bawol R, Friedman GD, Hoover R. Exogenous estrogen and breast cancer after bilateral oophorectomy. Cancer 1984; 54:139–44.
36. Kelsey JL, Fischer DB, Holford JR et al. Exogenous estrogens and other factors in the epidemiology of breast cancer. J Natl Cancer Inst 1981; 67:327–33.
37. Kaufman DW, Miller DR, Rosenberg L, Helmrich SP. Noncontraceptive estrogen use and the risk of breast cancer. JAMA 1984; 252:63–7.
38. Wingo PA, Layde PM, Lee NC, Rubin G, Ory HW. The risk of breast cancer in postmenopausal women who have used estrogen replacement therapy. JAMA 1987; 257:209–15.
39. Brinton LA, Hoover R, Fraumeni JF. Menopausal oestrogens and breast cancer risk: an expanded case-control study. Br J Cancer 1986; 54:825–32.
40. Thomas DB, Persin JP, Hutchinson WB. Exogenous estrogens and other risk factors for breast cancer in women with benign breast diseases. J Natl Cancer Inst 1982; 69:1017–25.
41. Dupont WD, Page DL, Rogers LW, Parl FF. Influence of exogenous estrogens, proliferative breast disease, and other variables on breast cancer risk. Cancer 1989; 63:948–57.
42. Bergkvist L, Adami H-O, Persson I, Hoover R, Schairer C. The risk of breast cancer after estrogen–progestin replacement. N Engl J Med 1989; 321:293–7.
43. Ewertz M. Influence of non-contraceptive exogenous and endogenous sex hormones on breast cancer risk in Denmark. Int J Cancer 1988; 42:832–8.
44. Gambrell RD. Role of progestogens in the prevention of breast cancer. Maturitas 1986; 8:169–75.
45. Anderson TJ, Fergusson DJP, Raab GM. Cell turnover in the resting human breast; influences of parity, contraceptive pill, age, and laterality. Br J Cancer 1982; 46:376–82.
46. Whitehead MI, Lobo RA. Progestogen use in postmenopausal women. Consensus Conference. Lancet 1988; ii:1243–4.
47. Abdalla HI, Hart DM, Lindsay R et al. Prevention of bone mineral loss in postmenopausal women by norethisterone. Obstet Gynecol 1985; 66:789–92.
48. Stoll BA. Effect of Lyndiol, an oral contraceptive, on breast cancer. Br Med J 1967; 1:150–3.
49. Stoll BA, Parbhoo S. Treatment of menopausal symptoms in breast cancer patients. Lancet 1988; i:1278–9.
50. Schottenfield D, Berg JW, Vitsky B. Incidence of multiple primary cancers. II. Index cancers arising in the stomach and digestive system. J Natl Cancer Inst 1969; 43: 77–86.
51. Weiss S, Darling JR, Chow WH. Incidence of cancer of the large bowel in relation to reproductive and hormonal factors. J Natl Cancer Inst 1981; 67:57–60.
52. Potter JD, McMichael AJ. Large bowel cancer in women in relation to reproductive and hormonal factors: a case-control study. J Natl Cancer Inst 1983; 71:703–9.
53. Davis FG, Furner SE, Persky V, Koch M. The influence of parity and exogenous female hormones on the risk of colorectal cancer. Int J Cancer 1989; 43:587–90.
54. Markland FS, Horn D. Steroid hormone receptor studies in a melanoma model system. J Supramol Struct 1980; 13: 35–46.
55. Walker MJ, Beattie CW, Briele HA, Patel MK, Das Gupta TK. Estrogen receptor in malignant melanoma. J Clin Oncol 1987; 5:1254–61.
56. Proctor JW, Auclair BG, Stockowski L. Brief communications; endocrine factors and the

growth and spread of B16 melanoma. J Natl Cancer Inst 1976; 57:1197–8.

57. Lopez RE, Bhakoo H, Paolini NS, Rosen F, Holyoke ED, Goldrosen MH. Effect on estrogen on the growth of B16 melanoma. Surg Forum 1978; 29:153–4.

58. Shaw HM, Milton GW, Farago G, McCarthy WH. Endocrine influences on survival from malignant melanoma. Cancer 1978; 42:669–77.

59. Pack GT, Scharnagel IM. The prognosis for malignant melanoma in pregnant women. Cancer 1951; 4:324–34.

60. Shiu MH, Schottenfield D, Maclean B, Fortner JG. Adverse effects of pregnancy on melanoma. A reappraisal. Cancer 1976; 37:181–7.

61. Sadoff L, Winkeley J, Tyson S. Is malignant melanoma an estrogen dependent tumour? Oncology 1973; 27:244–57.

62. Adler S, Gaeta J. Malignant melanoma. In: Helm F, ed. Cancer dermatology. Philadelphia, Lea and Febiger, 1979, 141–57.

Discussion

Studd: It may be that much of the apparent increase found with breast carcinoma may be one of increased surveillance in women who are having medical attendance, more palpation, more mammography. It may also be a problem of diagnosis in that in oestrogen-responsive tissues like endometrium and breast there is this grey area between atypical ductal hyperplasia, ductal carcinoma and invasive carcinoma, and this may be reflected in increased pick-up and increased diagnosis and decreased mortality, which two studies have shown.

I know that Professor Persson has answers to all of these questions.

Persson: The first question relates to detection and suggests that the women who is seeing her doctor for HRT has an increased likelihood of having a tumour detected. But it might operate in the other direction, because when she sees a doctor at her first visit she would be examined in the breast and in terms of risk factors for breast cancer, and those women who have a lesion in the breast – they might have mammography before starting treatment – would be screened out at that first visit. And so the women who are being put on oestrogens would be at a lower risk during HRT, in that population given HRT.

If there was a detection bias, I would expect it to be in the early phase of treatment and not by increasing duration, and there are good reasons to believe that there is little or no influence in our data of detection bias.

The second point referred to issues in endometrial histology. We do not believe that the problem of histology in the breast is much of an issue. Invasive breast carcinoma is quite easy to diagnose, in contrast to the lesions in the endometrium. The cases that we picked up in the foreword are those entered in the registry as invasive breast carcinomas and there is no doubt in our minds that these are real invasive carcinomas. And so we do not think there is a problem with endometrial cancer comparable with the problem with breast cancer.

However, it should be said that the associations for endometrial cancer cannot be explained away by this phenomenon. There have been extensive reviews of the pathology in most studies and that has not changed the results of the studies.

Studd: And the better survival? Is there now some doubt about that?

Persson: There are few data to say that the survival is improved but we are encouraged by our findings in the study of relative survival among the cohort of breast cancer cases as related to the background breast cancer cases. This is relative survival, the observed survival among these cases relative to that expected in the background population.

After 8 years of follow-up, those cases diagnosed within one year of cessation of HRT may have a better relative survival, but that could be due to other factors. It could be lead-time bias in such studies due to increased surveillance; no one really knows when the tumour started. And this method of measuring survival might also reflect an increased survival from other causes of disease besides breast cancer. It is a comparison with a background population and it might be that these women have less cardiovascular disease; which they do have because we have looked at it. It is not altogether easy.

In one study looking at mortality from breast cancer an increased incidence was found but a reduced mortality [1]. The argument is that at the onset of treatment, the women with a prevalent cancer or perhaps with risk factors for breast cancer are screened out, which means that from the start this is a population of women without any cancer, and a prolonged period of follow-up would be needed in order to see mortality increasing. That is what we have seen in the Swedish cohort. As yet there are no published data, but we have looked at mortality by years of follow-up. It is low at the start of the follow-up but it increses with follow-up time. So we need time to look at that.

Vessey: The same thing is true in the collaborative study which Kate Hunt and I co-ordinated. As reported, incidence was high and mortality was low, but with the passage of time mortality has risen. Those data remain unpublished but this may be due to initial selection bias, as Professor Persson has said.

There are two types of bias here. One is the initial selection bias which determines who gets into the cohort. We would expect, certainly in clinical practice although perhaps not in general practice, that people who have tumours would be screened out. That is one sort of bias. But then there is the suggestion that this rate of early detection might be further influenced by preferential mammography, preferential BSE, preferential screening by the doctors which might help them to boost the numbers of early tumours. That might tend to increase incidence without being reflected in mortality.

The point is that it is important to monitor mortality as well as incidence to try as far as possible to take care of those biases.

One of the advances of the late 1970s and early 1980s was the development of meta-analysis. Richard Peto has become a Fellow of the Royal Society for his brilliant work on meta-analysis in clinical trials, which has shown that if the effects of many clinical trials can be combined in a statistically sound way, a seeming random pattern makes sense in the field of small effects, and that this approach can resolve this difficulty of some studies which show no effect, some which show a positive effect and the odd one which shows no effect. Obviously this has been of tremendous importance in relation to aspirin and anticoagulants, and there are many other examples. But what does Professor Persson think about the application of meta-analysis and meta-aggression techniques to epidemiological observation studies as opposed to randomised controlled trials? I tend to approach things much as he does, putting up the risk and perhaps the confidence limits and looking at the pattern. One is so insecure about that variability of the design of the studies and so insecure about the ways in which they have been analysed and the different grouping intervals that it is very hard to produce any meta-analysis type overview. But obviously he has thought a lot about this.

Are there any views on that sort of unifying approach in relation to this kind of problem?

If we could carry out a meta-analysis, I am fairly confident, from Professor Persson's data, that we could come up with a small positive effect that was probably related to duration of use, and in some ways might be more satisfying derived from meta-analysis than derived from visual inspection plus commentary. I certainly never got into this field and I wondered whether he had thought about it.

Persson: No, I have not. I have heard the arguments, but in the context of studies on COCs and breast cancer. There was a meeting in London in 1989, both brothers Peto were there and there was strong argument from them to perform this meta-analysis on that issue. However, there was strong resistance, as far a I could gather, among the various authors of studies to doing that, because, as the studies were so different in their methodological aspects, it would not be meaningful. But I suppose that it would be feasible to look at the five cohort studies that I showed, to pool the data from these and to look at it.

All of the five cohort studies were consistent at present in showing this pattern or risk increase with increasing duration. But perhaps it would give much more power to the analysis and one might be able to do more subgroup analysis. However, there are very few studies on progestogens.

Ross: I guess my feeling in this regard is that meta-analysis would probably tell us no more than Professor Persson's summary. We can get a good picture from his duration of use data based on the cohorts he has looked at.

I tend not to like meta-analysis for observational studies.

Vessey: That was my view, but I was interested to see whether other people held the same view.

Ross: I tend to think it would not be very helpful.

I also do not agree with Professor Persson's view on prospective studies. I think the implication was that prospective studies are somehow inherently better in addressing questions such as oestrogens in breast cancer. With long latent periods, and with an exposoure after long-term use that is easily measured, case-controlled studies should provide as good an answer as prospective studies, and the balance of the evidence suggests that they have. And Professor Persson has given more or less the same answer to these questions.

Whitehead: I have some problems with Professor Persson's studies. His group in the same month published an interesting paper that seems to have been completely forgotten and on which nobody comments, on details of mammographic findings in these two groups of women [2]. My understanding of that paper is that the oestrogen users who subsequently went on to have breast cancer had more worrying types of pattern on Wolfe's scores than in the population not exposed to oestrogen. That is very important because it is a very important confounder.

Persson: It is true that there was a higher prevalence of the less-favourable mammographic pattern among those put on oestrogens and it seemed that this pattern did not change over time as treatment continued. We had two assessments of their mammography before and after treatment and they did have more of the unfavourable pattern. We are not sure what that means, but it is supposed, and disputed, that this pattern is a high-risk pattern for subsequent breast cancer. But this is not agreed by all authors.

Whitehead: Professor Persson is not sure what it means. I would suggest that that type of mammographic pattern identifies a high-risk group for breast cancer whether they take oestrogens or not, and that all that the researchers may be observing is the natural history of the type of mammographic pattern independent of oestrogen exposure in the group under study.

Persson: Which suggests that we have a selection bias; that those women who develop symptoms that make them want HRT are also at increased risk from the beginning. That is a possibility, but it is hardly likely

Whitehead: But it cannot be excluded?

Persson: No. But I can argue about it.
   We know from data from a case control study in Uppsala that women who have hot flushes are less likely to develop breast cancer. In other words it is likely that the women who have these indications may be more oestrogen-deficient than those who do not. If we believe in the hypothesis of oestrogens and breast cancer we would see the reverse. When controlling for confounding, we ended up with higher estimates. That means that the cohort women who developed breast cancer would rather be at a lower risk from the start regardless of oestrogen exposure than the others. That speaks against it but I agree that we do not know for sure and that they might be at an increased risk but I do not believe it.

Drife: I am concerned because the glandular component of breast tissue responds more readily to progestogens than to oestrogen in the normal cycle and I wonder what data there are on long-term exposure to opposed regimes of HRT and breast cancer incidence.

Persson: I did not say that, but the data showing the effects of the various regimens should be interpreted with great caution because they rely on small numbers. That is the problem with the cohort study. If we look at the various subgroups we end up with small numbers. That is the problem.
   But I wanted to show it because there is a pattern, and there is a pattern with increasing risk in all of these groups. We are saying that the risk increase seen after long-term oestrogen usage might not be eliminated, although I think it is an exaggeration to say that it might increase the risk. But we do not have very much power in our study to look at that. There are only ten cases in that cell of women taking combined treatment only for more than 6 years.

Drife: Were any of the 26 studies and the 16 studies related to long-term exposure to opposed regimes?

Persson: The only study that I can think of is Hunt and colleagues' cohort study [1]. The women in that study were on various different regimens. It states in the paper that 43% of the women were on some kind of combined treatment, but I do not recall exactly what it was. If they looked at some groups that combined, then Professor Vessey might be able to answer that.

Vessey: There were well over 100 different treatment combinations in that study. This is one of the difficulties in looking at HRT in any study in Britain because so many gynaecologists have their own particular combination. Kate Hunt and I coped with some 150 different treatment regimens. We were able to divide them between opposed and unopposed and it is certainly true that the majority of opposed regimens were not very strongly opposed, but beyond that it was difficult to draw any further conclusions.

We did a case control analysis at the end in which we compared the cases of breast cancer with controls and the treatment that really stood out was unopposed ethinyloestradiol. But it was very difficult to go beyond that.

Persson: One needs to understand the biology of the breast in relation to oestrogens and progestogens. There are different thoughts about that. Tom Anderson has clinical data on biopsy material from the breast and found that the mitosis rate in breast tissue, among breast cells, would be further increased in the luteal phase, suggesting that progestogens might act differently in the breast than the endometrium. But he has been challenged many times, specifically by the French group, who have shown, in in vitro studies with cell cultures, an antioestrogenic effect from progestogens on cell cultures with normal breast cells.

Studd: We can agree that with our present state of knowledge there is no logic at all in giving progestogens to protect the breast, as is the advice of very many people. That makes no sense at all.

Meade: I would not want to interrupt discussion about the relationship of progestogen to breast cancer but I do want to comment on the meta-analysis point that was under discussion. As Professor Ross was indicating, there is a difference between randomised controlled trials and observational studies. Randomised controlled trials have all the advantages of elimination of bias, provided they are done properly, and under those circumstances it is perfectly reasonable to get an overall estimate of the contributions of the separate trials, and people have to be altruistic and to accept that their own contribution will be merged with that of other people.

But the position is different with observational studies, where we are up against the problems of bias and by adding up the different effects we may simply be adding up a constant effect of a bias. So I would agree that what we need to do there is to display the data.

One principle that is common to both, whether it is randomised controlled trials or observational studies, that more and more people are accepting now, is that it is not reasonable to show the results of selected studies. One must show the results of all the studies that have dealt with a particular problem.

Ross: I believe Mr Cust concluded that cyclical combination therapy would bring endometrial cancer risk back to baseline: that is, the risk of a woman using no hormone replacement therapy at all. There does not yet seem to be a lot of data on that issue and I am wondering whether that is really a sensible conclusion. I ask because of the fact that typically, oestrogens are given for 14 or 15 days each month followed by oestrogens with a progestogen, and that period each month when the women gets oestrogens alone could be expected to raise the risk above and beyond the baseline risk of a women getting no therapy.

Cust: Yes. I would agree that there are not yet enough data to be able to say categorically that we shall be able to adduce baseline values from this. But, whilst oestrogen stimulation for 16 days or whatever will be higher than in the untreated postmenopausal woman, obviously the progestogen position will be much greater than in the postmenopausal woman for the subsequent 12 days. Whereas she may well have a low level of oestrogen stimulation continuously, the women who are on oestrogen therapy do still get progestogen changes for these 12 days.

Notelovitz: Could I ask a question about progestogens and the proliferative phase?
  If a patient who is on combination therapy maintains a proliferative phase without any atypia, what evidence is there that she will develop endometrial cancer? It is a very important question with relation to the potency of progestogens and the potential side effects in the cardiovascular system?

Cust: In other words, the woman who has a normal proliferative phase on unopposed oestrogen therapy?

Notelovitz: On opposed oestrogen therapy. If a patient who is on combination therapy, oestrogens plus progestogen, maintains a proliferative endometrium without any atypia, what evidence is there that she is at greater risk of developing endometrial cancer?

Cust: I do not think there is any evidence that she is at greater risk of developing endometrial cancer. The problem is the great inter-patient variation in response to progestogen, and whilst some women may respond very favourably to a very low dose of progestogen, some women obviously need a higher dose and in certain cases one may be able to identify that from the day of onset of her bleeding. But certainly the woman who maintains a normal proliferative endometrium may not be at increased risk.
  We biopsied the women on day 6, and it may be that if one went on to biopsy them later, they would have developed a secretory phase at that stage. We do not have those data.

Studd: In that Padwick [3] paper, some of that bleeding occurred before the end of the progestogen course. So what we are saying is that if we oppose it correctly the bleeding is meant to occur after she stops the progestogen. That is normal, and we are more anxious about any bleeding that occurs within the progestogen course. Is that all that it means?

Cust: It may be that women who bleed on day 11, i.e. the last one or two days of progestogen therapy, are as well protected as women who bleed after the end of their progestogen therapy, whereas the women who bleed much earlier in the cycle do not seem to be getting the same protection.

Studd: But the object is to create false periods after the progestogen course.

Stevenson: Two questions. The first relates to the potency of the oestrogens used.

How many cases of breast cancer in Professor Persson's study were taking ethinyloestradiol. He said that only 5% of the population were taking it, but how many cases of cancer were taking it?

Persson: Just as many as in the cohort, that is 5%. There is no difference in the distribution among the various compounds.

Both Dr Stevenson and Mr Whitehead are suggesting that the ethinyloestradiol compounds are more harmful than the others, but we have no evidence of that at all.

Stevenson: Is that because the numbers are not big enough?

Persson: Yes. It is an infrequently used drug and it has a diminishing presence in the market in Sweden.

Stevenson: My second question is about the confounding variables. What about the previous oestrogen usage in these women, whether it be hormone replacement therapy before they came into the study or oral contraceptive use premenopausally?

Persson: Oral contraceptives are not a problem for two reasons. First, there has been no report of an increased risk of breast cancer among menopausal women who have taken COCs. The literature is quite clear on that. The other reason is that these women were recruited into the cohort with a median age of 53. When COCs were introduced to the Swedish market their median age was 40 and they are unlikely to have been exposed to COCs.

We do not have those exact data, but I would not expect it to make any difference at all.

Stevenson: What about postmenopausal oestrogen use?

Persson: That was characterised from the questionnaires. The prescription data recruited the women into the cohort and then a sample of that cohort had questionnaires asking about their total intake of oestrogens. Half of them had started to take their oestrogens before the first date of recruitment, and we have estimates of total HRT intake.

Whitehead: But is that included in Fig. 14.3 showing duration of exposure?

Persson: Of course. That is the method of case cohort analysis. In other words, the cohort itself is characterised in detail by means of that sample questionnaire, and it is extrapolated to the whole cohort by means of statistical methods.

Kanis: There are very different confidence intervals in the various studies and so clearly there are sources of bias and very different relative risks together with different confidence limits. Would Professor Persson like to speculate?

Persson: I said briefly that every study has to be examined critically because of problems with that study. These are all observational studies. I did not have the time to go into it and it would be quite boring.

But we need to get some assessment of the whole picture. The more studies that there are, the more cohort studies that perhaps there are that are consistent in showing that risk, the more plausible would be the hypothesis that there is a relationship, a causal relationship. But bias or some confounding aspect can never be excluded.

Meade: The size of the confidence interval is simply a question of numbers.

Lindsay: The data were well presented but I always have a problem. Those who have an interest in breast cancer do themselves something of a disservice when they present their data, and Professor Persson may be guilty of this in that he presented the negative side of conjugated equine oestrogens by saying that he does not have enough numbers, but when he came to the progestogen issue he did not comment on the numbers issue, and it did not come up until the presentation. Nor did he comment on the relative risk of 1.6 in his paper in the women who claim not to have taken oestrogens.

Persson: That has been taken to say that the cohort women were selected in having an increased risk.

Among non-compliers, the women who said, in their questionnaires, that they had not taken the drug – some women – showed an increased relative risk. But it is a problem of classification. We had the opportunity to look at their medical records and to look at their prescription data, and we found that those breast cancer women who said that they had not taken anything were short-term users. But in the analysis, for the sake of consistency we used only the questionnaire data. However, when we discuss it we can say that these women who said they had not taken oestrogen were in fact short-term users, but we know it from the prescription data.

If we transfer the group of women who were takers to the group of early users, the increased risk among non-compliers disappears and the risk in the short-term usage group is at baseline.

References

1. Hunt K, Vessey M, McPherson K, Coleman M. Long-term surveillance of mortality and cancer incidence in women receiving hormone replacement therapy. Br J Obstet Gynaecol 1987; 94:620–35.
2. Bergkvist L, Persson, I, Adami HO, Schairer C. Risk factors for breast and endometrial cancer in a cohort of women treated with menopausal oestrogens. Int J Epidemiol 1988; 17:732–7.

3. Padwick ML, Pryse-Davies J, Whitehead MI. A simple method for determining the optimal dose of progestin in postmenopausal women receiving estrogens. N Engl J Med 1986; 315:19.

Chapter 16

Progestogens: Symptomatic and Metabolic Side Effects

J. C. Montgomery and D. Crook

Introduction

Oestrogen replacement therapy in postmenopausal women will prevent osteoporosis [1] and treat symptoms such as hot flushes [2]. First introduced over 50
years ago, postmenopausal oestrogen use did not gain popularity until the 1950s
and 1960s, with the USA at the forefront. In the 1970s reports emerged of an
apparent rise in the incidence of endometrial carcinoma in women given
unopposed oestrogen [3,4]. Although these studies documented a five- to
sevenfold increase in risk, the significance of this has been challenged. The
tumours were in general well differentiated and at an early stage, both factors
being associated with a good prognosis, suggesting an overdiagnosis of carcinoma
with an underdiagnosis of hyperplasia [5].

Recent studies have estimated the risk of endometrial carcinoma associated
with the use of unopposed oestrogens as a two- to threefold increase over the
expected rate [6,7]. Although it has been suggested that this was due to
continuous exposure to oestrogens, cyclical oestrogen therapy (3 weeks out of 4)
is still associated with a 7%–15% increased risk of hyperplasia [8].

The addition of a monthly course of progestogen decreases the incidence of
endometrial hyperplasia [8] and endometrial carcinoma [9]. Duration of progestogen use, rather than dose alone, appears to be the primary factor in the
prevention of endometrial hyperplasia. A 7-day course of progestogen will result
in a 5% incidence of endometrial hyperplasia whereas a 12–13 day course will
result in virtually a zero incidence [8].

Assuming a 12–13-day course, the daily oral doses of progestogen necessary to protect the endometrium vary from 200 to 300 mg (micronised progesterone), 10–20 mg (dydrogesterone), 10 mg (medroxyprogesterone acetate), 1 mg (norethisterone) down to 150 μg (levonorgestrel) [10,11].

Natural progesterone is poorly absorbed when given orally, although a micronised form is available (Utrogestan, Besins-Iscovesco, Paris). However, doses high enough to prevent endometrial hyperplasia are associated with drowsiness due to the action of progesterone as a central nervous system depressant.

Table 16.1. Classification of progestogens

I. *Natural* e.g. progesterone

II. *Synthetic*
a. Structurally related to progesterone e.g. medroxyprogesterone acetate, dydrogesterone
b. Structurally related to testosterone e.g. norethisterone, levonorgestrel
    1. Derivatives of norethisterone e.g. norethisterone acetate
    2. Derivatives of levonorgestrel e.g. desogestrel, norgestimate, gestodene

As a consequence of this, various synthetic progestogens have been developed for use in hormone replacement therapy (HRT) (Table 16.1). The pharmacology of these steroids has been reviewed recently [12]. Briefly, progestogens can be divided into two groups: those structurally related to progesterone, such as medroxyprogesterone acetate (MPA) and dydrogesterone, and those structurally related to 19-nortestosterone, such as norethisterone and levonorgestrel. There is a further division of this latter group into those derived from norethisterone, such as norethisterone acetate, and those derived from levonorgestrel, such as desogestrel, norgestrel and gestodene. This latter group – the "third generation" progestogens – are structural modifications of levonorgestrel in which unwanted androgenic characteristics of the parent compound have been reduced, leaving the progestational properties unchanged. These progestogens are already used in combined oral contraceptives and are currently undergoing trials to evaluate their suitability for HRT.

Use of Progestogens in Hormone Replacement Therapy

Progestogens are usually prescribed as a cyclical monthly course in combination with oestrogen therapy. However, a continuous dose of progestogens combined with continuous oestrogens may be used to prevent a monthly bleed in the majority of women [13]. Alternatively, progestogens may be used as a sole agent in women with a contraindication to oestrogen therapy, such as breast or endometrial carcinoma. Progestogens given alone have been shown to decrease hot flushes [14,15], albeit less efficiently than oestrogen therapy, and to prevent osteoporosis [16].

The progestogens used in HRT differ markedly in their progestagenic, androgenic and even oestrogenic activities. These characteristics may influence both symptomatic and metabolic side effects. The overall side effects of combined therapy will also depend on the dose (and hence bioavailability) of the progestogen, the route of administration and the balance between the oestrogen and progestogen components.

Symptomatic Effects of Progestogens

Most gynaecologists are aware that women given progestogens report adverse side effects, and that these may be so severe as to lead to discontinuation of therapy. Such symptoms include irritability, depression, headache, bloating and weight gain, symptoms typical of the premenstrual syndrome [17].

Although these problems are acknowledged on a practical basis, there has been a paucity of placebo-controlled studies on the adverse effects of progestogens, either when given alone or in combination with oestrogen. Such studies are essential given the importance of maintaining compliance with combined HRT.

Effects of Progestogens When Used Alone

Paterson [15] performed a randomised double-blind cross-over study which looked at the effects of norethisterone (5 mg per day) versus placebo in the treatment of menopausal symptoms. Patients assessed their own symptoms and side effects using a questionnaire. The women were followed for six months, with a crossover (active treatment/placebo or placebo/active treatment) occurring after 3 months. Norethisterone was significantly superior to placebo for the treatment of hot flushes, although not for other menopausal symptoms such as depression, anxiety or loss of energy. This study indicates that norethisterone given alone has few side effects. One major criticism of this relatively small (18 women) study is that the women were previously untreated and so any amelioration of their hot flushes may well have influenced their perception of adverse effects.

Effect of Oestrogen/Progestogen Combinations

There have been few placebo-controlled studies of the effects of progestogens given in combination with oestrogen therapy. Three studies have investigated the effect of a progestogen given cyclically to women receiving oestrogen.

Hammerbäck et al. [18] gave 22 postmenopausal women percutaneous oestradiol cream for 21 out of 28 days. Eleven of the group were also given 5 mg/day lynestrenol (a progestogen related to norethisterone) for days 10–21. Symptoms were assessed using a linear analogue scale. When compared to women given oestrogen alone, women given combined therapy had exacerbated negative moods and a decrease in positive moods. Breast tenderness and bloating were also significantly increased on combined therapy. These adverse symptoms appeared shortly after taking the progestogen, lasting several days into the treatment-free break (Fig. 16.1).

Magos et al. [19] designed a double-blind placebo controlled study to evaluate

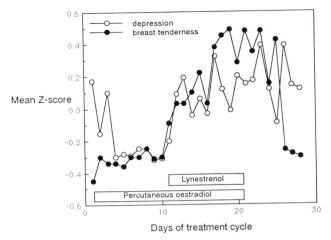

Fig. 16.1. Mean depression and breast tenderness scores in postmenopausal women given sequential oestrogen/progestogen therapy. Values are daily means obtained after six cycles of treatment. (After Hammerbäck et al. [18].)

the symptomatic effects of norethisterone in women receiving therapy for the treatment of menopausal symptoms. A total of 70 women receiving oestradiol and testosterone implants (mean duration 2.1 years, range 0.5–7.5 years) were allocated either 5 or 2.5 mg of norethisterone for one week out of five.

Physical, psychological and behavioural symptoms were measured using the Moos Menstrual Distress Questionnaire [20]. This quantifies eight clusters of symptoms: six negative, one positive and one control. Norethisterone at a dose

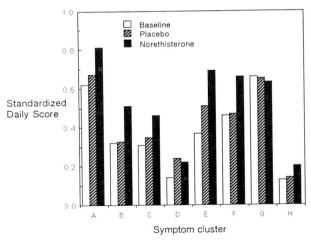

Fig. 16.2. Effects of placebo and norethisterone (5 mg/day) on symptom complexes in post-menopausal women receiving oestradiol implants. Symptom clusters: pain (A), loss of concentration (B), behavioural changes (C), autonomic reactions (D), water retention (E), negative effects (F), and arousal (G). H is a control cluster. (After Magos et al. [19].)

of 2.5 mg/day had no adverse effects when compared to placebo. When the higher dose (5 mg) was used, there was a significant deterioration in negative clusters such as depression, anxiety and irritability (Fig. 16.2).

In a recent placebo-controlled study of the effects of progestogens, Sherwin and Gelfand [21] evaluated MPA in combination with conjugated equine oestrogens (CEE). Ninety-five women were randomised into four groups: 0.625 mg/day CEE with 5 mg/day MPA or placebo, and 1.2 mg/day CEE with and without 5 mg/day MPA. The efficacy of symptomatic relief and the frequency and intensity of side effects were monitored during a pretreatment month and then during months 3, 6, 9 and 12 of treatment. Frequency of hot flushes was reduced in all groups, with MPA being indistinguishable from placebo. Similarly, daily ratings of nausea were low and not affected by the progestogen. Ratings of well-being energy level and sleep quality consistently showed deterioration in women given 0.62 mg CEE and 5 mg MPA when compared to those given 1.25 mg CEE and no progestogen.

The strategy of continuous combined therapy is attractive in that it involves lower daily doses of progestogen. Whitehead et al. [22] concluded that no continuous regimen has adequately demonstrated an improvement in side effects over sequential therapy.

Summary

There is an evident lack of information about the effects of progestogens on the symptomatic aspects of HRT. The few studies that have used placebo control indicate that progestogens may have adverse effects on both physical and psychological symptoms, although there is little evidence that one progestogen is better than another. Such comparative studies, reinforced by placebo control, are necessary if HRT is to achieve wider acceptance in women undergoing the menopause.

Metabolic Aspects of Progestogens

The lack of basic information about the effects of different progestogens on symptoms contrasts with the extensive body of data detailing the metabolic effects of oestrogens and progestogens.

Metabolic Risk

Oestrogens and progestogens affect many mebabolic processes aside from those concerned with the reproductive system. Over the past two decades there has been a growing awareness that apparently minor changes in areas such as insulin-mediated glucose handling or plasma lipid transport may be associated with risk of disease. These relationships hold even when the levels remain inside the range seen within the general population. Consequently, the evaluation of these metabolic changes has assumed increasing importance in the evaluation of the long-term safety of oestrogen/progestogen combinations, whether as oral contraceptives or as HRT.

This approach contrasts with the earlier view that metabolic parameters should be monitored solely to detect overt disease such as diabetes mellitus or hyperlipidaemia. Instead, the concept of biochemical risk markers has been introduced: factors that may relate to the possibility of future disease. These metabolic measurements have assumed a greater significance due to the recognition that risk markers relate to disease in a continuous and graded manner, contrasting with the older concepts of a threshold effect and "normal ranges".

The significance of metabolic risk markers is constantly under debate. Nevertheless, it would seem a prudent policy to formulate HRT so as to have minimal effect on risk markers, or perhaps to change them in ways which might reduce disease risk.

Effects on the Coagulation System

Oral oestrogens, especially synthetic oestrogens, increase the synthesis of clotting factors and other hepatic proteins. Accordingly, the doses of oestrogen used in oral contraception and in HRT has been minimised. Analysis of the impact of oestrogen replacement therapy is complicated by a lack of consensus over which aspects of clotting are the more important: steroid hormones affect both procoagulant and anticoagulant systems, and there may be some latitude for change as long as the balance is maintained. There are few data on the effect of combined HRT on coagulation factors and no evidence to suggest that concern about blood coagulation should influence the choice of progestogen.

Effects on Glucose and Insulin Metabolism

There are relatively few studies of the effects of HRT on glucose and insulin metabolism. Studies in users of oral contraceptives [23] indicate that oestrogen/progestogen combinations can reduce glucose tolerance and induce hyper-insulinaemia, and that these effects are mediated by the dose and androgenic nature of progestogen (and by the balance between the oestrogen and pro-gestogen components). It is not known how transferable these findings will be to the study of HRT. There is increasing interest in the involvement of hyper-insulinaemia in the cluster of metabolic disorders associated with cardiovascular disease [24] and there is a need for studies of glucose and insulin metabolism in users of combined HRT.

Effects on Lipid Transport

One of the most topical aspects of combined HRT is the effects of lipid metabolism. This interest derives from the observation that unopposed oral oestrogens protect against cardiovascular disease, and that this protection appears to be mediated through the plasma lipoprotein system [25]. It has been calculated that, for 100 000 women given combined HRT for 10 years, 4 to 5 times as many lives would be saved from ischaemic heart disease as would be saved by the complications of oesteoporotic hip fractures [26]. This saving would also far outweigh any putative deaths from breast cancer. Although there may be direct effects on the arterial wall [27], plasma lipoprotein metabolism, especially high density lipoprotein metabolism [25], has emerged as the candidate mechanism for this apparently protective effect.

In general, women taking unopposed oral oestrogens have lower levels of low density lipoprotein (LDL) and higher levels of high density lipoprotein (HDL) cholesterol levels than non-users, a profile which would be associated with protection from cardiovascular disease [28]. The interest in the metabolic effects of HRT progestogens is largely directed towards showing whether these steroids will oppose the apparently beneficial actions of oestrogens. If a combined HRT regimen does not lower LDL cholesterol and raise HDL cholesterol, then the protection from cardiovascular disease may be lost.

Accordingly, there have been numerous studies of the effects of combined HRT on lipid metabolism, often of considerable sophistication. Although this approach has increased our understanding of the pharmacological effects of HRT, the proliferation of measures of lipid metabolism may be intimidating. A recent review [29] of laboratory indices for evaluating oestrogen/progestogen effects on lipoprotein metabolism lists nearly 30 possible measurements, including lipoprotein fractions and subfractions (each measured in terms of their cholesterol, triglyceride, phospholipid or protein content) together with specific apolipoproteins and enzymes and permutations of these measurements, such as LDL/HDL cholesterol and apoB/apoAI.

Although many of these factors are of interest in understanding the precise mechanisms by which steroid hormones affect lipoprotein metabolism, we will concentrate on triglycerides, LDL, HDL and HDL subfraction cholesterol. Total cholesterol has been excluded as it is of limited use when considering the effects of HRT. Total cholesterol represents the sum of the cholesterol contained in metabolically different fractions, some of which relate to risk in opposite ways. For instance, a regimen which increased risk by lowering HDL, but did not affect other lipoproteins, would lower total cholesterol and could be misinterpreted as lowering risk. Nevertheless, the measurement of total cholesterol is obligatory as it allows estimation of LDL cholesterol [30].

Numerous reviews of the effects of oestrogens and progestogens on plasma lipoprotein metabolism are available [28,31,32]. Only sequential therapies are discussed here as continuous combined therapies have yet to demonstrate any clear advantage in terms of metabolic effects [22].

When considering these effects it is important to remember that the great majority of studies look at plasma lipoprotein metabolism during the phase of progestogen administration, where any adverse effects are likely to be accentuated.

Triglycerides

In addition to their role as fuel for delivery from the intestine and the liver to peripheral tissues, triglycerides are a structural component of lipoproteins. Although present in all lipoproteins, in the fasted state they are found primarily in very low density lipoproteins. The risk factor status of triglycerides is controversial, with the weight of epidemiological evidence failing to demonstrate an independent association with risk [33]. Such studies indicate that the high triglyceride levels seen in men and women who develop coronary heart disease (CHD) may be a consequence of their low levels of HDL, and are not in themselves causal. Nevertheless, it would seem reasonable to minimise the metabolic disturbance induced by combined HRT.

Natural oestrogens, and those given by non-oral routes, have little effect on triglyceride levels [34]. However, when synthetic or conjugated oestrogens are given orally, the liver responds to the first-pass delivery by increasing synthesis of triglyceride-rich lipoproteins, thus increasing plasma triglyceride concen-trations [28]. Progestogens, particularly those with androgenic properties, can lower triglyceride levels and have been used therapeutically for this purpose [35].

In combined HRT, many progestogens are able to oppose the oestrogen-induced increase, with the net effect of an increase, no change or decrease, depending on the balance between the two steroids [36,37]. How do we interpret the effects of a combination containing a progestogen such as dydrogesterone [38], which is unable to oppose the increase in triglyceride levels induced by oestrogen? Although the resulting elevated levels of triglyceride would not pose a problem according to current concepts of risk, it may be worthwhile to speculate on strategies which would avoid this increase. These include the use of progestogens with androgenic activities, in itself unattractive due to the effects of these agents on other aspects of lipid metabolism, the use of natural oestrogens, and use of hormones given by non-oral routes such as patches [39].

Low Density Lipoproteins

Depending on dose and type, oestrogens can lower LDL cholesterol, with the degree of lowering related to the initial levels [40]. Progestogens given alone can increase LDL cholesterol if given in sufficiently high doses [41]. When given in combination, the progestogen is able to oppose the LDL-lowering effect of oestrogen. The net effect will depend on the balance of the two components, with progestogens with androgenic characteristics more tenacious in their opposition to the oestrogen effect. Fortunately, few of the progestogens currently used in combined HRT are able to overcome the effects of oestrogen on LDL.

Thus, LDL levels are unchanged from pretreatment in postmenopausal women given levonorgestrel [36,37] or are lowered if the formulation contains a less androgenic progestogen such as dydrogesterone [38] or norethindrone acetate [42]. When given with percutaneous oestradiol, natural progesterone had no effect on LDL cholesterol [36]. Similarly, MPA had no effect when given with oestradiol valerate [37].

High Density Lipoproteins

Virtually all forms of oral oestrogen can increase HDL [28]. In the light of the Lipid Research Clinics Follow-up Study [25] and of more recent epidemiological support for the protective role of HDL in women [43], this effect is of considerable interest. However, the majority of currently prescribed regimens result in a net reduction in HDL cholesterol. Progestogens on their own can lower HDL cholesterol if given in sufficient doses [41]; when given in combi-nation, the net effect will depend on the balance between the oestrogen and progestogen components.

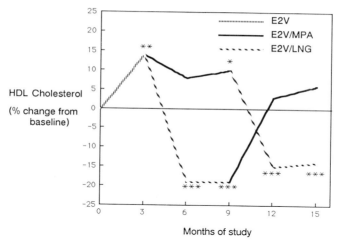

Fig. 16.3. Percentage changes in high density lipoprotein cholesterol in postmenopausal women given oestradiol valerate (E2V) with and without progestogen. After 3 months of unopposed E2V, the women were given medroxyprogesterone acetate (MPA) or levonorgestrel (LNG) in a double-blind design. After 6 months of combined therapy, the regimens were crossed over for a further 6 months. *P<0.05, **P<0.01, ***P<0.001 (differences from baseline values). (After Hirvonen et al. [37].)

The difference between progestogens in their effect on HDL cholesterol is demonstrated in Fig. 16.3. Hirvonen et al. [37] gave untreated postmenopausal women oral oestradiol valerate (2 mg/day) for 3 months, raising their HDL cholesterol by 15%. The women were then randomised to receive either MPA (10 mg/day) or levonorgestrel (0.25 mg/day), both given for 10 days/month, in addition to the oestradiol. After six months, the two progestogens were crossed over. Medroxyprogesterone acetate weakly opposed the oestradiol effect, with HDL levels still being higher than baseline. Levonorgestrel lowered HDL by nearly 20%.

Combinations containing norethisterone acetate [42] or dydrogesterone [38] maintain increased levels of HDL. Combinations of MPA and oral oestradiol valerate have been reported both to raise [37] and to lower HDL [44]. Preliminary data with a regimen containing desogestrel show a net increase in HDL [45].

High-density Lipoprotein Subfractions

HDL is not a single entity but is composed of a large family of lipoproteins, differing in density, size and chemical composition. HDL subfractions also differ in the range of enzymes and cofactors they carry. These various particles reflect different stages in the natural history of HDL, from the small, discoidal lipoproteins secreted by the liver to the large cholesterol-rich particles resulting from interaction with endothelial cells. This heterogeneity of function has led to the proposition that some HDL fractions may be of greater importance than others. Interestingly, the sex difference in HDL resides in the minor fraction, HDL_2; oestrogens increase HDL_2, and progestogens oppose this [28]. Studies in men indicate that HDL_2 may be the better indicator of risk [46]. However, there are virtually no comparable data in women (the historical lack of interest in CHD in women being compounded by the lack of a convenient assay) and prospective studies have yet to demonstrate that HDL subfractions may give more information than HDL alone.

Measurement of HDL subfractions may be important in the evaluation of the metabolic risk of HRT as it provides more precise information about HDL metabolism. Whether one subfraction is of greater importance than another awaits the results of further prospective studies, in particular those including women.

In women given combined oral contraceptives, HDL_3 is increased and HDL_2 decreased, according to the net androgenicity of the formulation [23]. There are relatively few data available on the effect of HRT on HDL subfractions, and the picture that emerges is confusing. When given to women receiving percutaneous oestradiol, levonorgestrel induced a decrease in both subfractions, whereas natural progesterone appeared to have more effect on HDL_3 [36]. MPA, in contrast, lowers HDL_2 when given to women treated with oral oestradiol valerate [44]. More studies are needed if the effect of HRT on HDL metabolism is to be fully understood.

Summary

The metabolic effects of oestrogen, such as the ability to raise HDL levels, appear beneficial according to current concepts of risk, and may protect women from cardiovascular disease. Progestogens tend to oppose these effects, depending on their androgenicity and dose. The net effect of a HRT combination will also depend on the characteristics of the oestrogen component, and the route by which the hormones are given. It would seem prudent to avoid potentially adverse actions, such as lowering of HDL, until there is good epidemiological evidence that the progestogen in combined therapies does not negate the cardiovascular benefits of unopposed oestrogen.

The introduction of third generation progestogens – desogestrel, norgestimate, gestodene – represents an exciting development in this area.

References

1. Lindsay R, Hart DM, Aitken JM, Macdonald EB, Anderson JB, Clarke AC. Long term prevention of postmenopausal osteoporosis by oestrogen. Lancet 1976; i:1038–44.
2. Studd JWW, Whitehead MI. Selection of patients for treatment. Which therapy and for how long? In: Studd JWW, Whitehead MI, eds. The menopause. Oxford: Blackwell, 1988; 116–29.
3. Ziel HK, Finkle WD. Increased risk of endometrial carcinoma among users of conjugated estrogens. N Engl J Med 1975; 293:1167–70.
4. Mack TM, Pike MC, Henderson BE, Pfeffer RI, Gerkins VR. Estrogens and endometrial cancer in a retirement community. N Engl J Med 1976; 294:1262–7.
5. Studd JWW. Oestrogens as a cause of endometrial carcinoma. Br Med J 1976; i:1276.
6. Hunt K, Vessey M, McPherson K, Coleman M. Long term surveillance of mortality and cancer incidence in women receiving hormone replacement therapy. Br J Obstet Gynaecol 1987; 94:620–34.
7. Persson I, Adami H, Bergkvist L, Lindgren A, Petersson B, Hoover R, Schairer C. Risk of endometrial cancer after treatment with oestrogens alone or in conjunction with progestogens: results of a prospective study. Br Med J 1989; 298:147–51.

8. Paterson MEL, Wade-Evans T, Sturdee DW, Thom M, Studd JWW. Endometrial disease after treatment with oestrogens and progestogens in the climacteric. Br Med J 1980; 1:822–4.
9. Gambrell RD. Estrogens and cancer. Int J Fertil 1986; 31:390–402.
10. Whitehead MI, Townsend PT, Pryse-Davies J, Ryder TA, King RJB. Effects of estrogens and progestins on the biochemistry and morphology of the postmenopausal endometrium. N Engl J Med 1981; 305:1599–605.
11. Lane G, Siddle NC, Ryder TA, Pryse-Davies J, King RJB. Effects of dydrogesterone on the oestrogenized postmenopausal endometrium. Br J Obstet Gynaecol 1986; 93:55–62.
12. Stanczyk FZ. Pharmacology of progestagens. Int Proc J 1989; 1:11–20.
13. Magos AL, Brincat M, Studd JWW, Wardle P, Schlesinger P. O'Dowd T. Amenorrhea and endometrial atrophy with continuous oral oestrogen and progestagen therapy in postmenopausal women. Obstet Gynecol 1985; 65:496–9.
14. Morrison JC, Martin DC, Blair R et al. The use of medroxyprogesterone acetate for the relief of climacteric symptoms. Am J Obstet Gynecol 1980; 138:99–104.
15. Paterson MEL. A randomized double blind cross-over trial into the effects of norethisterone on climacteric symptoms and biochemical profiles. Br J Obstet Gynaecol 1982; 89:464–72.
16. Abdalla I, McKay-Hart D, Lindsay R, Leggate I, Hooke A. Prevention of bone mineral loss in post menopausal women by norethisterone. Obstet Gynecol 1985; 66:789–92.
17. Magos A, Studd JWW. The premenstrual syndrome – a review. In: Studd JWW, Whitehead MI, eds. The menopause. Oxford: Blackwell, 1988; 116–29.
18. Hammerbäck S, Bäckström T, Holst J, Schoultz B, Lyrenäs S. Cyclical mood changes as in the premenstrual tension syndrome during sequential estrogen–progestagen postmenopausal replacement therapy. Acta Obstet Gynecol Scand 1985; 64:393–7.
19. Magos AL, Brewster E, Singh R, O'Dowd T, Brincat M, Studd JWW. The effects of norethisterone in postmenopausal women on oestrogen replacement therapy: a model for the premenstrual syndrome. Br J Obstet Gynaecol 1986; 93:1290–6.
20. Moos RH. Typology of the menstrual cycle symptoms. Am J Obstet Gynecol 1969; 103:390–402.
21. Sherwin BB, Gelfand MM. A prospective one-year study of estrogen and progestin in postmenopausal women: effects on clinical symptoms and lipoprotein lipids. Obstet Gynecol 1989; 73:759–66.
22. Whitehead MI, Hillard TC, Crook D. The role and use of progestagens. Obstet Gynecol (in press).
23. Godsland IF, Crook D, Simpson R et al. Relationship between oral contraceptive progestin content and disturbances in glucose, insulin and lipoprotein risk markers for coronary heart disease. N Engl J Med (in press).
24. Reaven GM. Role of insulin resistance in human disease. Diabetes 1988; 37:1595–607.
25. Bush TL, Barrett-Connor E, Cowan LD et al. Cardiovasculr mortality and non-contraceptive use of estrogen in women: results from the Lipid Research Clinics Program Follow-up Study. Circulation 1987; 75:1102–9.
26. Henderson BE, Ross RK, Lobo RA, Pike M, Mack TM. Re-evaluating the role of progestagen therapy after the menopause. Fertil Steril 1988; 49:9S–15S.
27. Sarrel P. Effects of ovarian steroids on the cardiovascular system. In: Ginsberg J ed. The circulation in the female from the cradle to the grave. Carnforth, England: Parthenon, 1989; 117–41.
28. Godsland IF, Wynn V, Crook D, Miller NE. Sex, plasma lipoproteins and atherosclerosis: prevailing assumptions and outstanding questions. Am Heart J 1987; 114:1467–503.
29. Chez RA. Clinical aspects of three new progestagens: desogestrel, gestodene and norgestimate. Am J Obstet Gynecol 1989; 160:1296–300.
30. Friedewald WT, Levy RI, Fredrickson DS. Estimation of the concentration of low-density lipoprotein cholesterol in plasma, without use of the preparative ultracentrifuge. Clin Chem 1972; 18:499–502.
31. Krauss RM. Effect of progestational agents on serum lipids and lipoproteins. J Reprod Med 1982; 27:503–10.
32. Whitehead MI, Fraser D. Controversies concerning the safety of estrogen replacement therapy. Am J Obstet Gynecol 1987; 156:1313–22.
33. Hulley SB, Rosenman RH, Bawol RD, Brand RJ. Epidemiology as a guide to clinical decisions: the association between triglyceride and coronary heart disease. N Engl J Med 1980; 302:1383–9.
34. Enk L, Samsioe G, Silfverstolpe G. Dose and duration effects of estradiol valerate on serum and lipoprotein lipids. Horm Metab Res 1986; 18:551–4.
35. Glueck CJ, Levy RI, Fredrickson DS. Norethindrone acetate, postheparin lipolytic activity and plasma triglycerides in familial types I, III, IV, and V hyperlipoproteinemia. Ann Intern Med 1971; 75:345–00.

36. Fahreus L, Larsson-Cohn, Wallentin L. L-Norgestrel and progesterone have different influences on plasma lipoproteins. Eur J Clin Invest 1983; 13:447–53.
37. Hirvonen E, Lipasti A, Mälkönen M et al. Clinical and lipid metabolic effects of unopposed oestrogen and two oestrogen–progestagen regimens in post-menopausal women. Maturitas 1987; 9:69–79.
38. Fletcher CD, Farish E, Dagen MM et al. A comparison of the effects on lipoproteins of two progestogens used during cyclical hormone replacement therapy. Maturitas 1987; 9:253–8.
39. Whitehead MI, Fraser D, Schenkel K, Crook D, Stevenson JC. Can progestogen be administered transdermally to postmenopausal oestrogen users? Lancet (in press).
40. Tikkanen M, Nikkila EA, Vartiainan E. Natural oestrogen as an effective treatment for Type II hyperlipoproteinemia in postmenopausal women. Lancet 1978; ii:490–1.
41. Silfverstolpe G, Gustafson A, Samsiöe G, Svanborg A. Lipid metabolic studies in oophorectomized women. Effects of three different progestogens. Acta Obstet Gynecol Scand 1979; Suppl 88:89–95.
42. Jensen J, Nilas L, Christiansen C. Cyclic changes in serum cholesterol and lipoproteins following different doses of combined postmenopausal hormone replacement therapy. Br J Obstet Gynaecol 1986; 93:613–18.
43. Jacobs Jr DR, Mebane IL, Bangdiwala SI, Criqui MH, Tyroler HA. High density lipoprotein cholesterol as a predictor of cardiovascular disease mortality in men and women: the follow-up study of the Lipid Research Clinics prevalence study. Am J Epidemiol 1990; 131:32–47.
44. Ottoson UB, Johansson BG, Schoultz B. Subfractions of high-density lipoprotein cholesterol during estrogen replacement therapy: a comparison between progestogens and natural progesterone. Am J Obstet Gynecol 1985; 151:746–50.
45. Samsioe, G. Progestagens and lipids. Int Proc J 1989; 113–17.
46. Miller NE. Associations of high-density lipoprotein subclasses and apolipoproteins with ischaemic heart disease and coronary atherosclerosis. Am Heart J 1987; 113:589–97.

Chapter 17

Oestrogen Replacement Therapy and Cardiovascular Disease

R. K. Ross, M. C. Pike, T. M. Mack and B. E. Henderson

Introduction

Loss of ovarian activity appears to result in an increased risk of cardiovascular disease. Men have higher mortality rates from cardiovascular disease at all ages, but the male to female ratio varies substantially throughout life [1]. The peak ratio occurs in conjunction with the female menopause and declines thereafer. In fact, in one large prospective study in which incident cardiovascular events were closely monitored, male and female rates of cardiovascular disease were indistinguishable by age 70 [2]. In the same study, at any given age women who were postmenopausal had substantially higher rates of cardiovascular disease than premenopausal women [3]. Furthermore, bilateral oophorectomy at a young age has long been known to result in premature development of atherosclerosis and an increased occurrence of its clinical outcomes [4,5].

These observations first suggested the possibility that oestrogen therapy administered to postmenopausal women might reduce the risk of cardiovascular disease. From a public health perspective it is clearly important to understand this possible relationship, as cardiovascular disease currently takes 650 000 lives annually in the United States alone and is the leading cause of deaths among postmenopausal women by a wide margin [6]. In the mid-1970s, oestrogen replacement had become one of the most frequently prescribed categories of drugs in the United States. Although prevalence if use decreased dramatically in the late 1970s in response to a series of studies showing that oestrogens cause endometrial cancer, the number of prescriptions of the most widely used brand of oestrogen replacement therapy (ERT) has since begun to increase rapidly once again [7].

Epidemiologists began seriously to explore the possible relationship between ERT and cardiovascular disease occurrence about a decade ago. Nearly twenty studies have subsequently been published which provide some useful information relevant to this hypothesis. These studies are summarised below. The various prospective studies are especially noteworthy by the consistency with which they demonstrate cardioprotection associated with oestrogen use, despite the diverse target populations under study. Furthermore, these observational studies, are strongly supported by available experimental data [8–10]. Nonetheless, in reviewing the epidemiological literature on this association, it becomes apparent that there is still much to be learned regarding dose–response effects, the interaction between duration and recency of use and cardiovascular disease risk, the degree to which oestrogen use interacts with other cardiovascular disease risk factors in modifying risk, and, most importantly, the precise mechanism of action to explain this relationship.

The following sections explore the current state of knowledge regarding each of these issues. The importance of cardiovascular disease to the overall risk to benefit equation for oestrogen replacement therapy is also discussed. Finally, a perspective is given on the impact on cardiovascular disease risk of the increasingly popular practice of adding a progestin cyclically or continuously to a monthly oestrogen regimen.

Retrospective Studies of ERT and Cardiovascular Disease

There have been ten published case-control studies which have reported on the association between postmenopausal ERT and cardiovascular disease risk [11–20]. These are briefly summarised in Table 17.1. Six of the ten [11,13,14,17–19] reported a reduction in risk in ERT users overall, but this effect achieved statistical significance only in the study by Ross et al. [11]. A seventh study reported a reduction in risk in three of the four summary categories (current users over and under age 45 and women with any past use under age 45) but not among women over age 45 with any past history of oestrogen use [16]. An eighth study [12] found a reduction in risk which seemed to be explained by differences between oestrogen users and non-users in the prevalence of other cardiovascular disease risk factors, so that the "adjusted" relative risk approached 1.0.

The ninth study, by Jick and colleagues, actually found a substantial elevation in cardiovascular disease among oestrogen users, but among all the reported studies was methodologically the least sound for addressing this issue [15]. In this study, non-contraceptive oestrogen use was compared between 14 previously healthy women aged under 46 years who had sustained a non-fatal myocardial infarction, and 21 previously healthy control women hospitalised for other reasons. Seven cases compared to four controls were oestrogen users at the time of admission. Not only was the study limited by the tiny sample size and young ages of the participants, but also because the association with oestrogen use was possibly confounded by the high prevalence of cigarette smoking among the

Table 17.1 Case control studies of oestrogen replacement therapy and coronary heart disease

Reference	Data source	Relative risk	
		Ever use	Current use
Rosenberg et al. [12]	Interviews	Not reported	1.0
Pfeffer et al. [13]	Pharmacy records	0.9	0.7
Jick et al. [15]	Interviews	Not reported	4.2
Rosenberg et al. [16][a]	Interviews	0.7	0.5
		1.5	0.9
Ross et al. [11][b]	Medical records	0.4	Not reported
		0.6	Not reported
Bain et al. [14]	Mailed survey	0.8	0.7
Adam et al. [17]	Doctor records	0.6	0.8
Szklo et al. [18]	Interviews	0.4	0.4
Croft and Hannaford [19]	Medical records	0.8	Not reported
Thompson et al. [20]	Medical records	1.1	Not reported[c]

[a]Rosenberg et al. reported results for women aged 30–44 years (top) separately from those for women aged 45–59 years.

[b]Ross et al. used two control groups for comparison: living controls (top) and deceased controls.

[c]Thompson et al. reported current use results for stroke and myocardial infarction combined; the relative risk estimate was 1.1, compared to non-users.

cases. The most recent study by Thompson et al. [20] in the United Kingdom also found a small statistically non-significant increase in risk among women who had used ERT, when adjusted for other cardiovascular disease risk factors (RR=1,1 compared to non-users). Like many of the case-control studies reported to date, the population under study was characterised by relatively short duration oestrogen therapy, and, in this particular study, most users had ceased taking oestrogens many years previously.

Prospective Studies of ERT and Cardiovascular Disease

Table 17.2 summarises the nine prospective studies which have evaluated the relationship between oestrogen replacement therapy and cardiovascular disease risk [21–29]. Eight of the nine show an inverse relationship between past use and risk, even though the various studies are characterised by markedly diverse target populations demographically and the measured cardiovascular disease outcomes differ somewhat from study to study.

The Kaiser Permanente Walnut Creek cohort study conducted in northern California, initially reported no association between ERT use and cardiovascular disease risk [30]. However, this well-designed study could provide little useful information at that time regarding this possible association, since virtually all the follow-up was limited to women under 50 years of age. Therefore, oestrogen use was uncommon and of short duration and the number of cardiovascular disease events available for analysis was small. In a longer follow-up of the same cohort, results are now consistent with the majority of epidemiological studies, demonstrating a substantial reduction in risk of fatal cardiovascular disease [26]. No reduction in risk has been observed for non-fatal disease, however.

Table 17.2 Cohort studies of oestrogen replacement therapy and coronary heart disease

Reference	Description of cohort	Endpoint	Relative risk
Burch et al. [27]	737 hysterectomised women	CHD	0.4
Hammond et al. [21]	610 hypoestrogenic patients	CHD	0.3
Bush et al. [27]	2269 white women	Fatal CHD	0.4
Wilson et al. [24]	1234 postmenopausal residents	CHD	1.9
Stampfer et al. [23]	32 317 postmenopausal nurses	CHD	0.5
Petitti et al. [26]	16 638 members of prepaid health plan	Fatal CHD[a]	0.5
Hunt et al. [29]	4544 postmenopausal British women	Fatal CHD	0.5
Henderson et al. [25]	8841 retirement community residents	Fatal MI	0.6
Criqui et al. [28]	1868 residents of planned community	Fatal CHD	0.7

[a]Non-Fatal CHD, RR=1.0

The one other study which has provided results which are inconsistent with the majority of prospective studies and the one which has created the greatest doubt about the validity of the hypothesis that oestrogens reduce risk of cardiovascular disease, is the Framingham cohort [24]. In that study, a 90% increased risk of cardiovascular disease was reported among oestrogen users, despite a generally more favourable cardiovascular disease risk profile among this group of women, compared to the remainder of the cohort. A series of criticisms has been directed at this analysis [31]. These have centred around the inclusion of "soft" endpoints, such as angina, as a substantial proportion of the measured outcomes, the failure to adjust for potentially important confounding variables such as age at menopause (early menopause is associated with a high risk of cardiovascular disease, as well as a high likelihood of being prescribed ERT), and inclusion of lipoprotein cholesterol levels (thought to be part of the mechanism for cardio-protection, as described below) in multivariate modelling. The authors have responded to each of these criticisms and none appear to explain entirely these discrepant results, although reanalyses excluding angina have demonstrated a significant protective effect in women under age 60, but not among older women [32]. It has previously been argued that, despite the enormous contributions made by Framingham toward understanding the epidemiology and aetiology of cardiovascular disease, the study is not particularly well-suited for studying oestrogen-related hypotheses [33]. Questions regarding oestrogen use were not part of the original study goals and, when oestrogen use histories were finally ascertained from the cohort, questions appear to have been casually asked and not followed-up. No duration or dose information was obtained and the timing of oestrogen use could not be related to the onset of menopause, or for that matter to any other specific event. Furthermore, no attempt was made to validate oestrogen use histories against medical records, as was done on at least a sample of patients in a number of the other studies.

In summary, the overall evidence from these epidemiological cohorts strongly suggests a beneficial effect of oestrogens on cardiovascular disease risk. More-over, the degree of protection appears to be very substantial – of the order of at least a 30%–40% reduction across al categories of oestrogen use.

Dose–Response Effects

Most of the available epidemiological data pertain to conjugated equine oestrogens. Table 17.3 summarises the currently available data on the possible modifying effect of dose of conjugated equine oestrogen on cardiovascular disease risk. There are clearly few and inadequate data confidently to assess this relationship. Understanding this important issue is further complicated by the tendency of many women to have used multiple doses, often each for substantial periods of time (in our own prospective study some of the women reporting any past history of conjugated equine oestrogen use also reported having taken multiple doses). The combination of recent trends towards lower preferred doses by physicians and patients alike and the apparent tendency of recent/ current users of ERT to have lower risk of cardiovascular disease than when they used ERT only in the distant past (see below), adds yet another degree of complexity.

Table 17.3 Summary of published data on the relationship between oestrogen dose[a] and risk of fatal or non-fatal cardiovascular diseases

Investigators	Reference	Dose category	Relative risk
Case-control studies			
Ross et al.[b]	11	None	1.0
		≤0.625 mg	0.4
		1.25+ mg	0.5
		None	1.0
		≤0.625 mg	0.8
		1.25+ mg	0.4
Pfeffer et al.	13	Cases: $\bar{x}$ dose=0.41 mg	–
		Controls: $\bar{x}$ dose=0.32 mg	–
Rosenberg et al.	16	None	1.0
		≤0.625 mg	0.7
		1.25+ mg	1.3
		Unknown	1.1
Cohort studies			
Henderson et al.	25	None	1.0
		≤0.625 mg	0.6
		1.25+ mg	0.6

[a]Conjugated equine oestrogen dose.
[b]Ross et al. utilized two comparison groups in their study; living controls (top) and deceased controls.

Keeping in mind these important limitations, there is currently no evidence to suggest that the cardioprotection associated with ERT is strongly dose-related. Since most current users are taking the lower of the two most frequently prescribed daily doses, they may appear, however, to have a low risk based on their recency of use rather than on their usual pill dose.

Duration of Use

Given the large and growing number of studies that have evaluated this hypothesis as it pertains to oestrogen use overall, there is also surprisingly little information available on the effects of duration of use on risk (Table 17.4). The few case-control studies which have provided any data on duration have been limited by the relatively brief average use in the study populations [16–18]. (The study by Thompson et al. in which the median duration of use was only seven months reported results by duration for stroke and myocardial infarction combined [20]). The nurses cohort study report [23] was also characterised by relatively brief use overall, but provided no suggestion that duration of use is strongly related to degree of protection. By far the most substantial data on duration of use come from the Southern California Leisure World cohort [25]. Long-term past oestrogen use is the norm in this community; the median duration of use is approximately ten years. Long duration of use appears to be associated with somewhat lower risk than short-term use, but the latter group of users still have reduced risk compared to lifetime non-users [34].

Table 17.4   Summary of published data on the relationship between duration of use of ERT and risk of fatal or non-fatal cardiovascular diseases

Investigators	Reference	Duration category	Relative risk
Case-control studies			
Adam et al.	17	None	1.0
		<2 years	0.7
		2+ years	0.6
Bain et al.	14	Cases: $\bar{x}$=7.0 years	–
		Controls: $\bar{x}$=4.8 years	–
Rosenberg et al.	16	None	1.0
		<2 years	1.1
		2+ years	0.7
Cohort studies			
Stampfer et al.	23	None	1.0
		<3 years	0.5
		3+ years	0.6
Henderson et al[a]	34	None	1.0
		< 4 years	0.6
		5–14 years	0.6
		15+years	0.5

[a]These are the most recent data on duration from the Leisure World study for fatal acute myocardial infarction only.

There remain a number of other important but inadequately addressed questions related to duration and the appropriate timing of postmenopausal oestrogen use to maximise the cardiovascular benefit for an individual patient. For example, Should use begin in the perimenopausal period? If use is delayed, will a woman realise a comparable benefit for comparable duration of use? Once use has begun, should it continue indefinitely? If use is discontinued is there retention of cardioprotection associated with the duration accumulated? The epidemiological literature again is insufficient to allow these questions to be suitably addressed.

Confounding/Interaction with Other Cardiovascular Disease Risk Factors

Several of the better designed epidemiological studies have been able to evaluate the possible confounding or modifying effects of other risk factors on the overall relationship between oestrogen use and cardiovascular disease.

There are important reasons to be concerned about confounding; such confounding could be related to the possibility that physicians use a variety of therapeutic criteria for oestrogen prescription, and also to the possibility that differences in access to medical care might affect the likelihood of receiving oestrogen therapy. For example, age at menopause, type of menopause and obesity are known to be associated with the prevalence of oestrogen use in various target populations and are also risk factors for cardiovascular disease; however, adjustment for the former two variables, if anything, would be expected to magnify any cardioprotection, since women with early menopause and/or surgical menopause are at high risk of cardiovascular disease and are more likely to receive oestrogens than are other postmenopausal patients. Thin women, on the other hand, are generally thought to be at low risk of cardiovascular disease but more likely to be prescribed oestrogens than their more obese counterparts. Women with a history of hypertension, previous vascular disease, or thromboembolic disorders, in particular (i.e., women at high baseline risk for cardiovascular disease), may be less likely than other women to be prescribed oestrogens, because of concern that the hypertension may be exacerbated or the oestrogens may further enhance risk of a thrombotic episode.

The evidence suggests that ERT is an independent cardioprotective factor, not explained by these or other cardiovascular disease risk factors [23,25,27,28]. A few studies have demonstrated that cardioprotection extends across numerous strata of women with and without cardiovascular disease risk factors, including women with and without hypertension and previous vascular disease, women of various weight categories, and women undergoing natural or surgical menopause at various ages [25,27]. There are some data to suggest that current cigarette smokers may achieve less protection with oestrogen use than past or lifetime non-smokers [23,25,27,28]. The explanation for this phenomenon is unclear; however, for unknown reasons, smokers have lower circulating oestrogen levels with comparable oral doses of conjugated equine oestrogens than do non-smokers [35].

Another important unresolved issue is the timing of oestrogen use relative to the development of other cardiovascular disease outcomes. For example, while it has been reported that oestrogens reduce cardiovascular disease mortality in women with a previous myocardial infarction or angina, it is unclear whether oestrogen use following these diagnoses results in a reduction of subsequent cardiovascular disease morbidity and mortality.

Current Versus Past Use

Most studies to date that have compared risk in current versus past users of ERT has found a lower risk, often a substantially lower risk, with current use (Table 17.5) [13,14,23,25]. There are some data to suggest that this effect is not due entirely to longer duration of use among the more recent users [34]. It is possible, but not yet tested, that the lower risk with current use is related to discontinuation of therapy in women who develop other cardiovascular disease risk factors (i.e., past users would be at inherently higher risk).

Table 17.5 Summary of published data on the relationship of cardiovascular disease risk to current versus past use of ERT

Investigators	Reference	Category of use	Relative risk
Case-control studies			
Pfeffer et al.	16	None	1.0
		Past	1.0
		Current	0.7
Bain et al.	13	None	1.0
		Ever	0.8
		Current	0.7
Rosenberg et al.	14	None	1.0
		Past	1.2
		"Recent"	1.0
Cohort studies			
Henderson et al	34	None	1.0
		Past	0.6
		Current	0.5
Stampfer et al.	23	None	1.0
		Past	0.7
		Current	0.3

Mechanism for Cardioprotection

The effects of oral oestrogen therapy on serum lipid and lipoprotein cholesterol levels are well established and provide the most probable mechanism for the reduction in risk of cardiovascular disease associated with ERT. Levels of serum low-density lipoprotein (LDL) cholesterol which are associated with an elevated risk of coronary heart disease are reduced by ERT, whereas levels of high-density lipoprotein (HDL) cholesterol, which are inversely associated with risk of heart disease, are increased.

Bush and Miller [36] have summarised the available literature on the effects of ERT and other steroid hormones on lipids and lipoprotein levels in postmenopausal women. Across all studies, daily use of 0.625 mg of oral conjugated equine oestrogen leads to an approximately 10% increase in HDL-cholesterol (roughly 6 mg dl^{-1} in postmenopausal patients) and a 4% decrease in LDL-cholesterol levels. These effects are dose related; the comparable changes in HDL- and LDL-cholesterol levels for a 1.25 mg daily dose are 14% and 8%, respectively. Data from large cross-sectional studies involving long-term users of ERT suggest even larger changes in lipid levels. The mean differences in HDL and LDL cholesterol levels in long-term users of ERT versus lifetime non-users in the Leisure World prospective study 25 are 13% and 16%, respectively.

Other than Framingham (which, as noted above, observed no cardioprotection with oestrogen therapy), the only other study to date to have lipid data available to include in multivariate analysis was the Lipid Research Clinics Follow-up Study. HDL cholesterol explained roughly half of the 60% observed reduction in cardiovascular disease mortality associated with use of ERT in that study [27].

It has been suggested that the beneficial cardiovascular effects of ERT may not be limited to those mediated by lipids; oestrogens may affect the prostaglandin/thromboxane system [37], causing vascular dilatation [38] and reducing platelet aggregation [39]. The reduced risk of cardiovascular disease in ERT users of short duration, as observed in several studies, combined with the apparently lower risk in current versus past users of ERT, may support such alternative mechanisms. On the other hand, women who have not used ERT for many years still maintain some degree of cardioprotection. The precise explanation for this effect remains to be determined, but it seems plausible that multiple mechanisms may actually be involved.

Possible Implications of Cyclic/Continuous Progestogen Therapy on Cardiovascular Disease Risk

Clinical studies of different progestogen regimens strongly suggest that the synthetic progestogens currently used with ERT have an effect opposite that of oestrogens on lipoprotein metabolism, resulting in an increase in LDL-cholesterol and a decrease in HDL-cholesterol levels [36]. If the beneficial effects of oestrogen use on cardiovascular disease risk are mediated entirely or in part by creating a favourable lipid profile, one can expect that at least some of this cardioprotection will be lost by adding a progestogen sequentially or continuously to oestrogen therapy alone.

These adverse lipid effects from the addition of a progestin to ERT are most evident with the 19-nortestosterone progestins [36], which are still widely prescribed as part of combination therapy to many postmenopausal women outside the United States. There are relatively few useful comparative data on the effects of adding a progesterone-derived progestin to ERT. Nonetheless, the published evidence suggests that such progestins also have adverse lipid effects. There have been five published studies in which a randomised or crossover design was implemented using such progestins, and HDL-cholesterol levels evaluated [40–44]. In each of these the addition of the progesterone-derived progestin decreased the benefit on HDL cholesterol levels observed with oestrogen alone. In the three studies using medroxyprogesterone acetate at the commonly prescribed dose of 10 mg for ten days out of 28, the effect, on average, was to return HDL-cholesterol levels to baseline [40–42]. The other two studies used 5 mg daily doses of a progesterone-derived progestin and, even though HDL-cholesterol levels remained substantially elevated over baseline levels, they were nonetheless lower than while on oestrogen alone [43,44].

These studies were small and none lasted more than a year. Recent cross-sectional data suggest that these deleterious effects may not continue in the long term, so it is clearly an area which demands clarification and further study [45]. However, the situation as it is currently understood provides a reasonable basis to conclude that, at commonly prescribed doses, all the widely used progestins in combination hormone replacement therapy today will decrease the beneficial effects of ERT on cardiovascular disease risk. Moreover, if the cardiovascular benefits of oestrogens are mediated through other mechanisms such as the prostaglandin/thromboxane system, thereby affecting vasodilatation and platelet aggregation, progestins are also likely to be harmful; oestrogens and progestins exert opposite effects on the prostaglandin/thromboxane system [37–39].

Routes of Administration/Type of Oestrogen

Virtually all the epidemiological data on the cardioprotective effects of oestrogen relate to orally administered conjugated equine oestrogens. If the beneficial effects of oestrogen are mediated through lipids, there is good reason to believe that other oestrogens (either natural or synthetic) will also reduce the risk of atherosclerotic cardiovascular disease. Bush and Miller [36] have recently reviewed and summarised the literature on the lipid changes associated with a variety of currently marketed oestrogens and all tend to create a favourable lipid profile. The magnitude of the observed changes associated with non-equine conjugated oestrogens are comparable to the equine-derived products; on average, the effect of synthetic preparations might quantitatively be somewhat greater even, but these preparations result in unwanted effects on coagulation profiles [46]. It is generally believed that much of the oestrogen-induced changes in lipids are due to a "first-pass" hepatic effect related to oral administration [47]. Nonetheless, it appears that HDL-cholesterol levels are also raised by non-oral (patch, pellet, cream) routes of administration. The five studies which have addressed this issue have been small and report a fairly wide range of HDL changes [47–51]. Therefore, it remains unclear whether non-oral routes of administration will achieve a comparable cardiovascular benefit as observed with oral therapy.

Risk/Benefit Analysis

While the evidence is strong that ERT leads to a reduced risk of cardiovascular disease (and, although not reviewed here, of occlusive cerebrovascular disease [34,52] as well), there also exist other well-established long-term benefits and hazards of such use. In terms of mortality, the outcomes of most interest are endometrial cancer and breast cancer, on the risk side of the equation, and osteoporotic hip fractures, on the benefit side [52].

In the Leisure World retirement community, where our own research on the risks and benefits of ERT has been conducted, the overall mortality in oestrogen users and non-users has recently been investigated. Primarily due to the substantial reduction in mortality from arteriosclerotic vascular diseases, the overall age-adjusted mortality rate was reduced by about 20% in women who had used oestrogens [34]. This mortality reduction was related to both recency and duration of use. The lowest mortality rate was observed among women who were current users of long duration (15 years or more). The mortality rate in these women was only 60% that of lifetime non-users.

It was considered important to develop a risk–benefit model for estimating the effects on mortality of oestrogen use in the population as a whole [52,53]. To do this, we first determined the annual mortality rates at various ages for the conditions of interest (endometrial cancer, breast cancer, ischaemic heart disease, occlusive stroke and osteoporotic hip fractures; for the latter, annual incidence rates and a case fatality rate of 15% were used, since adequate mortality rates were not available). We then estimated the relative risks for these five disease categories after ten years of use of 0.625 mg of conjugated equine oestrogens daily. These data were derived from a careful review of the epidemiological literature related to each association. For endometrial cancer, a case fatality rate for ERT-induced endometrial cancer estimated to be only one-eighth the normal rate was used. For breast cancer, a "worst case scenario" was presumed in which the estimated 37% increase in incidence after ten years of therapy would also result in a 37% increase in mortality. Our own data and those of several other groups suggest that the increment in mortality from breast cancer (if any) may not be as great as the increment in incidence [29,34,54].

An annual reduction in mortality for women 65–74 years of age of 302 lives per 100 000 non-hysterectomised women and 328 per 100 000 hysterectomised women was calculated. Similar conclusions were derived using other postmeno-pausal age groups. This theoretical predicted reduction in mortality represents a 15%–20% reduction in overall mortality in this age group.

Summary and Conclusions

This highly favourable risk–benefit equation argues for the routine use of ERT in the majority of postmenopausal women. Obviously such global recommenda-tions should only be made with considerable caution.

Much of the detail required to make such recommendations is regrettably lacking; the mechanism is not understood fully whereby ERT reduces risk of arteriosclerotic disease; there is an incomplete understanding of the effects of latency, dose, and duration of use as they relate to arteriosclerotic disease outcomes, especially, but also to other components of the risk–benefit equation; we remain largely ignorant about the degree to which ERT interacts with other risk factors for any of these disease outcomes of interest, much less all. Moreover, by considering only mortality as the index of therapeutic success or failure, other known or possible effects of ERT, which relate to quality of life or economic cost of illness are ignored. In fact, the risk–benefit model has recently been extended in an attempt to evaluate net changes in number of hospitalisations and cumulative number of days of disability to be expected with routine use of oestrogen therapy, and also to incorpoate some of these other known or suspected health effects (including the symptom complex of the climacteric, gallbladder disease and rheumatoid arthritis) [55]. The impact of incorporating these other conditions is negligible in terms of mortality. The net effect of ERT for hospitalisation and disability is one of slight risk rather than benefit, even without incorporating these other health outcomes.

Given the complexity of the issues and the uncertainty surrounding many details of these associations, we think it especially important that the postmeno-pausal patient should participate fully with her doctor in decisions regarding choice of therapy. Obviously, if the decision is to begin therapy, both doctor and patient must place high priority on surveillance for unexplained uterine bleeding and breast lumps, following use of any type of hormone replacement.

Acknowledgement. This work was supported by grant CA 17054 from the National Institutes of Health.

References

1. Ross RK, Paganini-Hill A. Estrogen replacement therapy and coronary heart disease. Sem Reprod Endocrinol 1983; 1:19–25.
2. Kannel WB, Hjortland MC, McNamara PM, Gordon T. Menopause and the risk of cardiovascular disease: the Framingham study. Ann Intern Med 1976; 85:447–52.
3. Gordon T, Kannel WB, Hjortland MC, McNamara PM. Menopause and coronary heart disease: the Framingham study. Ann Intern Med 1978; 89:157–61.
4. Robinson RW, Higano N, Cohen WD. Increased incidence of coronary heart disease in women castrated prior to the menopause. Arch Intern Med 1959; 104:908–13.
5. Parris HM, Carr CA, Hall DG, King TM. Time interval from castration in premenopausal women to development of excessive coronary atherosclerosis. Am J Obstet Gynecol 1967; 99:155–67.
6. Healthy People: The Surgeon General's Report on Health Promotion and Disease Prevention 1979. DHEW (PHS) Publication No. 79-55071, Washington, DC, US Government Printing Office, 1979.
7. Kennedy LD, Baum C, Forbes MD. Non-contraceptive estrogens and progestins: use patterns over time. Obstet Gynecol 1985; 65:441–6.
8. Pick R, Stamler J, Rodbard S, Katz LN. The inhibition of coronary atherosclerosis by estrogens in cholesterol-fed chicks. Circulation 1952; 6:276–80.
9. Adams MR, Clarkson TB, Koritnik DR, Nash HA. Contraceptive steroids and coronary artery atherosclerosis in cynomolgus macaques. Fertil Steril 1987; 47:1010–18.
10. Ludden JB, Bruger M, Wright IS. Experimental atherosclerosis – effect of testosterone proprionate and estradiol diproprionate on experimental atherosclerosis. Arch Pathol 1952; 33:58–62.
11. Ross RK, Paganini-Hill A, Mack TM, Arthur M, Henderson BE. Menopausal oestrogen therapy and protection from death from ischaemic heart disease. Lancet 1981; i:858–60.
12. Rosenberg L, Armstrong B, Jick H. Myocardial infarction and estrogen therapy in postmenopausal women. N Engl J Med 1976; 294:1256–9.
13. Pfeffer RI, Whipple GH, Kurosaki TT, Chapman JM. Coronary risk and estrogen use in postmenopausal women. Am J Epidemiol 1978; 107:479–87.
14. Bain C. Willett W, Hennekens CH, Rosenr B, Belanger C, Speizer FE. Use of postmenopausal hormones and risk of myocardial infarction. Circulation 1981; 64:42–5.
15. Jick H, Dinan B, Rothman KJ. Noncontraceptive estrogens and non-fatal myocardial infarction. JAMA 1978; 239:1407–8.
16. Rosenberg L, Slone D. Shapiro S, Kaufman D, Stolley PD, Miettinen OS. Noncontraceptive estrogens and myocardial infarction in young women. JAMA 1980; 244:339–42.
17. Adam S, Williams V, Vessey MP. Cardiovascular disease and hormone replacement treatment: a pilot case-control study. Br Med J 1981; 282:1277–8.
18. Szklo M, Tonascia J. Gordis L, Bloom I. Estrogen use and myocardial infarction risk: a case-control study. Prev Med 1984; 13:510–16.

19. Croft P, Hannaford PC. Risk factors for acute myocardial infarction in women: evidence from the Royal College of General Practitioners' Oral Contraception Study. Br Med J 1989; 298:165–8.

20. Thompson SG, Meade TW, Greenberg G. The use of hormonal replacement therapy and the risk of stroke and myocardial infarction in women. J. Epidemiol Community Health 1989; 43:173–8

21. Hammond CB, Jelovsek Fr, Lee KL, Creasman WT, Parker RT. Effects of long-term estrogen replacement therapy. I. Metabolic effects. Am J Obstet Gynecol 1979; 133:525–36.

22. Burch JC, Byrd BF, Vaughn WK. The effects of long-term estrogen on hysterectomized women. Am J Obstet Gynecol 1974; 118:778–82.

23. Stampfer MJ, Willett WC, Colditz GA, Rosner B, Speizer FE, Hennekens CH. A prospective study of postmenopausal estrogen therapy and coronary heart disease. N Engl J Med 1985; 313:1104–49

24. Wilson PWF, Garrison RJ, Castelli WP. Postmenopausal estrogen use, cigarette smoking, and cardiovascular morbidity in women over 50: the Framingham study. N Engl J Med 1985; 313:1038–43.

25. Henderson BE, Paganini-Hill A, Ross RK. Estrogen replacement therapy and protection from acute myocardial infarction. Am J Obstet Gynecol 1988; 159:312–17.

26. Petitti DB, Perlman JA, Sidney S. Postmenopausal estrogen use and heart disease (Letter). N Engl J Med 1986; 315:131.

27. Bush TL, Barrett-Conner E, Cowan LD et al. Cardiovascular mortality and noncontraceptive use of estrogen in women: results from the Lipid Research Clinics Program follow-up study. circulation 1987; 75:1102–9.

28. Criqui MH, Suarez L, Barrett-Conner E, McPhillips J, Wingard DL, Garland C. Postmenopausal estrogen use and mortality: results from a prospective study in a defined homogeneous community. Am J Epidemiol 1988; 128:606–14.

29. Hunt K, Vessey M, McPherson K, Coleman M. Long-term surveillance of mortality and cancer incidence in women receiving hormone replacement therapy. Br J Obstet Gynaecol 1987; 94:620–34.

30. Petitti DB, Wingerd J, Pellegrin F, Ramchuran S. Risk of vascular disease in women. Smoking, oral contraceptives, noncontraceptive estrogens and other factors. JAMA 1979; 242:1150–4.

31. Postmenopausal estrogen use and heart disease (Letters). N Engl J Med 1987; 315:1274.

32. Eaker ED, Castelli WP. Differential risk for coronary heart disease among women in the Framingham Study. In: Proceedings of the workshop on coronary heart disease in women. Bethesda, MD, National Institutes of Health (NIH Administrative RP no., 1987).

33. Ross RK. Progestogens and the cardiovascular system. Int Proc J 1989; 1:218–34.

34. Henderson BE, Paganini-Hill A, Ross RK. Decreased mortality in users of estrogen replacement therapy (in review).

35. Jenson J, Christiansen C, Rodbro P. Cigarette smoking, serum estrogens, and bone loss during hormone-replacement therapy early after menopause. N Engl J Med 1985; 313:973–5.

36. Bush JL, Miller VT. Effects of pharmacologic agents used during menopause: impact on lipids and lipoproteins. In: Mishell DR, ed. Menopause, physiology and pharmacology. Chicago, Yearbook Medical Publishers, 1987; 187–208.

37. Pitt B, Shea MJ, Romson JL, Lucchesi BR. Prostaglandins and prostaglandin inhibitors in ischemic heart disease. Ann Intern Med 1983; 99:83–92.

38. Ylikorkala O, Puolakka J, Viinikka, L. Vasoconstrictory thromboxane A_2 and vasodilatory prostacyclin in climacteric women: effect of oestrogen–progestogen therapy. Maturitas 1984; 5:201–5.

39. Mileikowsky GN, Nadler JL, Huey F, Francis R, Roy S. Evidence that smoking alters prostacyclin formation and platelet aggregation in women who use oral contraceptives. Am J Obstet Gynecol 1988; 159:1547–52.

40. Hirvonenu E, Malkonen M, Manninen V. Effects of different progestogens on lipoproteins during postmenopausal replacement therapy. N Engl J Med 1981; 304–560–3.

41. Ottosson UB, Johansson BG, von Schoultz B. Subfractions of high-density lipoprotein cholesterol during estrogen replacement therapy: a comparison between progestogens and natural progesterone. Am J Obstet Gynecol 1985; 151:746–50.

42. Hirvonen E, Lipasti A, Malkonen M et al. Clinical and lipid metabolic effects of unopposed oestrogen and two oestrogen–progestogen regimens in post-menopausal women. Maturitas 1987; 9:69–79.

43. Sherwin BB, Gelfand MM. A prospective one-year study of estrogen and progestin in postmenopausal women: effects on clinical symptoms and lipoprotein lipids. Obstet Gynecol 1989; 73:759–66.

44. Sonnendecker EWW, Polakow S, Benade AJS, Simchowitz E. Serum lipoprotein effects of conjugated estrogen and a sequential conjugated estrogen–medrogesterone regimen in hysterectomized postmenopausal women. Am J Obstet Gynecol 1989; 160:1128–34.
45. Barrett-Connor E, Wingard DL, Criqui MH. Postmenopausal estrogen use and heart disease risk factors in the 1980's. JAMA 1989; 261:2095–100.
46. von Kaulla E, Droegemueller W, von Kaulla KN. Conjugated estrogens and hypercoagulability. Am J Obstet Gynecol 1974; 122:688–92.
47. Chetkowski RJ, Meldrum DR, Steingold KA et al. Biologic effects of transdermal estradiol. N Engl J Med 1986; 314:1615–20.
48. Sharf M, Oettinger M, Lanir A, Kahana L, Yeshurun D. Lipid and lipoprotein levels following pure estradiol implantation in postmenopausal women. Gynecol Obstet Invest 1985; 19:207–12.
49. Jensen J, Riis BJ, Strom V, Nilas L, Christiansen C. Long-term effects of percutaneous estrogens and oral progesterone on serum lipoproteins in postmenopausal women. Am J Obstet Gynecol 1987; 156:66–71.
50. Notelovitz M, Johnston M, Smith S, Kitchens C. Metabolic and hormonal effects of 25-mg and 50-mg 17ß-estradiol implants in surgically menopausal women. Obstet Gynecol 1987; 70:749–54.
51. Stanclzdyk FZ, Shoupe D, Nunez V, Macias-Gonzales P, Vijod MA, Lobo RA. A randomized comparison of normal estradiol delivery in postmenopausal women. Am J Obstet Gynecol 1988; 159:1540–6.
52. Henderson BE, Ross RK, Lobo RA et al. Re-evaluating the role of progestogen therapy after the menopause. Fertil Steril 1988; 49:9S–15S.
53. Ross RK, Pike MC, Henderson BE, Mack TM, Lobo RA. Stroke prevention and oestrogen replacement therapy. (Letter) Lancet 1989; i:505.
54. Bergkvist O, Adami HO, Persson I, Bergstrom R, Kruseno UB. Prognosis after breast cancer diagnosis in women exposed to estrogen and estrogen–progestogen replacement therapy. Am J Epidemol 1989; 130:221–8.

Chapter 18

Oestrogens and Thrombosis

T. W. Meade

Introduction

There are a number of uncertainties and anomalies about the effects of oestrogens on thrombogenic pathways and thus on the incidence of clinical events that are due largely or partly to thrombosis – primarily ischaemic heart disease (IHD) and stroke. This chapter summarises the evidence on associations between oestrogen levels and thrombotic episodes and the apparent effects of these levels on thrombogenic mechanisms. It may be possible to resolve some of the anomalies observed, as least in part, by considering mechanisms protecting against thrombosis, as well as in those leading to it.

Thrombogenesis

On the arterial side, thrombotic vascular occlusion is due to the relatively rapid processes of platelet aggregation and fibrin deposition superimposed on the much more chronic process of atherogenesis. In the coronary arteries, it is usually the rupture of an atheromatous plaque that triggers thrombosis, although the occurrence of some arterial thrombi in the apparent absence of plaque rupture suggests that characteristics of the circulating blood (as well as of the vessel wall) are involved. Vessel wall changes are not, however, a marked feature of venous thrombi, in which fibrin deposition is usually much more obvious than platelet aggregation.

This chapter concentrates mainly, though not exclusively, on the acute, short-

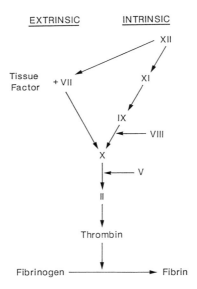

Fig. 18.1. A summary of the coagulation system.

term events in thrombosis rather than the longer-term processes involved in atherogenesis. While there is, of course, no doubt whatever about the central role of platelets in thrombosis, attempts to define "thrombotic tendency" in term of platelet function tests have so far been unrewarding, particularly in large-scale studies. Although some measures probably do suggest that thrombosis is occurring or may have taken place very recently, there is no consensus about methods for detecting people at high risk of future thrombosis on account of platelet sensitivity. The very considerable within-person and laboratory variation in tests of platelet behaviour [1] adds to the difficulties. For these and other reasons, the most useful studies on oestrogens and thrombosis have been concerned with the coagulation system. This is outlined in Fig. 18.1.

Besides its more familiar role in producing fibrin from fibrinogen, thrombin is a potent platelet-aggregating agent. Fibrinogen itself is an important co-factor in platelet aggregation [2,3]. The final common pathway of the coagulation system may be initiated by either the intrinsic or the extrinsic pathway, though these are not entirely separate, for example, the activation of factor VII by factor XII shown in Fig. 18.1. The extrinsic system is so called because its activation requires a component, tissue factor, not found (at least under usual circumstances) in the circulating blood. Tissue factor is likely to become available in large quantities when a plaque ruptures, and in smaller but nevertheless probably significant amounts as a result of the action of cytokines on endothelial cells and some white cells. In the presence of tissue factor, the level of factor VII activity, VII_c, is likely to exert a major influence on the rate of thrombin production.

There is now extensive evidence that high fibrinogen levels are strongly associated with an increased incidence of IHD in both men and women [4,5] and that, in men, high VII_c levels are also involved. The relationship between VII_c

and incidence in women has not so far been sought. Besides the associations of fibrinogen and VII$_c$ levels with the subsequent incidence of IHD, there is now considerable and rapidly growing evidence from other sources that these associations are likely to be of causal significance [4].

It is on VII$_c$ levels that oestrogens have most consistently been shown to have effects.

The pro-coagulatory system depicted in Fig. 18.1 may be countered by one or more systems with anticoagulatory effects. One of these is antithrombin III which, as its name suggests, neutralises thrombin, although it also reduces the activity levels of other clotting factors, mainly factor X. A second is the fibrinolytic system, whose function is to dissolve fibrin. A third (not considered further in this account) is the protein C and S system whose activation reduces coagulability and enhances fibrinolytic activity.

Before the effects of altering oestrogen levels are considered, an interesting physiological difference is the greater degree of platelet aggregability in women than men [2], which implies some kind of protective mechanism set at a higher level in women.

Oestrogens and Thrombosis

There are four main circumstances in which oestrogens may influence the risk of thrombosis. These are: (a) the use of oestrogens in combined oral contraceptives (COC); (b) their use in hormone replacement therapy (HRT); (c) the decline in oestrogen production associated with the menopause and (d) the use of oestrogens in men for the treatment of carcinoma of the prostate.

Oral Contraceptives

There is no reasonable doubt that the use of COC is accompanied by an increased risk of thrombotic events on both the arterial and venous sides, though the precise magnitude of these risks is still under discussion [6]. The most convincing evidence that the oestrogenic component of COC contributes to thromboembolism is that the higher the dose of oestrogen the greater the risk for both arterial and venous events [7,8]. Some caution is necessary in interpreting this apparent dose–response relationship since different types and doses of progestogen have been incorporated in the formulations containing the various oestrogen doses on which the studies in question have been based. However, there is little consistent evidence that the progestogenic component of COC affects the incidence of venous thromboembolism. The association between COC use and venous events can therefore be attributed with some confidence to the oestrogenic component. This in turn, lends support to the likelihood that the oestrogen also influences the incidence of arterial events. It has in fact been much easier to assess the progestogenic effects of COC, since two series of COC contain varying doses of the same progestogen (norethisterone acetate in one series, levonorgestrel in the other) at a constant dose (50µg or 30 µg) of the same oestrogen, ethinyloestradiol. There are clear dose–response relationships [9,10] for arterial events. It is probably through effects on blood pressure and blood lipid levels that the progestogens in COC exert their effect [11–13].

Table 18.1. Mean age-adjusted VII_c and fibrinogen levels in women using combined oral contraceptives (COC) according to dose of oestrogen [4]

	Not on COC ($n=243$)	COC oestrogen dose	
		30 µg ($n=15$)	50 µg ($n=63$)
VII_c (%)	83.0	96.6	121.1
Fibrinogen (g 1^{-1})	2.52	2.84	2.89

Table 18.2. Mean age-adjusted fibrinolytic activity (100/lysis time in hours) by smoking habit and COC use in 363 women [11]

	COC users	COC non-users
Smokers	30.3	26.3
Non-smokers	37.9	30.5

Both COC and smoking effects: $P<0.001$

Most coagulation studies in COC users that have included VII_c have found significantly higher levels than in non-users. Furthermore, the effect is dependent on the dose of oestrogen, as illustrated in Table 18.1 based on participants in the Northwick Park Heart Study (NPHS) [4]. Table 18.1 also suggests a dose-dependent relationship for fibrinogen levels. Some [14] but not all [15] studies suggest that COC may also lower antithrombin III levels. Perhaps surprisingly, COC use probably raises rather than lowers fibrinolytic activity. Table 18.2 summarises the effects of both COC use and smoking in NPHS participants [11], from which it appears that in both smokers and non-smokers, COC use is associated with more active fibrinolytic activity than in non-users. Although rather speculative, the explanation is probably a compensatory increase in one of the antithrombotic mechanisms to offset other, procoagulatory effects – in this case, the increases in VII_c and fibrinogen. There are other examples of this kind [15,16].

In summary, the oestrogenic component of COC increases the risk of thromboembolism, apparently by raising clotting factors whose levels are known to be associated with the risk of thrombotic events.

Hormone Replacement Therapy

Taken as a whole, the evidence from clinical, epidemiological and pathological studies suggests that oestrogens (taken as Premarin) confer some protection against IHD and, though there is rather less evidence available, against stroke as well [17–20]. The magnitude of these effects is uncertain, however. Much of the evidence comes from case-control studies in which it is possible that HRT may sometimes have been avoided in those considered to be at risk of thrombotic events, even though many of the studies in question have made extensive attempts to allow for potentially confounding characteristics. Conclusions from these studies that HRT dramatically reduces the incidence of IHD and stroke may therefore be over-optimistic. That this reservation is not just theoretical is well exemplified by comparing the results of randomised and non-randomised studies of the effects of oral anticoagulants on mortality following myocardial infarction, which shows that the benefit in the former is about 20%, compared with about 50% in the latter [21]. Almost certainly, the explanation for the contrast lies in the inability of non-randomised comparisons to allow fully for imbalances in characteristics other than treatment that are associated with a greater or lesser risk of experiencing an event.

Most women now using HRT take combined preparations which include a course of progestogen towards the end of each treatment cycle, to avoid the development of uterine cancer. While the dose of progestogens in combined preparations is not large, account must necessarily be taken of the effects of progestogens in COC unless and until clear evidence as to the effects of combined HRT formulations on the clinical incidence of thromboembolism is available. The rapid availability of new combined formulations and of new modes of delivery has to be taken into account and may make it hard to be sure about the cardiovascular effects of the opposed regimens mainly used over the next decade. Meanwhile, it is not justifable to assume, at any rate with any degree of certainty, that combined HRT formulations confer the same protection against IHD and stroke that is probably attributable to oestrogen-only preparations [22].

As with studies on the clinical cardiovascular effects of HRT, most of the work on coagulation changes has been based on oestrogen-only formulations. The most consistent coagulation change noted has been an increase in VII$_c$, possibly greater in those taking synthetic than natural oestrogens. Fibrinogen and factor X levels also probably rise, while antithrombin III levels fall [14].

In summary, oestrogen-only HRT probably does confer some protection against IHD and stroke, though quite possibly not as much as is often supposed. The coagulation changes produced by oestrogen-only HRT are similar to those caused by COC. There is an apparent anomaly between the clinical effects of oestrogens in COC and in HRT. A possible explanation is that, in the absence of adverse progestogenic effects on blood pressure and blood lipids in oestrogen-only preparations, the beneficial effects of these preparations on lipid profiles outweigh any adverse coagulation effects. Another possibility is considered later.

Menopause

There is little doubt that the incidence of IHD after the menopause rises over and above the increase associated with advancing age. It has been natural to consider the decline in oestrogen production as being responsible. This suggests another anomaly, i.e. the increase in thrombotic episodes associated with the oestrogen in COC compared with the decline of oestrogen production and an increased risk of thrombosis after the menopause.

Several recent studies have now provided remarkably consistent findings about the effects of the menopause on coagulability. Table 18.3 summarises clotting factor and cholesterol levels in women taking part in the Northwick Park Heart Study (NPHS), according to their menopausal status. The results in Table 18.3 are corrected for age. (The original publication [23] also gives actual values

Table 18.3. Mean age-adjusted clotting factor and cholesterol levels in 883 women according to menopausal status [23]

	Premenopausal (n=364)	Postmenopausal (n=469)
Factor VII$_c$ (%)	105.1	115.9
Fibrinogen (g l^{-1})	2.85	3.02
Cholesterol (mmol l^{-1})	5.91	6.26

All differences: $P=0.002$ or less

Table 18.4. Mean clotting factor and cholesterol levels during 6-year follow-up period by menopausal status [15]

	Continued periods (n=136)		Menopause			
			Natural (n=69)		Artificial (n=28)	
	Entry	Follow up	Entry	Follow up	Entry	Follow up
Factor VII$_c$ (%)	102.8	101.9	107.4	121.2[a]	99.5	106.6
Fibrinogen (g l^{-1})	2.76	2.80	2.84	3.31[a]	2.81	3.03
Cholesterol (mmol l^{-1})	5.46	5.34	6.05	6.69[a]	5.50	5.55

All changes with natural menopause: $P<0.0001$ (see also text)

in two-year age bands.) The difference in cholesterol levels was no longer significant after allowance was made for the correlation between VII$_c$ and cholesterol. The difference in VII$_c$ according to menopausal status has also been reported by others [24].

The cross-sectional findings in Table 18.3 have now been confirmed prospectively in women according to the occurrence or otherwise of the menopause during the six-year follow-up period [15]. The results are summarised in Table 18.4. In those who continued to have periods, there were no increases in VII$_c$ or fibrinogen. In those undergoing a natural menopause, there were highly significant increases in both clotting factors, and in cholesterol. Values for VII$_c$ and fibrinogen also appeared to have increased in the smaller number of women undergoing an artificial menopause, although the effects were not statistically significant at a conventional level. The difference between those experiencing a natural menopause and those experiencing an artificial menopause was significant ($P=0.03$) for fibrinogen but not significant at a conventional level ($P=0.3$) for VII$_c$. The difference was also significant ($P=0.007$) for cholesterol. Details of surgery were available for 22 of the 28 women whose menopause was artificial and revealed ovarian conservation in 18. This might partly explain the smaller average increase in clotting factors and cholesterol in these 28 women than in the 69 whose menopause was natural. The increase in cholesterol found in those undergoing the menopause in NPHS has also been described in an American group of women [25] in whom changes in high and low density lipoproteins (HDL and LDL) that would be expected to increase the risks of IHD were also found. Neither NPHS (unpublished observation) nor the American study found significant changes in blood pressure associated with occurrence of the menopause.

In summary, therefore, the menopause is associated with an increased risk of

IHD. From both cross-sectional and prospective studies, the coagulation and lipid changes observed are consistent with this increase. What has not so far been clearly demonstrated, however, is that it is only or even mainly the decrease in oestrogen levels at the menopause that is responsible for either the increase in clinical events or the changes in haemostatic and lipid characteristics. Could other hormonal changes such as the rise in gonadotrophin levels – although of shorter duration than the decline in oestrogens – be relevant?

Oestrogens in Prostatic Cancer

The increased incidence of thrombotic episodes in men undergoing oestrogen treatment for carcinoma of the prostate is well recognised. Much valuable information on clinical events and mechanisms has recently come from a Swedish randomised controlled trial of oestrogen and orchidectomy [26,27]. Oestrogen was given as polyoestradiol phosphate 160 mg intramuscularly every month for three months, and then 80 mg intramuscularly at monthly intervals. Patients also received ethinyloestradiol 1 mg by mouth daily for the first two weeks followed by 150 µg daily. The results are summarised in Tables 18.5.

Table 18.5. Major cardiovascular events (at 1 year) and coagulation changes (at 6 weeks) in trial of oestrogens in prostatic carcinoma [26,27]

	Oestrogens (n:53)	Orchidectomy (n:47)
Events	13	0
VII_c	+51%	+11%
Antithrombin III	−12%	+ 3%

There were 13 major cardiovascular events during the first year in those receiving oestrogens ($P=0.0008$). Seven of these events were arterial, four venous and two due to heart failure. During the first six weeks, oestrogen treatment was associated with a large net increase of some 40%, in VII_c and a net decrease of about 15% in antithrombin-III levels.

Clearly, an important feature of this and similar studies is the very large oestrogen doses used. Qualitatively, however, the effects of these oestrogens in men are similar to those of COC in women in increasing the incidence of both arterial and venous events and in raising the VII_c level. Despite the obvious differences between the context of oestrogens for prostatic carcinoma in men and HRT in women, the fact that the Swedish results come from a randomised comparison is perhaps an additioal reason for not unreservedly accepting the conclusion that unopposed HRT confers a very large benefit against arterial events.

Antithrombin III

Some progress towards resolving the anomalies that have been identified may be suggested by the findings in Fig. 18.2. This shows antithrombin III levels in

NHPS participants [15] using an improved method for antithrombin III by comparison with an earlier NPHS report on the menopause [23]. In men, there is a steady decline from the age of about 40 onwards which may imply diminishing capacity to deal with the increase in procoagulatory factors, including VII_c and fibrinogen, that occurs with advancing age. Among premenopausal women, values are lower than in men of the same age. It is clear, however, that the menopause is accompanied by a marked increase in antithrombin III levels so that postmenopausal women have the highest values of all. As the original paper points out, the decline in antithrombin III levels in postmenopausal women shown in Fig. 18.2, derived as it is from a multiple regression analysis of the data for all participants, may actually be less marked than shown here, or even absent. If so, the potential protection against thrombosis in postmenopausal women may be considerable and of some importance bearing in mind the marked increase in coagulability due to the menopause summarised in Table 18.4.

The higher values of antithrombin III in post- than premenopausal women have also been reported by others [28]. COC, which increase the risk of thrombosis, are used at ages when antithrombin III levels are relatively low. Consequently, there may be some impairment of capacity to counteract oestrogen-induced changes favouring thrombosis. HRT, on the other hand, is mostly used by postmenopausal women among whom antithrombin II activity levels are higher and may even, by counteracting the increased coagulability produced by HRT, allow oestrogen-only preparations to exert a protective effect through their influence on lipid profiles. Older men, among whom carcinoma of the prostate mainly occurs, have the lowest antithrombin III levels. The naturally low levels of antithrombin III in older men compounded by a further lowering of antithrombin III and an increase in coagulability due to oestrogens in the treatment of prostatic carcinoma may partly explain the increase in thrombotic

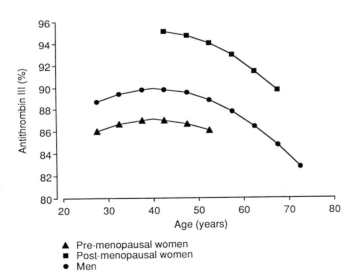

Fig. 18.2. Fitted values of antithrombin III levels in participants in NPHS [15]. ▲, Premenopausal women; ■, postmenopausal women; ●, men. (Reproduced with permission from *British Journal of Haematology.*)

events in these circumstances. Antithrombin III levels are probably of more relevance to venous than arterial thrombosis, but do also influence the latter [15].

Clearly, differences in dose and potency between COC, HRT and oestrogens used in prostatic carcinoma, and differences between the groups of subjects involved, unrelated to oestrogen administration, have to be recognised. As a possible way of reconciling some of the puzzling features of the relationship between oestrogens and thrombosis, however, the very different antithrombin III profiles summarised in Fig. 18.2 and their further implications seem to be worth considering. In clinical practice, a low antithrombin III level might, for example, be a reason for special care in presenting and monitoring HRT in a postmenopausal woman.

Conclusion

Table 18.6 summarises the effects of oestrogens on the haemostatic pathways and thrombotic events that have been considered. The findings for the menopause are shown both as a comparison of the findings in pre- compared with postmenopausal women (since it is in the former group that higher oestrogen levels occur, corresponding to the administration of oestrogens in COC, HRT and for cancer of the prostate) and as a comparison of post- and premenopausal women, which is the way the effects of the menopause are thought of.

Table 18.6. Summary of effect of oestrogens on coagulability and thrombotic events, and natural and/or oestrogen-induced antithrombin III levels

	Coagulability	Antithrombin III	Events
Oral contraceptives	↑	low	↑
Hormone replacement	↑	high	↓ [a]
Menopause:[b] pre v post	↓	low	↓
post v pre	↑	high	↑
Cancer of prostate	↑	low	↑

[a] Oestrogen-only preparations
[b] Effects assumed to be due to oestrogens

Any generalisation about oestrogens and thrombosis is clearly impossible. An approach based on antithrombin III levels that may help resolve some of the apparently anomalous observations has been suggested. The general assumption that the increase in thrombotic events after the menopause is solely due to oestrogen lack may be misleading. If so, more thorough investigation of the possible effects of other changes at the time of the menopause is indicated.

In clinical terms, perhaps the most important gap in present knowledge is the effect on thrombotic risk of opposed HRT formulations. Although like unopposed preparations, they might confer a degree of protection or be neutral so far as IHD and stroke are concerned, their adverse effects could even outweigh benefits if these assumptions turned out to be unwarranted.

Finally, turning to research implications, a more complete understanding of the reasons for the apparently differing effects of oestrogens in different circumstances would probably clarify pathways in the haemostatic system, with implications for a range of conditions in both women and men, as well as perhaps helping to rationalise the therapeutic use of oestrogens in different circumstances.

References

1. Vickers MV, Thompson SG. Sources of variability in dose response platelet aggregometry. Thromb Haemost 1985; 53:216–20.
2. Meade TW, Vickers MV, Thompson SG, Stirling Y, Haines, AP, Miller GJ. Epidemiological characteristics of platelet aggregability. Br Med J 1985; 290:428–32.
3. Meade TW, Vickers MV, Thompson SG, Seghatchian MJ. The effect of physiological levels of fibrinogen on platelet aggregation. Thromb Res 1985; 38:527–34.
4. Meade TW. The epidemiology of haemostatic and other variables in coronary artery disease. In: Verstraete M, Vermylen J, Lijnen R, Arnout J, eds. Thrombosis and Haemostasis. Leuven: Leuven University Press, 1987; 37–60.
5. Kannel WB, Wolf PA, Castelli WP, D'Agostino RB. Fibrinogen and risk of cardiovascular disease. JAMA 1987; 258:1183–6.
6. Vessey MP, Villard-Mackintosh L, McPherson K, Yeates D. Mortality among oral contraceptive users: 20 year follow up of women in a cohort study. Br Med J 1989; 299:1487–91.
7. Inman WHW, Vessey MP, Westerholm B, Engelund A. Thromboembolic disease and the steroidal content of oral contraceptives. A report to the Committee on Safety of Drugs. Br Med J 1970; 2:203–9.
8. Royal College of General Practitioners. Oral contraceptives and health. London, Royal College of General Practitioners, 1974.
9. Meade TW, Greenberg G, Thompson SG. Progestogens and cardiovascular reactions associated with oral contraceptives and a comparison of the safety of 50 and 30 μg oestrogen preparations. Br Med J 1980; i:1157–61.
10. Kay CR. Progestogens and arterial disease – evidence from the Royal College of General Practitioners' study. Am J Obstet Gynecol 1982; 142:762–5.
11. Meade TW, Chakrabarti R, Haines AP, North WRS, Stirling Y. Characteristics affecting fibrinolytic activity and plasma fibrinogen concentrations. Br Med J 1979; i:153–6.
12. Bradley DD, Wingerd J, Petitti DB, Krauss RM, Ramcharan S. Serum high-density-lipoprotein cholesterol in women using oral contraceptives, estrogens and progestins. N Engl J Med 1978; 299:17–20.
13. Khaw K-T, Peart WS. Blood pressure and contraceptive use. Br Med J 1982; 285:403–7.
14. Stanwell-Smith R, Meade TW. Hormone replacement therapy for menopausal women: a review of its effect on haemostatic function, lipids, and blood pressure. Adv Drug React Ac Pois Rev 1984; 4:187–210.
15. Meade TW, Dyer S, Howarth DJ, Imeson JD, Stirling Y. Antithrombin III and procoagulant activity: sex differences and effects of the menopause. Br J Haematol 1990; 74:77–81.
16. Meade TW. Epidemiology of atheroma, thrombosis and ischaemic heart disease. In: Bloom AL, Thomas DP, eds. Haemostasis and Thrombosis, 2nd ed. Edinburgh, Churchill Livingstone, 1987; 697–720.
17. Vessey M, Hunt K. The menopause, hormone replacement therapy and cardiovascular disease: epidemiological aspects. In: Studd J, Whitehead MI, eds. The menopause. Oxford, Blackwell Scientific Publications, 1988; 190–6.
18. Gruchow HW, Anderson AJ, Barboriak JJ, Sobocinski KA. Postmenopausal use of estrogen and occlusion of coronary arteries. Am Heart J 1988; 115:954–63.
19. Sullivan JM, Vander Zwaag R et al. Postmenopausal estrogen use and coronary atherosclerosis. Ann Intern Med 1988; 108:358–63.
20. Paganini-Hill A, Ross RK, Henderson BE. Postmenopausal oestrogen treatment and stroke: a prospective study. Br Med J 1988; 297:519–22.
21. Armitage P. Clinical trial in the secondary prevention of myocardial infarction and stroke. Thromb Haemost 1980; 43:90–4.

22. Thompson SG, Meade TW, Greenberg G. The use of hormonal replacement therapy and the risk of stroke and myocardial infarction in women. J Epidemiol Community Health 1989; 43:173–8.
23. Meade TW, Haines AP, Imeson JD, Stirling Y, Thompson SG. Menopausal status and haemostatic variables. Lancet 1983; i:22–4.
24. Scarabin PY, Bonithon-Kopp C, Bara L, Malmejac A, Guize L, Samama M. Increased factor VII reactivity in menopausal women. Thromb Haemost 1989; 62:56.
25. Matthews KA, Meilahn E, Kuller LH, Kelsey SF, Caggiula AW, Wing RR. Menopause and risk factors for coronary heart disease. N Engl J Med 1989; 321:641–6.
26. Henriksson P, Edhag O. Orchidectomy versus oestrogen for prostatic cancer: cardiovascular effects. Br Med J 1986; 293:413–15.
27. Henriksson P, Blomback M, Bratt G, Edhag O, Eriksson A. Activators and inhibitors of coagulation and fibrinolysis in patients with prostatic cancer treated with oestrogen or orchidectomy. Thromb Res 1986; 44:783–91.
28. Meilahn E, Kuller LH, Kiss JE, Matthews KA, Lewis JH. Coagulation parameters among pre- and postmenopausal women. Am J Epidemiol 1988; 128:908.

Discussion

Studd: Dr Meade spoke about hormone therapy being analogous to the combined oral contraceptive in some respects, and he spoke about the increased coagulability of oestrogen therapy. It makes one wonder what oestrogens he was talking about. Certainly with natural oestrogens there is no excess coagulability, although I seem to recall that the Northwick Park study did deal mostly with synthetic oestrogens.

Meade: When we look at the data as a whole, the effects do seem to be larger and more obvious with synthetic than natural oestrogens.

Studd: But are there data on natural oesrogens, the oestrogens we use in the menopause?

Meade: No, we have none. This is an overview of the studies that we did a few years ago and we did identify this as one of the problems. There was a wide range of preparations used in a wide range of different sorts of studies, but the conclusion we came to was that on these measures of coagulability, the use of HRT has fairly similar effects to those due to oral contraceptives.

Notelovitz: I should like to endorse that comment about the effect of so-called natural oestrogens, specifically conjugated equine oestrogens, and coagulation factors compared to the synthetic oestrogens and oral contraceptive usage. We have done studies in both populations using the same coagulation laboratory and see a big difference, specifically in relationship to antithrombin III. This has been confirmed by Howard Judd and his group when they did a study looking at the patch versus Premarin and found no change in antithrombin III activity. It is therefore, important to consider the type of oestrogens used, and within that context, the dosages used. The lower the dose of oestrogen, the less the effect seen on antithrombin III activity.

One other point was that as the patients are followed into the postmenopausal period, we found from the anticoagulation side they get an increase in plasminogen activity. Why this happens I do not know, but certainly it is statistically very significant. And that factor in turn is enhanced when these patients are given progestogens, and these progestogens can be either the 19-nortestosterone derivatives or medroxprogesterone acetate. We have done studies both with oral contraceptive users and with women taking natural oestrogens plus Provera and seen exactly the same effect.

The bottom line to this is the reproductive status of that individual, the type of hormone therapy they are getting, and the balance between the oestrogen and progestogen effect which will ultimately determine whether coagulation risk is really increased.

Meade: I think that Dr Notelovitz is right, and I think that the possibility that progestogens in the combined preparations might raise cholesterol levels and increase blood pressure, but at the same time increase fibrinolytic activity, simply makes the point more eloquently than anything else that we cannot solve what to me is perhaps the greatest question about HRT use at the moment, in other words what is the effect of combined preparations, in any other way than actually looking at what they do to the clinical events. Studying these mechanisms is very interesting and very important for all sorts of other reasons, but at the end of the day this problem will have to be grasped, preferably through a randomised controlled trial.

Studd: Can we firm up a view that we cannot extrapolate combined COC data with menopausal therapy, whether we are talking about strokes, heart attacks, lipids or anything? Certainly there are synthetic oestrogens and continuous progestogens that confuse the effect and that we have to work out.

Meade: It think that is right, but at the same time it is perfectly reasonable to look to what we know about COCs in the absence of firm evidence. I am not for a moment saying that because both progestogens and oestrogens in COCs appear to increase the risk of thrombosis, that is necessarily true of combined HRT. But I would be very foolish to overlook that possibility.

Vessey: We have just completed a three-year study of mortality in cardio-vascular diseases in England and Wales in women to age 39 years which looked specifically at COC use and it is nice to see that the relative risks are all very low in relation to cardiovascular disease, which does support the notion that modern pills used in a modern way have lower risks associated with them than older pills used in an older way. The risk for myocardial infarction is about 2.0 and for most of the other events it is between 1.0 and 1.5.

In relation to Professor Ross's presentation, the lack of data on dose and duration of use is intriguing, and is a pity. If one is postulating an effect through, say, serum cholesterol or HDL, one would expect to see dose relationships and one would expect to see duration of use relationships, and if they were not seen one would be very suspicious that there were collective mechanisms operating that were tending to generate the low relative risk, i.e. low-risk women were being selected into the group to be given HRT, which could pose a problem.

Nearly all the studies come from the United States and they nearly all relate to Premarin, and therefore I personally feel more comfortable with Premarin as a therapy than I do with any of the other combinations or products about which we know nothing. It is rather nice to know something about at least one product.

But I get tired of saying that all the data relate to Premarin and relate to unopposed Premarin. We know that Premarin is being opposed with medrox-yprogesterone acetate (MPA) in the United States. I do not know how slow physicians in the United States were to get on to opposing Premarin with MPA, but there must be a lot of it around now. I take it there are no data on opposed Premarin in the Leisure World study, but is anything known about the opposition of Premarin with MPA in the United States and is there some definitive case-controlled study that could be done in the United States that would generate data not just about unopposed Premarin but at least about Premarin plus MPA?

Ross: There is essentially no use of combination therapy in Leisure World. It is strictly related to the age of the population, when they went through the menopause and what was popular practice at that particular time.

We did a survey of gynaecologists in the Los Angeles area a couple of years ago to try to find out how their hormone replacement therapy prescribing practices had changed over time. Most said that they were using combination therapy fairly routinely for their postmenopausal patients. That disagrees greatly with what we found in a case-controlled study in breast cancer of perimen-opausal and early postmenopausal women aged 50–60 years that is ongoing in Los Angeles County, and we are really trying to address the issue of combina-tion therapy and breast cancer risk. Ever use in a fairly large number of controls is in the neighbourhood of 5% in any history of any past use of combination therapy, and long-term use – long-term being more than three years – is considerably less common than that.

We do get women who say their doctors have told them to take combination therapy and they do not like it, so they simply do not comply with the recommendation by their physician. They do not like to bleed and so they do not take it.

I cannot really answer the question directly. There certainly is evidence that the prevalence of prescriptions of Provera in particular is rising in the United States fairly dramatically. Doctors in Los Angeles say they are using them, and gynaecologists say they are using them routinely in postmenopausal patients. The data from what is essentially a sample of the upper social class in Los Angeles suggest that they are not in very common use, and so there is conflicting information.

There was a question about dose–response relationships and the fact that we really have very few data. I mentioned in passing that we see no evidence for dose–response effect for the cardiovascular disease outcomes in Leisure World, and that is certainly true. However, it is not straightforward trying to evaluate dose effects in Leisure World, because of trends in prescribing practices and the apparent reduced risk with increase in users. Women who stayed on oestrogen therapy through the endometrial cancer reports in the mid-1970s have tended to change their dose and to move from higher dose to 0.625 mg, so virtually all the recent users and current users, are taking the lower of the two doses, which really complicates evaluation by dose response.

Persson: We have looked at myocardial infarct outcome in the cohort (unpub-lished results). We do not have the same level of detail in the analysis for that outcome simply because we do not have the question and data from the cases that have accrued. We have associations with oestradiol compounds in this cohort, that is the main type of oestrogen, and overall we find a protective effect in the order of 30%.

Studd: With oestradiol valerate?

Persson: Yes. But we could look at the subgroup from prescriptions, the subgroup of compounds with oestradiol 2 mg plus levonorgestrel 250 µg, because that was a fixed brand that was recognised on the prescriptions. And in that subgroup there is also a protective effect.

The data are very preliminary and it could be that these women had been on oestradiol before that. We do not know the exact duration because these are only prescription data. But it is an indication that they do not get rid of the whole of the protective effect by having that particular progestogen, for 10 days in that combined trial. I must stress that these are unpublished data.

Whitehead: In the groups on the combination therapy – that risk was reduced by 30% as well?

Persson: At least 30%.

Whitehead: As much as for oestrogen by itself?

Persson: Yes. But that relies on prescription data from a three-year period and there is considerable misclassification anyway.

Whitehead: And the combination of oestrogen plus progestogen is in one tablet?

Persson: Right. So we could catch that from the prescriptions. In that subgroup of the cohort, in those who had ever been prescribed that compound there was still a protective effect.

Whitehead: And it is not as though the patient could have taken the oestrogen component and not taken the progestogen?

Persson: No. It is in one tablet.

Hart: As far as the effect of progestogens on lipids is concerned, a long-term study of micronised oestradiol plus norethisterone – Trisequens – and continuous micronised oestradiol 2 mg plus 1 mg norethisterone as Kliogest (and we now have some women who have 5 years of Kliogest), showed that both these preparations require that the women take a progestogen. But what appears to happen is that as time goes by, changes revert to baseline, so that after a year on Trisequens and certainly two years on Kliogest the actual cholesterol fraction changes and we are more or less back to baseline. However, with continuous oestradiol and norethisterone there seem to be some apolipoprotein changes co-existing.

So it does look as if some of the worries about the effects of androgen-derived progestogens counteracting oestrogens are based on 6 months, or 3 months or so, and that with the passage of time things do seem to revert to baseline.

There is another interesting point. Giving dihydrogesterone with conjugated equine oestrogen, and on the other hand the androgen derived norgestrel with conjugated equine oestrogen, we found that there was not so much difference as one might have expected between the so-called favourable dihydrogesterone and the norgestrel, because the norgestrel prevented some of the rise of triglyceride and the norgestrel depressed low-density lipid cholesterol. A back-up to that is that from the long-term 3-year lipid study on implants, the oestradiol plus testosterone implant at 3 years showed a decrease in low-density lipid cholesterol, which was the only significant change seen at that length of time.

Studd: Were the changes on this preparation, the Kliogest, beneficial?

Hart: The changes were basically a decrease in high-density lipid. They were deleterious changes taking away part of the benefit of the oestrogen.

But the good news was that as time went by, certainly by two years on continuous therapy these potentially harmful changes had returned to baseline. But of course that is not as good as getting the positive benefits of unopposed oestrogen.

Can anyone comment on the place of aspirin 75 mg/day as a prophylactic in patients who may have superficial venus thrombosis, or perhaps the occasional patient whose life is being made impossible by flushing and sweating a long time after a deep-vein thrombosis and who is very keen to go on to oestrogen?

Studd: Could I first ask Dr Montgomery to comment on the lipid information.

Montgomery: I agree with Dr Hart. The progestogens do appear to oppose oestrogen, and obviously a lot of the studies that have been done have looked at short term effects at 3 months or 6 months, and the feeling is that presumably long term there will be a balance. As he says, there might be a return to baseline, but that presumed cardioprotective value of oestrogens alone is lost.

Whitehead: In Portugal in July 1989, Brian Henderson presented data on supposed beneficial lipid changes with oestrogen by itself showing that where therapy is initiated with oestrogen alone there is an increase in HDL and suppression of LDL, but three years after initiation of oestrogen-only therapy those beneficial changes had completely disappeared; they were transient.

Ross: I am not quite sure that that is what he presented.

In Leisure World, where we have just cross-sectional data, not clinical data with crossover or control data, we can detect no differences in lipid profiles between oestrogen users and that small group of women who we have been able to get samples on who were using combination therapy. I said there is no combination therapy; there is very very little, not enough to give us any useful information as to outcomes.

Whitehead: But I am talking about oestrogen by itself.

Ross: I showed data from Leisure World, which I believe are the only data which he has available to him, which are the cross-sectional data for oestrogen alone, during my presentation, and there is a very favourable influence on HDL.

Whitehead: Which is maintained long term?

Ross: These are long-term users by and large. That is correct. I guess I misunderstood the question. We see no evidence in Leisure World, again based on cross-sectional data, that those lipid changes deteriorate at all, even after many years.

Anderson: Could Dr McKay Hart or Dr Montgomery comment on the changes in relation to the stage of the cycle – the progestogen dose at the time in the cycle that they are on in relation to the progestogen.

Hart: In our publication we have taken blood samples during the progestogen phase. We have looked at the two phases of the cycle and in fact the lipids do not change so rapidly. At one stage we had ladies attending for 10 weeks having blood taken on Trisequens in an attempt to see whether we could confirm Klaus Christianssen's data some years ago suggesting that there was a better effect in mineral metabolism during the combined phase as compared to the oestrogen-only phase. We re-ran that study and in fact could not confirm it. But we did lipids weekly and there was no up-down, up-down, up-down. A week or half a week is too short a time to get a change.

   If we are talking about combined therapy, then we are looking at the mean of a fortnight on oestrogen, a fortnight on oestrogen plus progestogen, and we did not see a significant change, up-down, up-down, up-down, from week to week.

   In answer to Mr Whitehead's question about the long-term effect: in 40 women on mestranol at 10 years and 32 women who had been taking nothing for 10 years, LDL was significantly down, HDL up, the good thing about it being that it was mainly HDL II-fraction that was up. That was after 10 years – still the same protective or beneficial effect. Yes, the triglyceride was still raised, but the cholesterol changes were infinitely better and more protective than the slight change in triglyceride.

   So I would maintain that if women take the therapy for a long time, and at an average 23 μg mestranol daily, they do not lose the effect.

Whitehead: I just misinterpreted the data. I am sorry.

Montgomery: I talked about different doses and different types of progestogens and I suggested that maybe these new third-generation progestogens might be of interest. I did hint at the route of administration of progestogens and I wondered if any member of the Group might care to suggest what effect giving the progestogen percutaneously might have on lipoprotein metabolism.

Studd: Does it make a difference?

Whitehead: In a small study to be published soon, we were not able to show any effect at small doses of transdermally administered norethisterone. In a larger study we do see some, but we do not see an increase in HDL. Whether that is because transdermal administration of oestrogen does not cause an increase in HDL we really do not know. But there is not a lot going on.

Stevenson: It is fair to say that giving progestogens transdermally does not necessarily abolish any adverse metabolic effects.

Selby: Thinking about routes of administration, is it not rather strange that we should be thinking that to give oestrogen either transdermally or by subcutaneous pellet might totally abolish any beneficial effect on lipoprotein profiles if we are saying at the menopause the lipoprotein changes are adverse and they are not getting oestrogen into their portal circulation premenopausally? Mr Studd has done subcutaneous implants in many patients. Does he have any data coming up on cardiovascular mortality?

Studd: It is coming up as regards lipid data, and it is as good as with oral oestrogen in producing an elevation of HDL. But we have no data on events and death rates.

In Martin Vessey's study started six or seven years ago, one-third of the patients were implants, and given time we should get the answer from there.

Meade: Can I give my view on aspirin. Dr McKay Hart asked about the use of aspirin in somebody who is on opposed HRT.

Hart: Who is on any sort of therapy. Whether or not she has had a hysterectomy would be irrelevant.

Also we know that quite a number of the patients are referred to the menopause clinics by their cardiac physicians, patients who have had coronary bypass operations. I tend to put them all on to aspirin if they are not already on it. But I wonder am I kidding myself? Are the platelets less important, or vascular wall events?

Meade: The evidence that aspirin has much effect against venous thrombosis is very slim. I would certainly think that is the right way to go about it for patients who had had arterial events, but not venous events.

Studd: It is a very important point, previous deep-vein thrombosis and pulmonary emboli. Certainly in deep-vein thrombosis I would give oestrogens, and with great confidence that they are safe.

Anderson: Percutaneous or subcutaneous?

Studd: It does not matter. Particularly if they are post-hysterectomy and there is no need for progestogen. If a woman post-hysterectomy has some sort of thrombosis, a vague diagnosis years in the past, and that women is severely ill with menopausal symptoms, I certainly would not deny her oestrogens and I believe it is absolutely safe.

Hart: The quality of life can be so miserable that women sometimes say they would prefer to take the risk of dying from a thrombosis. And I, like Mr Studd, do not think there is a significant risk.

Studd: But where Dr McKay Hart has it in mind to give aspirin, I would give them oestrogens.

Hart: As well as oestrogen.

Purdie: We have to be very careful to make a distinction between a previous deep-venous thrombosis which is secondary to a known event which predisposes to it, and spontaneous deep-venous thrombosis. I am extremely suspicious, even allowing for the difficulties in clinical diagnosis, of a recollected deep-venous thrombosis which was in fact spontaneous. Any woman who gives such a history must have a very thorough evaluation of her haemostatic mechanism before considering oestrogen for her.

Studd: But would this thorough evaluation tell us anything 10 years after the event?

Purdie: In a recent case we found an isolated antithrombin III deficiency.

Whitehead: I have had one like that as well.

Notelovitz: The question of aspirin is very important. There is a good pharmacological basis for this, the effect that low doses of aspirin have – and that is the key – on the synthesis of prostacyclin in relationship to thromboxane. At the dose that Dr Hart was suggesting we would see a relevant predominance of prostacyclin over thromboxane.
   I think that one should give these patients low-dose aspirin when they are put on combination hormone therapy. It is quite important.

Meade: From a point of view of arterial events?

Notelovitz: Arterial events, yes. But nothing to do with venous thrombosis.

Meade: From Professor Vessey's FPA study [1] with his rather reassuringly low but still slightly raised RRs, he must presumably be able to get some idea about whether the risks have changed over time with the change in the use of different preparations.

Vessey: The data are not presented in that report which was concerned with mortality, and based on small numbers of events, and was largely concerned with overall risk and benefit. We have published studies of morbidity and they all suggest lower risks with which I would call modern oral contraceptives rather than the older high doses.

Studd: The other question was a previous heart attack, or previous bypass. Professor Ross's group has data there and there is another study showing the decreased mortality with oestrogen users on patients who have had previous heart attacks. In a way that is not a contraindication for therapy but an indication for oestrogen therapy. Would we agree with that?

Hart: I was really asking whether they should be given aspirin as well.

Selby: There is certainly a lot of evidence from the lipid people that I work with that if we do not get these people's lipids right, they will run into problems with closure of their grafts. If we have a simple measure like giving oestrogen that will put lipid back towards the levels that we would feel happier with, then we ought to be doing it.

Studd: Should we give these patients oestrogens unopposed? Are we justified in giving these patients the cyclical unopposed oestrogens knowing what is at stake, heart attacks, which can be fatal, when they may develop hyperplasia of the endometrium, which is harmless? Are we justified in doing this?

Hart: I think so.

Vessey: What does one do when one finds they have got hyperplasia? I think this is a very interesting idea and I am glad we are discussing it. We do not know a lot about progestogens and we are quite worried about some of them, and therefore perhaps we should be going back to low-dose oestrogens much more than we thought in the past. One of the things that worries me is that somebody starts off on oestrogens and a year later she is found to have endometrial hyperplasia, what is to be done then?

Studd: Correct it. We correct it with progestogen, for 2 months. It is very simple.

Hart: 200–300 mg of progesterone.

Vessey: For how long?

Studd: Two or 3 months for 15 days a month.

Vessey: And then start all over again?

Hart: I am very much in favour of the trend towards continuous combined oestrogen and progestogen. That does not work very well with implants because of the higher oestradiol levels and the fact that the oestradiol level is varying and going up and down. But with oral therapy perhaps 70% of women will not bleed if they are given the Kliogest preparation, which unfortunately is not on the market in the UK, or if they get conjugated equine oestrogen plus 1 mg norethisterone daily, or 200 or 300 mg progesterone I am sure would do too. So what I would be tempted to do in that case would be to give the progesterone continuously, because if it is not having an adverse cardiovascular effect and the oestrogen is having a beneficial effect and the patient is then bleeding at all and has got endometrial protection, she has really got the best of all worlds.

What I would like would be a totally harmless progestogen which gave good endometrial bleeding control so that we could abolish cyclical therapy and all women with a uterus could have combined continuous oestrogen/progestogen and get the benefits without the undoubted nuisance of having bleeds.

Ross: At a meeting in Naples, Florida, a year or so ago, Malcolm Pike and I raised the idea of something that gained attention in the 1970s, the use of the progesterone-containing IUD. It would presumably totally prevent endometrial cancer, it would deliver progestogen to the only organ that really likes it, and presumably there would be no problem with breast cancer or with cardiovascular disease.

It was dismissed as another crazy idea from those guys from Los Angeles and there was very little discussion about it, but I keep coming back to this possibility.

Studd: But in the USA who would make it and which clinicians would be brave enough to insert it?

Notelovitz: We proposed a study like this to ALZA Laboratories about 10 years ago and we were funded for the programme. Unfortunately Ciba–Geigy bought them out two or three months later and so the study was never done, and then we had the IUD controversy.

The situation at the moment in the United States is that we can use IUDs, but there is a 5–10-page informed consent to be completed beforehand, and consequently they are not used nearly as often as they should be. But they are available for use, both the copper-T, the equivalent of the copper-T, and the Progestosert, which is what Professor Ross referred to.

I think it is an excellent idea. Especially for women as they come into the perimenopausal period when it would be relatively easy to put in one of these IUDs.

Anderson: A progestogen-containing IUD or an androgen-containing IUD?

Notelovitz: Progestogen.

Baird: Both are available. There are those that contain pure progesterone and those that have levonorgestrel.

Notelovitz: The Population Council has a levonorgestrel type of IUD but the one that ALZA make has natural progesterone. They have done studies in the premenopausal woman showing that a little of this progesterone is linked into the systemic circulation. So it really is a good idea.

Boyde: In view of the known association of prostaglandins in bone resorption, is there not a relationship of the aspirin question to osteoporosis and HRT? Indeed, have any of the studies which we have heard about this morning looked at the bone in the same patients?

Kanis: No. But we do know that both oestrogens and progestogens are bone sparing. With respect to prostaglandins it is really disappointing in the sense that there is no good evidence that the modulation of prostaglandin synthesis in vivo has any effect whatsoever on bone resorption in vivo. The reasons are not immediately obvious, but one of the reasons may be that we cannot get enough aspirin or similar drug to the relevant site.

Brincat: In defence of progesterone, I find it difficult to accept that an ordinary cycling female producing progesterone each month has got a good lipid picture, and that once she is menopausal and we try and replace her hormones, progestogens become bad. This must surely be due to the fact that we still do not have the correct pharmaceutical preparation of a progestogen available, and that pure progesterone as such is probably not harmful from a cardiovascular point of view, although the little work that has been done on pure progesterone might suggest otherwise.

I also find it difficult to accept the idea that progesterones are only of use to the uterus. We have had a study on up to 300 mg tid of progesterone as an antihypertensive which showed that pure progesterone itself has an antihypertensive effect in those patients who are hypertensive. Certainly it is an area that still needs to be explored.

Finally, I would hope that once and for all we can bury the idea that HRT as it is currently used is hypertensive and may have a deleterious effect on blood pressure. Could we hear views on the point that HRT, as it is currently used, has no effect on blood pressure one way or the other, and need not be contraindicated for hypertensives.

Studd: From the Leisure World data it would seem that hypertension would be an indication for oestrogen therapy.

Ross: I have never done any work in this area but it is my understanding that HRT as it is currently used has no effect on blood pressure in the population as a whole. I have heard talk about an idiosyncratic reaction in a tiny proportion of women, but by and large any change in blood pressure would be insignificant. Among those subgroups of women who had and had not a history of hypertension, we find evidence of cardioprotection in both groups.

Meade: But this discussion refers to oestrogen-only preparations. I want to reiterate this once more. I can see that over the next few years, decisions as to which preparations to use will be made on the basis of very poor and incomplete knowledge so far as the progestogenic question is concerned. But the crazy ideas could go on, and on, and on. The possibility of using progestogen inserts has just been discussed. I was told the other day, I do not know whether it is true but it shows the way people are thinking, that some women in the United States are now having a hysterectomy in order to go on to unopposed HRT.

These questions have got to be answered, but the basic question is what do these preparations actually do. Unless people grasp the nettle now and take whatever steps are necessary to get the answer, I think we could find ourselves in five or ten years time with a wide range of most extraordinary procedures.

Studd: There are many studies under way within this Group to answer the question.

Meade: Good. That is reassuring.

Fogelman: In terms of trying to come to any conclusions, the one big unanswered question is the long-term clinical effect of opposed oestrogen. We know how there is almost a consensus about the effect of oestrogen in bone. There seems to be a consensus about breast cancer. But the big question in terms of advising patients is the effect on the myocardium, and I think that has to be addressed.

One further point. It has come up several times that progestogens are bone sparing. Are all progestogens the same? Norethisterone seems to protect against bone loss, but norgestel, for example, does not, and not all progestogens have the same effect on the skeleton.

Lindsay: The reason is that it is very difficult to give norgestrel to non-oestrogenised women.

Selby: But at the doses that we would normally use, MPA has little effect on bone and native progesterone has little effect on bone, and if there is an effect, it appears to be limited to the 19-nortestosterone derivatives.

Lindsay: There are several studies which show that MPA in doses of between 10 and 20 mg have effects on skeleton.

Selby: But that is getting above the sort of dose that most people use.

Anderson: At that level MPA is a mild goucocorticoid and it could well have adverse effects.

Baird: If I might infuse a note of caution about progestogen IUDs as being the panacea. The problem with progestoserts which release progesterones is that they induce a very high incidence of spotting and menstrual episodes. For that reason they are extremely unpopular and they have had no commercial success even though they are licensed for use in the UK. If a progestogen-releasing IUD such as the one developed by the Population Council is to be used, the amount of progestogen which is released per day is quite significant. In order to deliver enough progestogen to the endometrium to induce endometrial atrophy, some significant systemic absorption of progestogen would still occur. It may be less than would have to be given in order to convert the endometrium systemically, and ovulation would not have to be suppressed at the same time, but there would be some systemic effect.
  It is worth exploring, but it is not a panacea.

Notelovitz: I agree entirely. The spotting issue is a very worrisome one, especially in perimenopausal patients: is it due to the IUD or is it due to something more suspicious? But on the other hand, it has to be tried and I think it is worth taking further.

Purdie: I would not like the record to show, that we think that HRT and oestrogen, opposed or otherwise, is a treatment for hypertension. It is very important that we agree that patients who we discover to be hypertensive in their evaluation prior to HRT are investigated and treated first. I do not regard mild or moderate hypertension as a contraindication, but I do regard it as a contraindication to beginning immediately.

Hart: Bruno de Lineures at the Naples, Florida meeting addressed the issue of whether there is an adverse effect of progestogens, and he gives quite a number of references and quite a bit of information suggesting that in the doses used in hormone replacement therapy, progestogens and oestrogens have no adverse effect on hypertension and that hypertension is not a contraindication to their use.
  Of course somebody with hypertension must be treated for their hypertension, but we must be careful to put the message over clearly that hypertension is not a contraindication to HRT. I get numerous letters to the menopause clinic, "This lady has a blood pressure of 150/100 therefore I am not prepared to give her hormone replacements", and we very definitely must get over the message

that mild hypertension, treated hypertension, is not a contraindication to cyclical unopposed HRT of any sort.

Persson: Would it then be an advantage to give percutaneous treatment because there is less of a metabolic effect by the liver? There would be no effect on the renin substance. Theoretically it would be an advantage to give it percutaneously.

Whitehead: But the forms of renin substrate increased by oral oestrogens have not been shown to be the forms of renin substance which are involved in the genesis of hypertension.

Persson: This brings up another point which I want to make. It has been said before that the end-point data should be studied when the effects of combined treatment are investigated. What are we looking at? We are looking at markers, that is the lipids. These are really markers for cardiovascular disease in those without treatment. Giving treatment causes a metabolic change via the liver and there will be changes in the lipid profile. Is that the same as saying that this is a marker for changes in the disease? Nobody knows that. Maybe we should stop thinking of these markers as the truth and really look at clinical trials.

Meade: What studies are in progress to settle the question?

Studd: Mr Whitehead's and my own. David Cooke has several going on.

Meade: What are they doing? Are they intermediate measure studies, in which case I would agree with what Professor Persson has just said, or are they end point studies?

Studd: Both.

Meade: But an end-point study would have to be very very big.

Studd: And very long. It will take a long time.

Meade: I would be very interested to hear what the study is.

Studd: First of all, we are using the correct hormones. We are using oestradiol, and not stilboestrol, mestranol or ethinyloestradiol, and we are using low-dose progestogens. We have serial studies looking at the clotting factors and lipids. And they are now in their ninth month.

Meade: But not end points. Not on a randomised basis in a large number of people looking at end points.

Whitehead: We desperately need clinical end point data from big epidemiological studies, because I remain unconvinced that progestogen effects in lipids would actually negate oestrogen benefits.

Meade: I agree.

Whitehead: Look at the monkey colony, the work of Thomas Clark. An androgenic progestin can be given in combination with an oestrogen, with total suppression of HDL, the LDL can be greatly increased, and yet when those animals are killed they are protected against atheroma formation as compared to an untreated group. And it may be that the benefits of oestrogens are so overrriding.

I would just add this as a word of caution, because my impression from what has been said is, "Progestogens will be bad. Progestogens work through lipids." It is all hypothesis.

Meade: They may be bad. That might be right and it might be wrong. There is only one way to find out.

Whitehead: But we need epidemiological data.

Notelovitz: There is a very important study that has not been mentioned so far, the study by Stampfer et al. [2] in which a 20-year follow-up study of oral contraceptive usage showed no adverse effect of combination oral contraceptive usage. So it bears out that point.

Although we are measuring certain obvious bad changes that have taken place in the lipid lipoprotein profile, what does it really mean when two preparations are in use, one of which is having a positive effect while the other is having a negative effect? When a potent oestrogen is used, it seems to me, based on the Clarkson data, that it is overriding this bad potential effect that we see. We see the same thing in oral contraceptive studies where the HDL2 levels were reduced to about 40% of what they should be, and we are not seeing atherogenic disease.

Whitehead: The lipoprotein profiles in men are being extrapolated to disease risk in women when men and women are fundamentally different; one has a large amount of oestrogen and the other does not.

Notelovitz: We are also dealing with a person who has an endogenous disease versus a healthy person being treated with sex steroids where cause and effect are slightly different!

Drife: It is not only us, but also the consumers, i.e. the GPs, who are very hung up on blood lipid profiles, and that is because that kind of data is used very extensively by drug firms to sell their product as opposed to somebody else's. The GPs certainly are now schooled into believing that HDL data mean cardiovascular mortality.

Studd: And it is probably meaningless.

When it boils down to it, the great problem with progestogen is producing a bleed every month, and this is the one downside I give the patients, that the benefits will be this, that and the other and the real problem for them will be a regular bleed that may be heavy, that may be painful, and they may have premenstrual tension as well.

And we are leaving out breast cancer. That is not something that many of us discuss much with our patients. And the question of screening. Should all patients pre-HRT have mammography? I guess so. There would be no dissent, would there?

Hart: There would be from the radiologists. That is the one problem.

Vessey: We now have national screening programmes.

Studd: Precisely. And there are quite a few breast surgeons, experts, who would not agree with routine screening.

Hart: I get a lot of criticism from the radiologists for sending too many patients from the menopause clinics.

Vessey: Most patients are in the right age group, 50 to 64 years, and they may well get it. If they do not get it before starting they should get it then.

Hart: Medicolegally they should probably have a mammogram before starting, providing they are 40 years and upwards. However, there would be resistance with the present state of availability, but that is not to say it should not be done.

Vessey: I have one comment that is relevant to breast cancer as well as to cardiovascular disease.

It is important to record that none of these small clinical studies we have been discussing will answer these questions. What we need are more epidemiological studies. But the Medical Research Council is looking carefully at doing another big epidemiological study in Britain along the lines of the RCGP oral contraceptive study and has a working party exploring why they are doing such a study. One of the difficulties is that there are still too few people using HRT in Britain to make such a study easy, and most of them use it for a short time, and nobody will embark on a 30 000 or 40 000 person cohort study if they expect to find that 75% of those recruited as takers have discontinued two years later. It would be a mammoth waste of a couple of million pounds. Nonetheless, that is the sort of study that is needed if the balance of benefit and risk is to be sorted out definitively, and if we are to get this question of how HRT preparations containing progestogen behave.

The other difficulty will once again by the multiplicity of preparations. But I do not think there is any substitute, to mirror what other members of the group have said. We must have end-point studies. They are the only thing anybody will believe, and certainly the only thing I shall believe.

Cardozo: It has been my understanding until fairly recently that previous oestrogen-dependent tumours which had been treated made further oestrogen replacement therapy in that individual taboo. Certainly one of our foremost breast surgeons now feels that if hormone replacement therapy is indicated in someone who has had breast cancer it should not be withheld. I do not know what the present view would be but it is quite important to discuss oestrogen-dependent tumours and oestrogen replacement therapy.

Whitehead: There is no evidence that if such patients are given HRT it increases the risk of recurrence.

Meade: There is no evidence it does not.

Studd: There is work from Creasman concerning oestrogen therapy with endometrial carcinoma. The study was uncontrolled, but it showed better survival in the oestrogen treated patients.

Anderson: Following on Professor Vessey's suggestion and the need for these cohort studies, patients referred to menopause clinics are generally a highly motivated group who as a group I would predict would continue for much longer on HRT than any other group.

How is this working party thinking of tackling this, and have they considered establishing or linking up with 20 or 30 such clinics as being at least likely to provide a cohort of patients that will go on for a very long time? They will not be representative of all postmenopausal individuals.

Vessey: That was what Kate Hunt and I were doing in collaboration with 20 or 30 such people. That study has been useful. But one problem is that the people at menopause clinics are very selective and we are uncertain as to the generalisation of data from those individuals. It is also hard to find controls. So those are two difficulties, but it has been useful.

Meade: One of the other things that that same MRC group is doing is finding out from general practitioners what they would be prepared to consider in terms of trials of different HRT preparations in either hysterectomised or non-hysterectomised patients. That would be a much more unselected population.

Studd: What the MRC study refused to do is to look at patient acceptability and to ask 1000 patients in their MRC practices if they were offered this, what would be the uptake.

References

1. Vessey MP, Villard-Mackintosh L, McPherson K, Yeates D. Mortality among oral contraceptive users: 20 years follow-up of women in a cohort study. Br Med J 1989; 299:1487–91.
2. Stampfer MJ, Willett WC, Colditz GA, Speizer FE, Hennekens CH. A prospective study of past use of oral contraceptive agents and risk of cardiovascular diseases. N Engl J Med 1988; 319:1313–17.

Section IV

Therapeutic Potential

Chapter 19

Population Screening and the Prevention of Osteoporosis

D. W. Purdie and A. Horsman

Introduction

The existence of the condition called osteoporosis and the realisation that both it and its attendant fractures are susceptible of prevention, leads naturally to an enquiry as to whether it is clinically possible and logistically feasible to discover that sector of our population which is at risk. The field of screening, however, is littered with the wreckage of schemes which failed due to inadequacies in the scientific design of the project or in its applied marketing to the population. As we can have no prior knowledge of the outcome of such a complex operation, it seems prudent to carry out a mathematical simulation of the screening process together with geographically limited clinical trials, on the sound principle of Clausewitz that times spent in reconnaissance is rarely wasted. This chapter will bring together the North Humberside Osteoporosis Screening Project based on the English cities of Hull and Beverley, and the mathematical modelling work of the MRC Bone Mineralisation Group based at Leeds University.

We will examing the suitability of the disease, of the test and of the various interventions which may be used in a screening programme, together with the likelihood that the population will accept screening and that the State will pay for it. At all stages it will be emphasised that rigorous quality control must be exercised through the validation of procedures and the acquisition of usable data.

Above all, and in the light of past experience, it will be necessary to recall the dictum of Sir Walter Raleigh that it is not in the inception, but rather in the prosecution of any great matter until it be thoroughly finished, that yields the true reward.

Suitability for Screening

The Disease

Osteoporosis robs old ladies of their lives and of their independence. In the opinion of many sufferers the loss of the latter is of greater moment than loss of the former, but the common antecedent, fractured neck of femur (FNF), must be a prime preventive target of any screening programme. It is possible, that femoral neck osteoporosis is a Gompertzian condition, i.e. one of early onset, multiple aetiology, relentless progression and resistance to therapeutic intervention [1]. Nevertheless, such resistance is not absolute and interventions have been described which appear to reduce substantially the incidence of FNF [2,3]. The second target of a screening programme must be spinal osteoporosis, which results both in the clinical distress of acute vertebral crush fracture and in the social distress of progressive height loss and stoop due to multiple wedge deformities. It is admitted at the outset that there is substantial evidence that FNF and spinal crush fracture may have different natural histories, but both operate through the final common pathway of reduced bone mineral density (BMD). We will later examine whether osteoporosis, defined via BMD, is appropriate for examination through a screening programme.

Prevalence

The usefulness of any screening is broadly proportional to the prevalence of the condition, provided that the condition itself exposes the affected individual to significant morbidity. It must be clearly stated that screening, as envisaged in the following discussion, is not screening for osteoporosis itself, but for predisposition to later osteroporosis through present relative osteopenia. It is therefore analogous to screening plasma lipid profiles for predisposition to ischaemic heart disease, in that a continuously distributed variable is sought which is itself capable of protective change by means of therapeutic intervention.

The prevalance of osteoporosis is substantial among the ranks of elderly women. In order, at this point, not to enter the controversy over the definition, either of osteoporosis or of fracture thresholds, prevalence will be defined in terms of age-related fractures alone. The incidence of the classical Colles' fracture due to a fall on the outstretched hand, begins to rise linearly at about age 45 and effectively levels out by age 60. The age-adjusted rate in women over 35 is 409 per 10^5 patient-years in the United States [4] and 309 per 10^5 patient-years in the United Kingdom [5].

Spinal fractures are of two types, the acutely painful crush fractures seen in the "young elderly" and the more prevalent silent wedge fracture of the "old elderly". A Danish study [6] found that in 70-year old women, the percentage exhibiting spinal fractures, 44%, was partitioned 4 : 1 in favour of wedge fracture. The overall age-adjusted prevalence of spinal fracture in Rochester, Minnesota is put at 1540 per 10^5 patient-years [4]. As with Colles' fracture, the incidence of spinal fracture begins to rise in the perimenopause but, in contrast to radial fracture, the rate continues to rise without abatement into extreme old age.

FNF data indicate that the incidence shows an exponential rise from the perimenopause into extreme old age, the age-adjusted incidence in Oxford in 1983 being 259 per 10^5 patient-years [7]. This translates into an estimated 40 000 cases of FNF in the United Kingdom in the present year. Hence it can be clearly appreciated that oesteoporosis-related fractures have an aggregate incidence such that their prevention would materially enhance the public health.

Personal and State Implications

The prevalence alone of a disease is insufficient to warrant the institution of a screening programme. The common cold, for example, is prevalent and un-pleasant, but is rarely a major threat to life or limb. Osteoporosis, however, may threaten both. The disease has its more violent impact on personal welfare through FNF. It has been calculated that a woman sustaining such a fracture has a 50%–20% obligatory excess risk of death in the ensuing 12 months [8] and c. 50% of the survivors do not return to functional independence in their own homes [9]. The personal or psychosocial cost of such an event cannot easily be quantified and it is equally difficult to assess the revenue consequence for the state, i.e. the NHS in Great Britain. A non-attributable statement from the Department of Health (1990) put the cost in care plus aftercare of osteoporosis-related fractures at £500–750 million per year. In the USA, FNF alone will cost $30 billion by 2020 AD, assuming 3% constant inflation and present demo-graphic trends [10]. Still more ominous is the clear indication that the incidence of FNF is rising even after allowance is made for the demographic expansion of the population at risk. Between 1954–8 and 1983 the age-specific rate of FNF in women over 65 years in the city of Oxford rose by 100% [7]. Similar trends are reported both from Europe and the United States [11]. Thus the overall severity of osteoporosis and related fractures together with its present secular change can be adduced as evidence in favour of a screening programme targeted on prevention.

Natural History

No screening programme aimed at prevention is of the least value unless the target condition, or a predisposition to it, exists in a demonstrable form and sufficiently in advance of the clinical onset for prophylactic measures to act. With regard to osteoporosis this criterion would seem to be satisfied through the behaviour of BMD and of certain biochemical parameters of mineral metabolic function in the immediate postmenopause. Peak bone density may be achieved as early as the late second decade of life [12] and loss of both cortical and trabecular bone is well established by the time of menopause. Women ultimately destined to develop fracture of spine or hip are likely to be among those whose BMD at menopause is low, although precise prediction especially in respect of FNF is not yet possible [13]. Nevertheless, two recent studies have strongly suggested that perimenopausal decrements of BMD compared to age-matched controls, are predictive of ultimate fracture risk both in the spine and at the femoral neck [2]. The long steady attrition of bone mineral in the postmenopause makes it likely that a single measurement of BMD may be sufficient to place an individual in an appropriate category regarding intervention. Such would not be the case if osteoporosis were of acute onset or if the accuracy of BMD measurement were low.

The Test

The qualities which determine applicability of a test to a screening programme differ substantially from those whch may be acceptable in the investigation of an individual patient. The attributes of the test are seen from different perspectives by the patient and the investigator.

The general opinion of the patients which will ultimtely determine the success or failure of the programme are as follows:

It shall not hurt
It shall not embarrass
It shall be safe
It shall be quick
It shall be once

The requirements of the investigator are necessarily of a more statistical nature but there is substantial overlap with the patients' needs.

It shall be quick
It shall be robust
It shall be precise
It shall be accurate
It shall be valid

The speed of measurement and the robustness of the instrument are necessary to ensure continued high throughput of the population to be screened. The measurements must be precise so that a true comparison can be made with subsequent examinations, and accurate so that management decisions based on them will be secure. Above all, the test must be valid with its sensitivity protected by a low number of false negatives and its specificity protected by a low number of false positives.

Biophysical Screening

Comparison between the various techniques for BMD measurement is shown in Table 19.1.

The single photon absorptiometry (SPA) technique though accetable to patients, relatively cheap and capable of rapid throughput, suffers from the difficulty of extrapolating appendicular measurements to the axial skeleton [14]. Although correlation between distal radial BMD and total body mineral is reasonable [15], correlation is poor with both spinal [16] and femoral neck BMD [17,14]. Even the more highly trabecular ultradistal radial site (60%–70%) or indeed the os calcis (80%) are unable to deliver close correlation with the axial sites [19,20].

Table 19.1. Features of BMD measurement techniques: axial measurements of hip and spine

	Site	Precision (%)	Accuracy (%)	Time (min)	Cost
SPA	Appendicular	1–2	5	10	x
DEXA	Axial	<1	3–5	25	1.5x
QCT	Axial	1–2	5–10	30	2.0x

Abbreviations: SPA, single photon absorptiometry; DEXA, dual-energy X-ray densitometry; QCT, quantitative computed tomography.

The quantitative computed tomography (QCT) technique delivers high precision and extremely high sensitivity in the spinal BMD measurements [21] and throughput is comparable though somewhat lower than with DEXA (see below). The technique suffers, however, from a relatively high radiation exposure – 300–500 mrem depending on the system [22]. It must also be noted that QCT is currently rather more expensive than alternative systems.

Table 19.2. Unit cost of DEXA screening

	£
Capital equipment	
DPX at £60 000 for a 7-year life	
Depreciation	8570
Maintenance control at 12% of CE	7200
Minor equipment depreciation	500
	16270
Staff	
Scientific Officer 0.2 whole-time equivalents (wte)	4600
Technical Officers 1.0 wte MTO3	14500
1.0 wte MTO3	10800
Secretary 0.1 wte	800
(All inclusive of National Insurance Superannuation)	
	30700
Consumables	
Computer accessories	300
Printer accessories	500
Stationery	250
Communications	825
	1875
Area maintenance	
Equipment supply	200
Building maintenance £14/m²	432
Energy £5/m²	300
Cleaning £24/m²	840
	1822
Total	50667

Annual throughput ≡ 8 patients/session × 8 sessions/week × 50 weeks/year
≡ 3200 patients/year
Estimated cost per patient = £15.83

Dual-energy X-ray densitometry (DEXA) delivers rapid throughput, with up to 3200 patients per year obtaining measurements of spine and femoral neck in an eight-session working week. The technique is acceptable to patients and our experience with the "DPX" system has allowed us to verify in the United Kingdom both its safety and, in particular, the manufacturer's claim for a precision of < 1%. It is thus ideal for serial comparisons when these are required.

The radiation exposure for each examination is 3–5 mrem and the system delivers an accuracy of 2%–3% in measurement of lumbar spine (L2–L4 inclusive) and of the proximal femur where data are available, from the femoral neck, from its base (Ward's triangle) and from the intertronchanteric area.

Given that our intention is to measure BMD at the femoral neck and spine in each patient, the cost of the system now installed in the Princess Royal Hospital is shown in Table 19.2. First, it must be re-emphasised that DEXA is a tailor-made technique for high-volume screening in that it is non-invasive, painless, safe and quick. The problems of invasiveness and of post-examination discomfort which affect cervical cytology and mammography respectively do not apply to DEXA.

Biochemical Screening

In 1987 it was proposed by Christiansen [23] that women losing radial BMD at > 3% per year could be identified with virtually 80% sensitivity and specificity using one biophysical measurement (fat mass) and three biochemical measurements (urinary calcium, urinary hydroxyproline and serum total alkaline phosphatase). The four results in each patient were then combined to assign each patient to an appropriate classification.

The obvious attraction of such an approach is the ability to add a measure of current loss rate to a densitometric measure of current bone mass at specific sites. The cost of the biochemical screen is £12.00 at 1990 prices. Addition of a measurement of plasma osteocalcin to the function will raise the sensitivity to 88% but will also raise the price to £17.00. This unit cost is little different from the unit cost of one DEXA screen but the essential procedural difference between the techniques lies in their convenience and simplicity for patients. DEXA can be performed at any time of day and is indifferent to the fasting state. The biochemical approach requires a patient in the fasting state, discarding of the rising urine specimen, production of the test specimen two hours later and a 48 hour abstinence from meat or gelatin in order to protect the hydroxyproline measurement. It is also technically invasive in that a venepuncture is required. Were the parameters to be refined so as to eliminate the requirements for a fast and the dietary restrictions, the sample could be taken at any time of day. Given the achievement of high specificity, i.e. the few false positives who would be offered HRT, and given competitive costing through economies of scale, the biochemical approach might well have a place in a screening programme. This might lie in clarifying that range of BMD immediately above that which mandates an offer of HRT. Further developments in the area of biochemical screening are awaited with interest.

The Treatment

There is little purpose in accurately identifying those at risk even of a highly prevalent and morbid disease, if no effective treatment can be offered to those so identified. A full discussion of the pharmacology of the agents used to conserve bone mineral is beyond the scope of this section, so a brief review of each must suffice. Of great importance to any screening programme, however, are three central aspects of any drug regimen; its efficacy, its safety and its cost.

Oestrogen ± Progestogen

It is beyond any reasonable doubt that members of the C_{18} group of steroids, collectively known as oestrogens, inhibit bone loss in the human postmenopause. Oestrogen receptors have now been identified in cells of the osteoblast lineage [24] and there is evidence of an oestrogen effect on mineral metabolism via the calcitropic hormones, particularly 1,25-dihydroxyvitamin D [25] and calcitonin [26]. Oestrogens, given in an appropriate dosage such as 0.625 mg conjugated equine oestrogens, 2 mg oestradiol valerate or 0.50 mg transdermal oestradiol, will effectively halt bone loss for as long as the regimen is given. Efficacy in bone mineral conservation is evident for at least 10 years of continuous medication [27]. The bone loss of the early natural or surgical postmenopause is highly oestrogen-sensitive and treatment at this point may be attended by a modest gain in bone mineral [28]. Treatment with oestrogen has been shown to be associated with a reduction in the rate of both spinal [2,27] and femoral neck fractures [4].

Women with an intact uterus require cyclic addition of a progestogen to protect the endometrium from overstimulation. There has been evidence for some time that certain of the 19-norprogestogens also inhibit bone loss [29] and may in fact promote bone formation [30] an observation supported by the recent demonstration that progestogen receptors are also present in cells of the osteoblast lineage [24]. Hence the addition of progestogens appears to have no adverse effect on the efficacy of oestrogen, at least in terms of skeletal protection.

The safety of oestrogen preparations in HRT is dealt with elsewhere in this volume. From the point of view of a screening programme however, it can be said that, after a competently-taken history and a clinical examination to uncover any absolute contraindication or major relative contraindication, oestrogen may be safely and confidently prescribed by family practitioners for prolonged periods of time to women shown to be at risk of osteoporosis. However, such prescription should be attended by at least an annual face-to-face review. The place of mammography before or during such long-term treatment remains to be determined.

The cost of some oestrogen-containing HRT preparations are as follows:

Oestrogen as Prempak C £49.00

Oestrogen as Cycloprogynova £40.00

Oestrogen as Estrapak £103.00

Calcitonin

This hormone is licensed by the Food and Drug Administration in the United States but is not available for clinical use in the United Kingdom. As it is a polypeptide, synthetic salmon calcitonin cannot be administered orally and, as an injectable preparation, is clearly unsuitable for prophylaxis in healthy women. Recently, however, two studies have indicated that given by intranasal spray it is capable of preventing loss of bone mineral from the spine in the postmenopause [31,32].

The drug is well tolerated and to date serious side effects have not been reported. Nevertheless, the basic NHS cost of treatment, presently unknown, is likely to be high and in the first instance it will probably find a place in the prophylactic treatment of those women in whom oestrogen-containing HRT is contraindicated or unsuitable.

Diphosphonates

These agents first found a place in the clinical management of Paget's disease where they were found to reduce bone turnover. Recently it has been reported [33] that, if given in the early postmenopause, a diphosphonate (Tiludronate) was capable of preventing loss of spinal BMD. The effect was still present some six months after cessation of six months' treatment and side effects were no different from those found in palcebo-treated controls. The diphosphonates are reasonably inexpensive and, if the above data are confirmed, may yet supply a useful alternative to HRT in postmenopausal prophylaxis.

Thus given the present availability of tried HRT delivery systems and the likely flexibility in future from calcitonin and the diphosphonates, therapy is not a barrier to the institution of a screening programme for osteopenia in postmenopausal women.

Use of a Mathematical Model to Predict Outcome of Screening

The implemention of a screening programme, however well planned, necessitates a thoroughly alarming number of clinical and behavioural assumptions. It is not enough to know that the target condition is prevalent, the screening sensitive and the intervention effective. If possible additional information should be sought on the likely effect of the intervention on the disease, specifically on fracture incidence, and on the long-term financial implications for both the primary care and the hospital care sectors of the health district involved Such assumptions are extremely difficult to quantify in the absence of any previous district-based screening data and it is here that mathematical modelling may play a role.

In 1985 Horsman, Marshall and Peacock [34] described a stochastic model which showed the behaviour of an ageing cohort of women in the United Kingdom based on the hypothesis that the risk of femoral neck fracture was

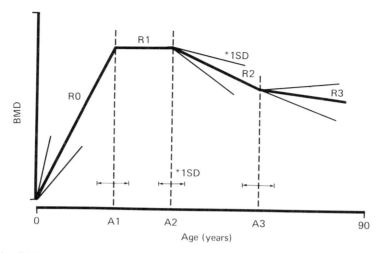

Fig. 19.1. BMD behaviour in an ageing cohort. Ages are: A1 (20 years); A2 (35 years); A3 (60 years). Rate of change between ages are shown as R values. All variables normally distributed.

primarily determined by the ambient bone mineral density of the femoral neck. Using the model it was possible to demonstrate that the risk of fracture after a fall increased exponentially with decreasing BMD. The model's prediction of the mean BMD deficits in patients sustaining FNF when compared to age-matched non-fracture cases was consistent with observed values. Later extensions of the model took account of falls [35]. Bone mineral density in the femoral neck was regarded as an estimator of the risk of hip fracture due to a fall [36].

Fig. 19.1 shows the age-related changes in BMD. All variables are assumed to be normally distributed and the ages of peak bone density attainment, onset of loss and deceleration of loss are 20, 35 and 60 years respectively. The resulting mean values of BMD in members of the cohort who had not sustained fractures at any given age, were in close approximation to published cross-sectional data on femoral neck BMD in non-fracture cases [37].

Falls were assigned to 50–60-year-old members of the cohort according to the data of Aitken [38] whereas those occurring in patients over 60 years old were assigned with a frequency based on data supplied by Dr Cyrus Cooper. An age at death was allocated to each individual based on DHSS mortality tables derived from the 1981 UK census. No member of the cohort was permitted to survive beyond 100.

The model was implemented by first assigning to each individual, data describing her lifetime variation in BMD. Each was then allocated falls on the basis of the known risk of falls as a function of age. For each individual all falls which occurred were examined and a decision, based on ambient BMD, was taken on whether or not to associate a fracture with the fall. No-one was allowed more than two femoral neck fractures. The age-specific incidence of fractures predicted by the model was computed by summing the number of fractures occurring at yearly intervals. This incidence was then compared to the true incidence shown in Fig. 19.2.

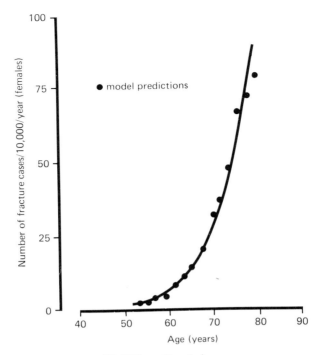

Fig. 19.2. Number of fracture cases/10 000/year (females).

Simulations

These were performed on a suite of programs written in compiled BASIC on an IBM-compatible PC. A 30 megabyte hard disk was used to store data for retrospective analysis. Cohorts of 50 000 women were simulated over 12 hours of computing time.

Results

In each cohort member sustaining a fracture reference was then made to that individual's peak bone density (PBD). It was found that fracture cases partitioned between the peak bone density quartiles as shown in Table 19.3.

Table 19.3. Origin of FNF by peak bone density quartile

PBD quartile	% of FNF
Upper	3.1
Upper mid	9.3
Lower mid	22.1
Lower	65.5

The other determinant of BMD in the elderly is rate of bone loss. Women sustaining a fracture were also classified according to their loss rate in the initial (35–60) bone loss sector. The fractures partitioned between the loss rate quartiles as shown in Table 19.4.

Table 19.4. Origin of FNF by BMD loss rate quartile (35–60)

BMD loss rate quartile	% of FNF
Upper	31.1
Upper mid	26.1
Lower mid	23.1
Lower	19.7

Table 19.5. Effect on FNF incidence by T years of effective prophylaxis against BMD loss. Cohort depleted by UK mortality

T	FNF	FNF prevented	% FNF prevented	Py/FNF prevented
0	5368	0	–	–
10	3853	1515	28	316
15	3168	2200	40	325
20	2425	2943	55	321

For abbreviations see text.

The next task set for the model was to simulate the effect on fracture incidence of a delay in the onset of bone loss (Table 19.5). To this end the simulation programs were repeated with a value (T) added to the previous breakpoints describing BMD behaviour. For each value of T the total number of fractures occurring was computed as the cohort aged from birth to death, allowance being made for death before and during treatment. The fractures predicted could then be compared to the known number in the untreated cohort and the investment in patient years (Py) to prevent one fracture could be calculated. It was assumed that the treatment had no effect on the risk of falling, or on mortality.

The programs were then re-run to determine the effect of preventing bone loss in selected sections of the cohort defined by their peak bone density (PBD) in relation to the mean for the whole cohort (Table 19.6).

Table 19.6. Predicted effect of FNF incidence of 15 years' prevention of bone loss in all women from a cohort of 50 000 whose peak BMD is below the indicated limit

PBD limit	% treated	FNF	% FNF prevented	Py/FNF prevented
None	100	3168	40	325
Mean	50	3466	35	192
−1SD	16	4328	19	111
−2SD	2	5173	4	75

PBD, peak bone density.

Discussion

The model has been shown to generate age-specific incidences of FNF which match real observations. Up to the age of 70 years fracture risk rises exponentially as BMD declines, and the risk of fracture after a fall rises by a factor of about 4.0 for each BMD reduction of one standard deviation (SD). Interestingly, above the age of 70 years the model indicates that an age-related factor independent of BMD is operating. The nature of this factor or the components which determine it are unknown.

The particular value of the model is to provide a reconnaissance of the field of BMD screening in perimenopausal healthy UK women, since from it we can plan a screening strategy which will eliminate the necessity of prolonged and expensive preliminary clinical trials. Thus it can be seen that 66% of FNF occur in women whose peak bone mass falls within the low quartile of the distribution. Prophylaxis should be targeted on this quartile. The rate of bone loss in middle age appears to be less predictive and the lifetime risk of FNF for a given survival period appears to be dominated by the BMD attained in youth.

Practical Applications: The North Humberside Project

The present rising prevalence of osteoporosis and related fracture in the UK, together with the human and financial costs of the condition, mandate that a serious and multicentre attempt be made to tackle the problem by prevention.

The data presented here are being used to plan a screening programme involving the 500 000 people who live in the Health Districts of Hull and East Yorkshire, under the direction of D. W. Purdie and Dr Sheelagh Doherty. A population education campaign is under way and, with co-operation from the Family Practitioner Committee, women aged 50–55 years will be invited, through their general practitioners, to attend for bone screening by DEXA. Those falling into the low quartile at spine or hip will be offered, again through their GPs, dietary advice, exercise advice and HRT. The project will be subject to rigorous quality control and the end-points, which will be behavioural, financial and clinical, will be subject to statistical assessment in advance to ensure that the various study designs within the project are of satisfactory statistical power.

At present we simply do not know if women want screening for osteoporosis, if they will accept advice on its prophylaxis based on screening or if they will comply with this advice in the long term. Equally, we do not know if the cost of the programme and the investment in prophylaxis will generate a meaningful return in terms of fracture prevention, or in the case of HRT, in increased protection against stroke and myocardial infarction. Collaboration with the Centre for Health Economics at York University will aid us to uncover the broader financial implications of the screening programme.

The initiative of the RCOG in convening this study group is to be welcomed. Osteoporosis has long been a clinical orphan in desperate need of two adoptive professional parents who will take on responsibility for the critical area of prevention. It is proposed that the gynaecologist and the general practitioner should be these two guardians, just as the physician, rheumatologist and orthopaedic surgeon are responsible for the management of the established disease.

The climacteric is a time of great uncertainty among women as they look ahead to old age, the prospect of which may indeed by drear [39]. It is plainly the duty of all who care for women to look ahead with them and to identify, if possible, trouble looming. It is their duty to make available the means to allow the individual to remain unbowed and straight, and to end her days with as much independence as she herself may determine.

References

1. Melton LJ, Riggs BL. Further characterisation of the heterogeneity of the osteoporotic syndromes. In: Kleerekoper M, Krane SM, eds. Clinical disorders of bone mineral metabolism. New York: Liebert, 1989; 145–52.
2. Ettinger B, Genant HK, Cann CE. Long-term estrogen therapy prevents bone loss and fracture. Ann Intern Med 1985; 102:319–24.
3. Hutchinson TA, Polansky JM, Feinstein AR. Postmenopausal oestrogens protect against fracture of hip and distal radius. Lancet 1979; ii:705–9.
4. Melton LJ, Riggs BL. Epidemiology of age-related fractures. In: Avioli LV, ed. The osteoporotic syndrome: detection, prevention and treatment. New York: Grune and Stratton, 1983; 45–72.
5. Knowelden J, Buhr AJ, Dunbar O. Incidence of fractures in persons over 35 years of age: a report to the MRC Working Party on fractures in the elderly. Br J Prev Soc Med 1964; 18:130–41.
6. Chen TL, Feldman D. Distinction between alpha-fetoprotein and intracellular estrogen receptors: evidence against presence of estradiol receptors in rat bone. Endocrinology 1978; 102:236–44.
7. Boyce WJ, Vessey MP. Rising incidence of fracture of the proximal femur. Lancet 1985; i:150–1.
8. Cummings SR. Osteoporotic fractures: the magnitude of the problem. In: Christiansen C, Johansen JS, Riis BJ, eds. Copenhagen: Osteoporosis, vol. 2. Osteopress, 1987; 1193–6.
9. Nickens HW. A revies of factors affecting the occurrence and outcome of hip fracture, with special reference to psychosocial issues. J Am Geriatr Soc 1983; 31:166–70.
10. Cummings SR, Nevitt MC. Epidemiology of hip fractures. In: Kleerekoper M, Krane SM, eds. Clinical disorders of bone and mineral metabolism. New York: Liebert, 1989; 231–6.
11. Melton KLJ, O'Fallon WM, Riggs BL. Secular trends in the incidence of hip fractures. Calcif Tissue Int 1987; 41:57.
12. Meunier P, Courpron P, Edouard C, Bernard J, Bringuier J, Vignon G. Physiological senile involution and pathological rarefaction of bone. Quantitative and comparative histological data. Clin Endocrinol Metab 1973; 2:239–56.
13. Mazess RB. On aging bone loss. Clin Orthop 1982; 165:239–52.
14. Mazess RB, Peppler WW, Chesney RW, Lange TA, Lindgren U, Smith E Jr. Does bone measurement on the radius indicate skeletal status? J Nucl Med 1984; 25:281–8.
15. Gotfredsen A, Borg J, Nilas L, Tiellesen L, Christiansen C. Representativity of regional to total bone mineral in healthy subjects and anticonvulsive treated epileptic patients. Measurements by single and dual photon absorptiometry. Eur J Clin Invest 1986; 16:198–203.
16. Laval-Jeantet A-M, Roger B, de Vernejoul MC, Laval-Jeantet J. Testing of dual-energy postprocessing method of QCT densitometry. J Comput Assist Tomogr 1985; 9:616–17.
17. O'Duffy JD, Wahner HW, O'Fallon WM, Johnson KA, Muhs J, Riggs BL. Mechanism of acute lower extremity pain syndrome in fluoride-treated osteoporotic patients. Am J Med 1986; 80:561–6.
18. LeBlanc AD, Evans H, Jhingran S, Johnson P. High resolution bone mineral densitometry with a gamma camera. Phys Med Biol 1984; 29:25–30.
19. Mazess RB. Advances in single-and dual-photon absorptiometry. In: Christiansen C, Arnaud CD, Nordin BEC, Parfitt AM, Peck WA, Riggs BL, eds. Osteoporosis, Proceedings of the Copenhagen International Symposium on Osteoporosis. Glostrup, Denmark: 1984.

20. Wasnich RD, Ross PD, Vogel JM. Evaluation of a screening test for fracture risk prediction: a prospective study of bone mineral content and fracture incidence. West Regional SNM, 1985.
21. McBroom RJ, Hayes WD, Edwards WT, Goldberg RP, White AA. Prediction of vertebral body compressive fracture using quantitative computed tomography. J Bone Joint Surg 1985; 67:1206–14.
22. Kalender WA, Klotz E, Suess C. Vertebral bone mineral analysis: an integrated approach with CT. Radiology 1987; 164:419–23.
23. Christiansen C, Riis BJ, Rodbro P. Prediction of rapid bone loss in postmenopausal women. Lancet 1987; i:1105–8.
24. Eriksen EF, Berg NH, Graham ML et al. Multiple sex steroid receptors in cultured human osteoblast-like cells. International Symposium on Osteoporosis, Aalborg, 1987. Abstract 67.
25. Stevenson JC. Vitamin D in postmenopausal women. In: Duusma SA, Sluys Veer JVD, eds. Vitamine D 43055. Utrecht: Wetenschappelijke uitgeverij Bunge, 1983.
26. Morimoto S, Tsuji M, Okada T, Kumahara Y. The effects of oestrogens on human calcitonin secretion after calcium infusion in elderly female subjects. Clin Endocrinol 1980; 13:135–43.
27. Lindsay R, Hart DM, Forrest C, Baird C. Prevention of spinal osteoporosis in oophorectomized women. Lancet 1980; ii:1151–4.
28. Lindsay R, Aitken JM, Anderson JB, Hart DM, MacDonald EB, Clark AC. Long-term prevention of postmenopausal osteoporosis by oestrogen. Lancet 1976; i:1038–41.
29. Lindsay R, Hart DM, Purdie D, Ferguson MM, Clark AS, Kraszewski A. Comparative effects of oestrogen and a progestogen on bone loss in postmenopausal women. Clin Sci Mol Med 1978; 54:193–5.
30. Christiansen C, Riis BT, Nilas L, Rodbro P, Deftos L. Uncoupling of bone formation and resorption by combined oestrogen and progestagen therapy in postmenopausal osteoporosis. Lancet 1985; ii:800–1.
31. Reginster JY, Denis D, Albert A et al. 1-year controlled randomised trial of prevention of early postmenopausal bone loss by intranasal calcitonin. Lancet 1987; ii:1481–3.
32. Overgaard K, Riis BJ, Christiansen C, Hansen MA. Effect of calcatonin given intranasally on early postmenopausal bone loss. Br Med J 1989; 299:477–9.
33. Reginster JY, Lecart MP, Deroisy R et al. Prevention of postmenopausal bone loss by tiludronate. Lancet 1989; ii:1469–71.
34. Horsman A, Marshall DH, Peacock M. A stochastic model of age-related bone loss and fractures. Clin Orthop 1985; 195:207–15.
35. Horsman A, Burkinshaw L. Stochastic models of bone loss and fracture risk. In: Ring EFJ, Evans WD, Dixon AS eds. Osteoporosis and bone mineral measurement. York: IOPSM, 1989; 15–30.
36. Horsman A, Birchall MN. Assessment and modification of hip fracture risk – predictions of a stochastic model. In: Proceedings of Steenbock Symposium on Osteoporosis, Madison (in press).
37. Mazess RB, Barden H, Ettinger M, Shultz E. Bone density of the radius, spine, and proximal femur in osteoporosis. J Bone Miner Res 1988; 3:13–18.
38. Aitken M. Osteoporosis in clinical practice. Bristol: Wright, 1984.
39. Burns R. To a Mouse. In: Poems, chiefly in the Scottish dialect. Kilmarnock: J Wilson, 1786, 22–3.

Chapter 20

Long-term Follow-up of Women on HRT

D. M. Hart

Hormone replacement therapy (HRT) has caught the attention of the lay population and the media, but discussion is often emotional rather than rational, with claims of the elixir of youth on one hand and warnings of impending doom, mainly in the form of cancer, on the other hand. Long-term follow-up of women taking HRT, comparing them with untreated women matched for age and time from menopause, gives valuable information. It is, of course, difficult for one clinic to follow a very large number for a very long time and the commencement of new long-term random allocation placebo-controlled studies is no longer justifiable.

The Glasgow Study

Commencing in 1968, 217 women were recruited to a random allocation study and were asked to take 40 µg mestranol daily, or a matching placebo. Forty eight women commenced six weeks after hysterectomy and bilateral salpingo-oophorectomy for non-malignant disease, 127 were three years from operation and 42 were six-years post-surgery (Fig. 20.1). The series continues to the present and this permits results of up to 21 years of continuous follow-up to be reported here.

The original object of the study was to compare the effects of active and placebo therapy on bone density, and using a single photon absorptiometry (SPA) technique on the middle metacarpal [1,2], it was noted that active therapy, when commenced within two months of oophorectomy, prevented bone loss (Fig. 20.2). When treatment was commenced three years after oophorectomy, by which time there had been loss of bone mineral, there was

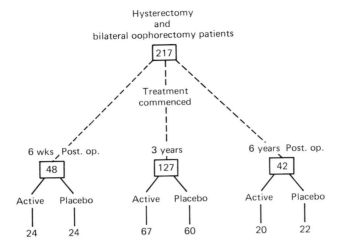

Fig. 20.1. The Glasgow mestranol study.

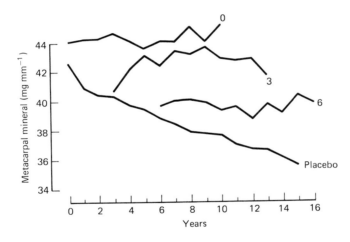

Fig. 20.2. Metacarpal mineral in subjects commencing mestranol 6 weeks (0) 3 years (3) and 6 years (6) after hysterectomy and bilteral oöphorectomy and in placebo group.

significant increase in mineral content. Mestranol therapy, commenced six years after operation, prevented further loss, but did not replace lost bone mineral. The average daily dose taken was 23 µg. Using a radiological technique [3] the gain in mineral content of the metacarpal was shown to be due to increased cortical thickness.

After a median follow-up time of 9 years, there was significant loss of height in the placebo group, but not in those receiving mestranol [4]. The placebo group

Table 20.1. Distribution of spine scores

	No of women with scores of:						
	0	1	2	3	4	5	Mean*
Oestrogen	41	13	2	1(1)			0.35
Placebo	14	8	7(1)	8(2)	3(1)	2(1)	1.62

*$P<0.01$.

Figures in parentheses indicate numbers of patients with vertebrae considered by measurement to have crush fractures.

had a higher spine score (scoring wedging as 1 and collapse of vertebral body as 2), larger wedge angle and lower central vertebral height than the active therapy group when the second lumbar and ninth thoracic vertebral bodies were examined by lateral radiography (Table 20.1). the significant difference in metacarpal densitometry, as measured by SPA, which had been demonstrated at five years, was maintained (Fig. 20.3). Thus, protection of central as well as peripheral bone was demonstrated with reduction of vertebral compression. Similar metacarpal protection after 10 years of conjugated equine oestrogen therapy was reported by Nachtigall et al. [5]. Bone density in untreated subjects was most closely related to time since oophorectomy.

At ten years of therapy no impairment of liver function was found and significant protective effects were still present in the mineral metabolic screen. No correlation could be found between basal calcitonin level or calcitonin reserve and change in bone density in 54 subjects at ten years of active or placebo therapy [6].

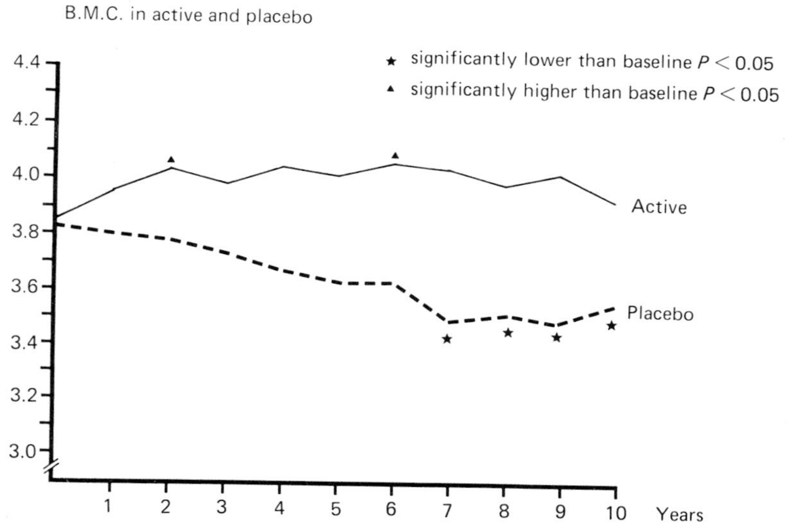

Fig. 20.3. Metacarpal mineral in subjects who commenced mestranol or placebo 3 years after hysterectomy and bilateral salpingo-oöphorectomy.

A total of 14 subjects who had received active mestranol ceased therapy of their own accord after four years. When metacarpal densitometry was repeated after four years of therapy, significant bone loss had occurred [7]. Christiansen et al. [8] demonstrated bone loss when cyclical hormone therapy was withdrawn after two years.

When we acquired dual photon densitometry (DPA) in 1985 (Lunar Radiation DP3) a comparison was made between spine density and femur density at a median of 15 years in 26 mestranol-treated and 25 placebo-treated subjects. They were well matched for age at oophorectomy, time since oophorectomy, height at recruitment and measurement and weight at recruitment and measurement. Significant projection against loss of bone mineral was demonstrated in the spine (Fig. 20.4) and in femoral neck and Ward's triangle (Fig. 20.5) [9].

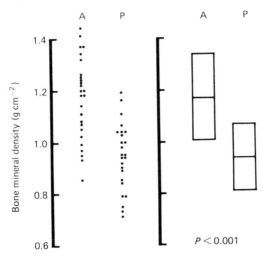

Fig. 20.4. Lumbar spine density by dual photon absorptiometry after 15 years of mestranol or placebo (p).

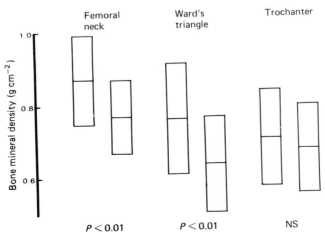

Fig. 20.5. Femoral bone density by dual photon absorptiometry after 15 years of mestranol or placebo (b).

By using a new gamma ray computed tomography scanner in 21 of the active and 19 of the placebo group, trabecular and cortical bone density of radius were measured separately [10]. Protection against bone loss was demonstrated at all sites in the mestranol group (mean 26 µg/day) with the greatest difference between active and placebo present in trabecular bone (Fig. 20.6). Repeat measurement after one year showed no further loss in the placebo group but a 1.2% increase ($P > 0.01$) in cortical bone in the treated group. At 15 years posto-ophorectomy one would not expect significant loss in a single year.

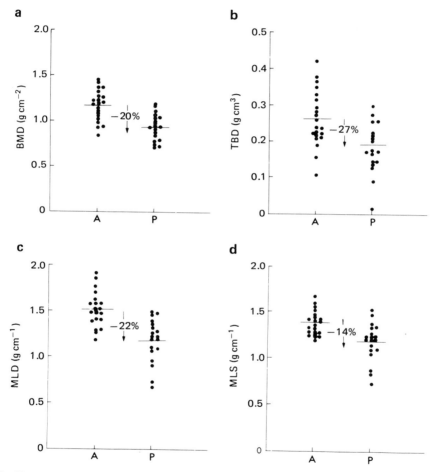

Fig. 20.6. Bone density after 15 years mestranol (a) and placebo (p) in lumbar spine: **a**, distal radius, **c** (both sites mixed cortical and trabecular bone), in central 50% of ultra-distal radius (pure trabecular bone) **b**, and in mid-shaft radius (cortical bone), **d**.

The protection against bone loss confirmed here is, of course, important, but other causes of morbidity and mortality are numerically more important (Fig. 20.7). Deaths from coronary heart disease and cerebrovascular accidents are responsible for the majority of deaths in women and it is important to know what effect long-term hormone replacement has on these. The numbers in the Glasgow series are not large enough for the incidence of major cardiovascular events to reach significance, but a number of relevant factors have been

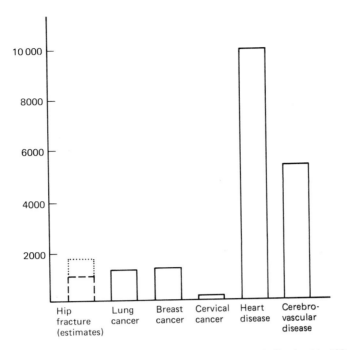

Fig. 20.7. Relative incidence of causes of death in women in Scotland in 1986.

investigated. With regard to blood coagulation, factor X was not significantly different in active and placebo-treated patients up to seven years, but factor VII was significantly elevated at one to six years on mestranol, though not alarmingly [11]. Oestrogens with a 17-ethinyl group such as mestranol are thought to have a greater effect on coagulation factors than have natural oestrogens, but in 20 women taking 30 μg of mestranol daily (calculated from the returned dispensary cards) or placebo at a median of 15 years from oophorectomy, no significant difference was found in prothrombin time, partial thromboplastin time or in antithrombin III level [12]. The commonest vascular incidents were leg cramps (Table 20.2) when 1030 women years of mestranol therapy were compared with 950 woman years of placebo. No other event showed a significant difference in incidence between the two groups.

Table 20.2.   Vascular incidents during mestranol and placebo therapy

	Mestranol	Placebo
Cramps in legs	19	2
Cerebral	3	2
Deep vein thrombosis	3	4
Myocardial infarction	1	3
Superficial vein thrombosis	6	7
Treatment years	1030	950
No. of patients	207	202

Aspects of the Oliver coronary risk score have been investigated [11]. No adverse effect on blood pressure was detected, though systolic and diastolic blood pressures had risen after three years in obese patients on placebo therapy. No significant rise was seen in weight-matched mestranol subjects. Patients on antihypertensive therapy and taking mestranol were not significantly different from those on antihypertensive therapy and placebo (H. I. Abdall, unpublished data). With regard to weight the majority of those who lost weight were on active therapy and the majority of those who gained weight were on placebo. Thin patients fared no differently on active or placebo, but patients over standard weight for height tended to lose weight on mestranol and gain weight on placebo. Mid-triceps fat-fold thickness increased on placebo and decreased on active therapy.

With regard to lipoprotein risk factors, mestranol treatment was associated with a significant fall in serum cholesterol and a significant rise in serum triglyceride after one year [13]. In 40 actively treated women and 32 placebo controls after ten years of therapy [14], the mestranol was associated with increased serum triglyceride, decreased low density lipoprotein (LDL) cholesterol and increased high density lipoprotein cholesterol (HDL). The cardioprotective HDL_2 fraction constituted the main component of the increased HDL suggesting that the long-term mestranol therapy had a beneficial effect on serum lipoproteins (Table 20.3). It is of interest that when 61 bilaterally oophorectomised women who had received implants of oestradiol or oestradiol plus testosterone for three years were compared with 67 matched controls, the only significant finding was a reduced LDL cholesterol in the oestrogen/testosterone group [15]. This suggests that long-term parenteral therapy may not have the cardiovascular protective effect of oral therapy.

Table 20.3. Serum lipoprotein concentrations (mean ± SD) in mestranol and placebo treated subjects

No. of patients	Treatment	Age	Total triglyceride ($mmol l^{-1}$)	Total cholesterol ($mmol l^{-1}$)	VLDL cholesterol ($mmol l^{-1}$)	LDL cholesterol ($mmol l^{-1}$)	HDL cholesterol ($mmol l^{-1}$)
40	Mestranol	58 ± 3	1.94 ± 0.65[a]	6.52 ± 1.08	0.62 ± 0.23	3.87 ± 1.00[b]	2.03 ± 0.46[a]
32	Placebo	60 ± 3	1.48 ± 0.74	6.60 ± 1.30	0.52 ± 0.23	4.46 ± 1.20	1.59 ± 0.33

[a]Significantly different from placebo group $P<0.001$.
[b]Significantly different from placebo group $P<0.05$.

Detailed cardiovascular assessment of the active and placebo groups is at present being carried out using electrocardiography, echocardiography, exercise tolerance and non-invasive isotope techniques. De Lignieres [16] has indicated that oestrogens and progestogens as used in HRT are not likely to affect blood pressure adversely and that hypertension is not a contraindication to the use of HRT.

Many general physicians and endocrinologists have a belief that HRT elevates prolactin above the normal range. To investigate this, 51 subjects taking mestranol and 37 taking placebo for a mean of eight years, had prolactin measured and 17 of the active group and 13 controls had basal resting prolactin and an HRT stimulation test [17]. There was no significant difference between random prolactin levels in the active and placebo groups. The basal resting prolactin was lower in the placebo group, but in both groups the level was within the normal range. The percentage prolactin increment in response to HRT was the same in the active and placebo groups and was within normal range. It is therefore incorrect to attribute an abnormally high prolactin level to oestrogen therapy.

Conclusion

It is my belief that duration of hormone replacement therapy should depend on the reasons for the therapy, including risk factors for osteoporosis and cardio-vascular disease, the acceptability of the therapy to the patient and the possibility of adverse effects. One must beware of fluid retention syndrome and treat it, preferably with calorie restriction (800 or 1000 kcal diet) though diuretics may be necessary. Premenstrual syndrome symptoms may occur on cyclical therapy and bleeding may be unacceptable in a patient with an intact uterus. Liver-mediated adverse effects and malignancies must be avoided if possible and screening during long-term follow-up should include regular breast examination (both self-examination and medical examination) and mammography according to local recommendations and availability. Blood pressure must be monitored regularly, as blood pressure tends to rise with age. Endometrial sampling in patients with a uterus on cyclical or combined continuous oestrogen/progestogen therapy is indicated if there is inappropriate bleeding and hysteroscopy has a role to play here. Full blood count and urea, electrolytes and liver function tests help detect the heavy smoker, the alcohol abuser and the occasional intercurrent disease.

References

1. Aitken JM, Hart DM, Lindsay R. Oestrogen replacement therapy for prevention of osteoporosis after oophorectomy. Br Med J 1973; iii:515–18.
2. Lindsay R, Aitken JM, Anderson JB, Hart DM, MacDonald EB, Clarke AC. Long-term prevention of postmenopausal osteoporosis by oestrogen. Evidence for an increased bone mass after delayed onset of oestrogen treatment. Lancet 1976; i:1038–41.
3. Lindsay R, Anderson JB. Radiological determination of changes in bone mineral content. Radiography 1978 XLIV; 517:21–6.
4. Lindsay R, Hart DM, Baird C. Prevention of spinal osteoporosis in oophorectomised women. Lancet 1980; ii:1151–4.
5. Nachtigall LE, Nachtigall RH, Nachtigall RD, Beckman M. Estrogen replacement therapy I: a 10 year prospective study in the relationship to osteoporosis. Obstet Gynecol 1979; 53:277–81.
6. Leggate J, Farish E, Fletcher CD, McIntosh W, Hart DM, Somerville JM. Calcitonin and postmenopausal osteoporosis. Clin Endocrinol 1984; 420:85–92.
7. Lindsay R, MacLean A, Kraszewski A, Hart DM, Clark AC, Garwood J. Bone response to termination of oestrogen treatment. Lancet 1978; i:1325–7.
8. Christiansen C, Christensen MS, Transbol I. Bone mass in post menopausal women after withdrawal of oestrogen/gestagen replacement therapy. Lancet 1981; i:459–61.
9. Al-Azzawi F, Hart DM, Lindsay R. Long-term effects of oestrogen replacement therapy on bone mass as measured by dual photon absorptiometry. Br Med J 1987; 294:1261–2.
10. Hosie CJ, Hart DM, Smith DAS, Al-Azzawi S. Differential effect of long-term oestrogen therapy on trabecular and cortical bone. Maturitas 1989; 11:137–45.

11. Hart DM, Lindsay R, Purdie D. Vascular complications of long-term oestrogen therapy. Front Horm Res 1978; 5:174–91.
12. Al-Azzawi F, Smith D, Parkin D, Hart DM, Lindsay R. Blood coagulation profile in long-term hormone replacement therapy with mestranol. Maturitas 1989; 11:95–101.
13. Aitken JM, Lorimer AR, Hart DM, Lawrie DDV, Smith DA. The effects of oophorectomy and long-term mestranol therapy on the serum lipids of middle-aged women. Clin Sci 1971; 41:597–603.
14. Hart DM, Farish E, Fletcher CD, Howie C, Kitchener H. Ten years post-menopausal hormone replacement therapy – effect on lipoproteins. Maturitas 1984; 5:271–6.
15. Fletcher CD, Farish E, Hart DM, Barlow DH, Gray CE, Conaghan CJ. Long-term hormone implant therapy – effects on lipoproteins and steroid levels in post-menopausal women. Acta Endocrinol 1986; 111:419–23.
16. de Lignieres B. Progestogens in the climacteric: mechanisms of action-water, salt metabolism and blood pressure. In: Lobo RA, Whitehead MI, eds. Consensus development conference on progestogens. Int Proc J 1989; 1:93–9.
17. Barlow DH, Beastall GH, Abdalla H, Elias-Jones J, Lindsay R, Hart DM. Effect of long-term hormone replacement on plasma prolactin concentrations in women after oophorectomy. Br Med J 1985; i:589–91.

Discussion

Anderson: Can I raise the question of cost, and of Professor Purdie's dismissal of ethinyloestradiol and presumably mestranol? It presumably would make an enormous difference to the calculations if maybe a smaller dose than people have used of ethinyloestradiol was effective.

It seems to me that there are a number of confused issues. The drug companies have really strong motives for not having something as cheap as ethinyloestradiol being effective.

Purdie: My natural preference is to go for oestradiol, the natural hormone.

Anderson: Orally?

Purdie: Not necessarily. By transdermal transmission as well.

Anderson: But that is a separate issue.

Purdie: I am spending a lot of time trying to persuade my GPs that it is better to give patients a natural human hormone rather than a synthetic hormone like ethinyloestradiol/mestranol. I would find it very difficult to reverse track now and to persuade them that perhaps we might be using a synthetic oestrogen.

In general terms, the family care physicians in our area by and large are prescribing oestradiol-containing compounds at the present time, or Premarin.

Hart: I have shown a lot of data produced on mestranol which theoretically is not a good agent to use, with its 17-ethinyl group and its 3-methyl ether. It does not seem to be doing a lot of harm. I feel that it is probably even safer to use natural agents. I cannot swear that I have proof that is safer to use natural oestrogens, but my own preference is to use the natural oestrogens.

We do not put any patients other than study patients on mestranol, and mestranol is not available.

Without knowing precisely why, I do prefer either oestradiol or conjugated oestrogen. However, it appears that the Department of Health is suggesting ethinyloestradiol should be used. Ethinyloestradiol is the cheapest preparation available, and if we are going purely on cost, it is probably not unreasonable to use ethinyloestradiol. But personally I have been subjected to so much information from so many people suggesting that natural oestrogens are safer that I cannot help believing it, although I have shown a lot of data suggesting that mestranol is not unsafe.

Anderson: But there is a lot of confusion between giving it by a non-oral route, in which case I can see the sense in using oestradiol in one form or another, and giving some "natural compound" by an abnormal route.

Dr Hart is saying he has been brainwashed to some extent.

Hart: Yes. I strongly believe that oral therapy should be used in the first instance. The biggest problem is the cardiovascular problem, and if by giving oral therapy we get the best effects on the cardiovascular system, I think we should use oral therapy unless there is reason to do otherwise.

I am a little apprehensive about transdermal oestradiol plus oral norethisterone. We have a long-term study on this which we are not yet ready to analyse but I am waiting with interest to see whether that has a good, a neutral or a bad effect on lipids.

I certainly would use an oral natural oestrogen in the first instance, and if at all possible, i.e. in women who have had a hysterectomy, I would use unopposed oestroen. If there was a bad personal or a very bad family history of coronary heart disease, then I would be thinking in terms of unopposed cyclical oral oestrogen with careful endometrial surveillance.

Baird: I can see that there are good grounds for thinking that an orally administered preparation might have a different effect, through first pass through the liver on liver enzymes, etc., than preparations which bypass that either by the transdermal or the vaginal route. But if we think of the way oestrogens act in the body, I know of no evidence that they act on any target organ other than by interacting with their steroid receptor. Is there really any evidence that there is any difference at all in the chain of events which is initiated following the administration of an oestrogen, oestradiol-17ß, ethinyloestradiol, mestranol or the equine oestrogens? Is there any difference in the chain of events which follows that stimulation by any of these oestrogens?

I think it is relevant, and not only in respect of the cost. If one is to mount any form of a trial and not treat all the oestrogen preparations as an oestrogen preparation, the analysis of the trial will be impossible. There are 30 or 40 different HRT therapies available and those would have to be broken down into the different components, which is impossible.

Is this the appropriate point to discuss this? We should have some evidence if there are differences other than the mode of administration.

Hart: I have a suspicion that a lot of the worry about oestrogens or the 17-ethinyl group stems from one paper, that of Gow and MacGillivray many years ago, which showed a frightening incidence of deep-vein thrombosis in people on mestranol [1].

Wolf Utian spoke out quite strongly about that paper. He was in Aberdeen at the time and knew the background. Many of these ladies were elderly, some of them immobilised, some of them with orthopaedic problems, and he was very strongly of the opinion that that was not a representative group of pepole to be on any oestrogen.

Drife: What the *British National Formulary* says specifically at the beginning of that section is that there is no evidence that the so-called natural oestrogens have any benefit above ethinyloestradiol. That is what the GPs are reading, and what they would regard as an authoritive source. If we describe ethinyloestradiol and the pill as "pharmacological" and oestrogens in HRT as "psychological" – and I should like to know what that means – then we shall lose credibility. Those who try to persuade GPs that HRT is safe without having the data to back up what they are saying will sooner or later lose credibility.

Hart: Can anyone say why micronised oestradiol is not used in oral contraceptives?

Baird: It is impossibly expensive to prepare enough oestradiol to get it through the liver. The major breakthrough in synthetic chemistry was to get orally active oestrogens and gestogens which could be administered. We have known since the discovery of oestradiol and progesterone back in 1923 that we could inhibit ovulation, but it was not until we had an orally administered active synthetic compound that it became practical to do it.

Drife: The other consideration is the relative potencies regarding FSH suppression and other organs. Ethinyloestradiol has a particularly high potency in FSH suppression which is needed with the pill, but that is not to say that it is therefore more potent, or much more potent in other organs.

Whitehead: It is no accident that the ethinyl group is in the 17 position. The first principal intracellular metabolism of oestradiol occurs there, and adding an ethinyl group there renders that substance no longer a substrate for the dehydrogenase group of enzymes.

But I accept totally that once the substance reaches the genome, a preprogrammed set of responses is initiated. But if the cell cannot metabolise ethinyloestradiol as rapidly as it can metabolise oestradiol-17ß, and that metabolism probably takes place over milliseconds or over a few seconds, the nuclear retention time of ethinyloestradiol will be much longer and therefore we can predict that potency will be enhanced. That is the mechanism.

From the data looking at hepatic markers, or a weight for weight basis ethinyloestradiol in terms of induction of certain hepatically derived proteins in globulins is between 200 and 1000 times more potent than oestrone or oestrone sulphate.

There are a lot of biochemical data indicating that synthetic oestrogens do cause much greater hepatic derangement.

Drife: We have just heard a presentation of the world's longest follow-up of women on synthetic oestrogen which concluded that it had no adverse effects.

Whitehead: But with the greatest respect to the authors, the study population is so small and the events that people are worried about occur so infrequently that one would not see these events occurring in this size of population.

Baird: Let us take the situation where we want a beneficial effect on liver enzymes. The way that any oestrogen induces these changes in liver enzymes is by interacting with nuclear receptors in the liver. Of course ethinyloestradiol and those with the substitution groups at position 17 would be more potent, which is why we give so much less of them.

But I do not know of any evidence that to give the same biological response a differential response would be achieved – potency for potency. And that was why I was asking for information.

Is there any evidence that 3 mg Premarin, which is what is required to suppress ovulation, has the same effects on the coagulation system as 20 or 25 μg ethinyloestradiol, which is also what would be needed to suppress ovulation? Do they produce the same effects on the pelvic system?

Meade: It is difficult to give an answer because of the nature of the studies, the small numbers, the wide range of preparations that have been used and some potency issues as well.

Whitehead: But in terms of bone conservation, it seems that 0.625 mg Premarin most probably gives similar bone effects to about 15 μg or 18 μg/day ethinyloestradiol. But they give different hepatic effects. We need to give about 15 μg/day of ethinyloestradiol to get bone conservation. Hepatic effects are more marked with that dose, which is a minimum bone-sparing dose, as compared to 0.625 mg of conjugated oestrogens.

Lindsay: There are no long-term data looking at doses of much less than the doses that Dr hart and I used in Glasgow. The way in which the efficacy was determined related to dose in that study was related to the returning of postcards, so that people who did not take a 20 μg tablet a day in essence were not taking ethinyloestradiol every day. It is not the best way to do a dose–response type of study.

On the other hand, the dose-responsivity for Premarin was calculated based on daily dosing of those individuals right down to 0.15 mg/day.

So, although we can talk of the short-term changes on ethinyloestradiol, I doubt in the long term if we have the data to know whether or not there is a bone-sparing effect at doses of much less than 10–20 μg/day. On the other hand, I have to agree that in terms of the effects on bone there is no difference between any of the oestrogens and all that matters is that one gives enough of that oestrogen to get an effect. If urine hydroxyproline is reduced and urine calcium is reduced, we see an effect on skeleton in that study, and if enough of an oestrogen is given to get those biochemical effects, then the bone effect will occur.

Kanis: Some of the comments were related to the fact that oestrogens act through oestrogen receptors. In other areas of steroid metabolism there is quite a lot of evidence now for extra-genomic effects of corticosteroids and occupation of receptors other than the authentic receptor for that hormone. In other words, it has weak affinity for other receptor sites. And so one does not necessarily need to lock on the fact that all oestrogens are equal on that basis, because they all act through a common factor.

Baird: I know of no evidence for oestrogen. The only evidence I know for progesterone relates to the central nervous system, the anaesthetic effects of progesterone, and on the oocyte of the frog. But I know of no evidence, biochemical or otherwise, of oestrogen acting other than through interaction with this nuclear receptor.

Kanis: With some of the corticosteroids there seems to be.

Baird: They may. I do not know.

Kanis: And in the case of the vitamin D analogues.

Anderson: Mr Whitehead said 200 to 100 times more potent. If we calculate 10 μg/day ethinyloestradiol and say that is equivalent to a 50 mg oestradiol implant, which is probably not that far off, and that the 50 mg lasts a year, it is only a tenfold or a fifteenfold difference. One is comparing an extremely potent oral steroid where most of it is metabolised first time through with something which is not metabolised at all first time through, and that potency comparison of between 200 and 1000 times more potent is hardly fair.

Whitehead: Why should it be unfair?

Anderson: It is inaccurate.

Whitehead: It depends on the end points.

Anderson: But it is not reasonable to compare a steroid which is highly potent and is not metabolised in the liver to one which is in any case an oestrone sulphate or oestradiol valerate. Oestrone is an extremely low-potency oestrogen in the first place, and to conjugate it and to put it in through a route where it gets metabolised, it would need to be given in kmols.

I do not want to dwell on it, but in any comparison of the relative potency of oestradiol and ethinyloestradiol given by equivalent routes, it is certainly not of that sort of order.

Whitehead: I think there are data coming up with a relative potency irrespective of route on rat hepatocytes of about 1000 to 1 for ethinyloestradiol versus oestradiol-17ß. It is all very well having theoretical concerns, but one has to take into account how the body will handle the steroids that are administered, irrespective of route.

Reference

1. Gow S, MacGillivray I. Metabolic, hormonal, and vascular changes after synthetic oestrogen therapy in oophorectomized women. Br Med J 1971; ii:73–7.

Chapter 21

Effects of Oral, Percutaneous and Transdermal Oestrogens on Postmenopausal Bone

M. I. Whitehead

Introduction

Osteoporosis is a serious consequence of the menopause and a major public health issue. Within the UK, unlike many European countries, there is at present no clearly defined subspecialty of metabolic bone disease. Therefore, counselling of women requesting information on osteoporosis, fracture risk and preventive measures will involve general physicians, endocrinologists, rheumatologists, orthopaedic surgeons, family doctors and gynaecologists. The latter are increasingly becoming involved because the recent Consensus Development Conference on prophylaxis and treatment of osteopoprosis concluded that oestrogens are "currently the only well established prophylactic measure that reduces the frequency of osteoporotic fractures" [1].

This chapter reviews some of the studies which have reported the effects of exogenous oestrogens on postmenopausal bone. The aim is not only to provide the prescriber with the background to the Consensus Development Conference statement [1], but also to draw attention to areas of ignorance.

Routes of Administration

Types of Oestrogen

The title of this chapter is somewhat inappropriate. It implies that oestrogens, when prescribed by different routes, may exert dissimilar effects on the skeleton and that perhaps, only some may achieve bone conservation. This is a physiological nonsense.

The precise mechanism(s) whereby oestrogens protect the postmenopausal skeleton still require further elucidation and a review of them is beyond the scope of this chapter. It is however, most probable that oestrogens act through some form of steroid-receptor mechanism. Although there are differences between the various oestrogens with respect to their affinity for the intracellular receptor, all oestrogens – provided that the dose is adequate – are capable of binding to the oestrogen receptor. Following nuclear translocation they will then produce an identical response. Thus, it can be confidently predicted that provided the plasma oestrogen concentration is above an, as yet undefined, threshold, all routes of oestrogen administration will protect against postmenopausal bone loss. Therefore, the most important issue is not the route of administration but the plasma oestrogen concentration that is achieved within the individual woman.

Evidence for this is already available. Postmenopausal osteoporosis is due principally to the loss of endogenous oestradiol which is directly secreted into the systemic circulation. However, orally administered oestrogens, as will be discussed, are potent bone conservers. As the oral dose is decreased, benefits are reduced and the protective effects on the skeleton of oral oestradiol at a dose of 1 mg day^{-1} are less than 2 mg day^{-1} which, in turn, are less effective than 4 mg day^{-1} [2].

What is not clear is whether the protective bone effects observed with both oral and non-oral routes of administration are due more to the oestradiol or to the oestrone concentration that is achieved in the plasma. Many studies have reported that irrespective of whether oral oestrone sulphate (Harmogen: Abbott Laboratories) or oral oestradiol valerate (Progynova: Schering) is administered, the principal product in plasma is oestrone and the elevation in plasma oestradiol is less. Non-oral administration of oestradiol as a subcutaneous pellet or implant (Organon), as a percutaneous gel (Oestrogel: Laboratoires Besins-Iscovesco) or transdermally via a skin patch (Estraderm: Ciba-Geigy) preferentially increases plasma oestradiol but plasma oestrone concentrations also rise significantly [3–5]. The principal site of the interconversion between oestradiol and oestrone is not known; it could be within hepatic tissue or within plasma which contains the interconverting enzymes, the dehydrogenases. Even within the postmenopausal endometrium, the principal active oestrogen is oestradiol [6]. It is likely than oestradiol is the more potent oestrogen with respect to postmenopausal bone conservation but this has not been demonstrated conclusively. Thus, the contribution that oestrone may make to reduction in fracture risk is unknown. Therefore, it would be unwise to dismiss oestrone as being irrelevant because it is biologically active in other tissues. For this, and other reasons to be discussed, caution should be exercised in recommending that a certain plasma oestradiol value is necessary to achieve bone protection.

Oestriol, unlike oestradiol and oestrone, is not bound in plasma to a globulin or albumin but circulates largely in an unbound or "free" form. Thus, unlike oestradiol and oestrone, oestriol is primarily excreted via the kidney and its half-life is much shorter. Most of a loading dose of oral oestriol is excreted within 8 hours. Therefore, to achieve a biological response similar to that observed with oestradiol, oestriol has to be administered either at high dose, in a vehicle which allows sustained release, or frequently. There is a substantial literature reporting that under these conditions oestriol produces effects identical to those of oestradiol in oestrogen-dependent tissues in lower mammals. Data on the skeletal effects of oestriol in postmenopausal women are sparse; high doses of oestriol hemisuccinate, 12 mg day^{-1}, administered orally were not effective in one study [7], and the effects of vaginally administered oestriol do not appear to have been determined. Oestriol will not be considered further in this review.

The oestrogens referred to previously are described as "natural" because they give rise in plasma to oestrogens identical to those produced by the human ovary. Conjugated equine oestrogens (Premarin: Wyeth-Ayerst Laboratories) is also included in this group. Approximately 65% of conjugated equine oestroen is oestrone sulphate and the remainder is a complex mixture of equine oestrogens. The importance of the latter with respect to bone metabolism is not known. "Synthetic" oestrogens which are derivatives of oestradiol are also available; this group includes ethinyloestradiol and mestranol. Their place in modern-day practice is controversial. Studies in vivo have shown that these synthetic oestrogens, on a weight-for-weight basis, possess a much greater potency than their natural counterparts with respect to induction of various hepatically derived proteins [8]. For example, ethinyloestradiol is approximately 230 times more potent than oestrone sulphate at inducing renin substrate. Although synthetic oestrogens have the advantage of being cheaper, their more pronounced hepatic effects and anxieties about potentially greater adverse fibrinolytic and coagulation changes have resulted in their use in postmenopausal women declining dramatically during the last 10 years in the United Kingdom. Because many of the early studies on the effects of oestrogens on postmeno-pausal bone mass were performed with synthetic oestrogens they will be reviewed.

Limitations of Published Studies

Because this chapter is aimed at the prescribing doctor, it is important that the limitations of the currently available literature be fully appreciated. Statements such as "the minimal effective dose of oral short-acting oestrogen is 0.625 mg of conjugated equine oestrogens, 2 mg of 17ß-oestradiol, or 0.25 mg of ethinyl oestradiol" have appeared in prestigious reports such as that of the Consensus Development Conference [1]. The unwary, who accept this statement at face value, may then prescribe the recommended minimal effective dose in the belief that it will be beneficial in all women and at all relevant skeletal sites. However, various factors must be taken into account when considering any study of the effects of oestrogens upon the postmenopausal skeleton. These will now be briefly discussed.

The Skeletal Site

Methods for determining bone density accurately are a relatively recent develop-ment. The pioneering studies from the Glasgow group instituted in the early 1970s used photon absorption measurements of the third metacarpal [9]. Single photon absorption (SPA) measurement of the wrist was developed in the late

1970s [10], and was followed by spinal measurements, first using quantitative computed tomography (QCT) [11] and then dual photon absorptiometry (DPA) [12]. Refinements to DPA so that it can accurately measure the femoral neck are most recent: indeed, they are so new that no prospective studies of the effects of oestrogens at this skeletal site are currently available, and only one cross-sectional study (which used synthetic oestrogens) has been published [13]. The lack of data about the hip is to be regretted becaue this is the most important site of fracture with respect to morbidity, mortality and costs [14].

The most recent development is that of dual-energy X-ray absorptiometry (DEXA). This is similar in principle to DPA but the energy source is an X-ray tube. The greater photon flux results in improved precision and a shorter scanning time.

Understandably, there are no long-term prospective data comparing the effects of ageing and menopausal status on bone density in the spine and hip. Recently published cross-sectional data indicate that spinal bone density is relatively well preserved in premenopausal women but declines dramatically after the menopause [15]. This emphasises the importance of ovarian status in determining bone density at this site. The data for three sites at the hip (femoral neck, Ward's triangle and trochanteric region) were slightly different; an age-related decline was observed during the reproductive era and was most marked at Ward's triangle and in the femoral neck. Thus, factors other than the oestrogen status appear to influence hip bone density. However, there was a further reduction after menopause at all three sites in the hip [15].

Further cross-sectional data which compared bone density in the wrist, forearm and spine in early postmenopausal women reported that whereas correlations exist between the different anatomical sites, these are not strong [16]. The different response to ovarian failure seen in the various anatomical sites may not be surprising because the different sites contain dissimilar amounts of cortical and trabecular bone. The metabolism of trabecular bone varies from site to site [16]. The response to oestrogens may also vary at the different anatomical sites. It is well recognised that metacarpal and radial rates of bone loss are correlated significantly with vertebral bone loss [11], but there is considerable dispersion about the regression line. Thus, in an individual woman taking oestrogens, it is not possible to use metarcapal and radial measurements to predict vertebral bone loss accurately [11].

The conclusions, for clinical practice, from these studies are that site-specific skeletal measurements are necessary to predict fracture risk at a given site; that conservation of appendicular (metacarpal and wrist) bone mass with oestrogens does not imply that vertebral conservation is also being achieved, and that the spine and hip may not respond in an identical fashion to postmenopausal oestrogen therapy.

The Study Population

Various genetic and lifestyle factors influence skeletal mass in women. Some of the lifestyle factors include alcohol tobacco intake [15], and the effect of the latter may be mediated through lowering plasma oestrogen concentrations [17]. As little as one or two standard alcoholic drinks per day reduces bone density in Ward's triangle by approximately 5% in premenopausal women; more than two standard drinks per day results in a 12% reduction [15]. Additionally, the type of menopause cannot be discounted because bone loss in castrated women may be greater than in those who have undergone a natural menopause. One group of investigators, using identical methods in both groups, reported a 5% mean annual rate of loss of spinal bone in women after natural menopause [18], and almost a 9% annual loss after oophorectomy [11].

No data are available on how much these factors influence the skeletal response to oestrogen therapy. However, it would not be surprising if the minimal effective oestrogen dose required for skeletal protection in a small, thin, sedentary, heavy tobacco and alcohol user who had undergone castration was shown to be higher than that required by a heavier woman with none of these risk factors.

The importance of these potential confounding factors must be allowed for when the effects of any oestrogen preparation are to be determined, and they should be equally distributed in the treatment and control groups. Only then can the effects of therapy be determined in a scientifically valid manner. However, exclusion of women with risk factors means that the study population may no longer be representative of the general population. This must always be borne in mind when results from highly selected groups of women are applied to the individual patient who may possess a different spectrum of risk factors.

Many studies have reported that the design was "double-blind and placebo controlled". Whilst this is scientifically valid, the aims of the design (particularly with respect to blinding the investigator) may be difficult to achieve in practice. Symptomatic women will report improvements in menopausal symptoms: furthermore, women with an intact uterus will bleed. Therefore, fulfilment of the aims of this type of design requires the study of asymptomatic, hysterectomised women, or a protocol whereby the doctor monitoring overall patient well-being and compliance (especially if bleeding diary cards are used) should not perform the bone mass measurements.

Methods of Measurement

Longitudinal studies to determine the effects of oestrogens upon the skeleton require good precision, usually expressed as a coefficient of variation (CV). These values range around 1%–2% for distal forearm measurements using SPA; around 1.5%–2% for spinal measurements using QCT or DPA, or around 1% using DEXA; and for the three sites measured in the proximal femur are around 1.5% for the femoral neck, and 2.5% for Ward's triangle and the trochanteric region. If the annual rate of bone loss at a particular site approximates the CV, then obviously studies of longer than 12 months duration must be performed. Furthermore, the greater the CV the larger the number of patients that must be enrolled for the study to possess sufficient statistical power to provide a meaningful result. Short-term (6 month) studies of small numbers of women utilising a method with a large CV are of little value.

All of the methods of measurement that have been developed have inherent problems. For example, spinal DPA may provide a falsely high (good) result by including aortic calcification or vertebral osteophytes within the measurement. However, the most important drawback with photon absorptiometry is source decay. The principle of the measurement is to pass a photon beam through the bone under investigation and to measure the radiation that is not absorbed but appears upon the other side. The source used in DPA is gadolinium-153 which has a half-life of approximately 242 days. Source decay, over a 12-month period, is such that bone density will appear to have increased by approximately 4%. Some DPA systems automatically correct for source decay, and this particular problem does not apply to DEXA. It has often been stated, perhaps unkindly but not unfairly, that the best way to demonstrate a positive effect with any therapeutic modality is not to include a control group in the study. The use of a control or referent group is currently believed essential for the study to be valid. For this reason, uncontrolled studies will not be considered here.

Expression of Results

For ease of display and comprehension, it has become customary to present the results of a study as a mean of the absolute values or as a mean of the percentage change from baseline. This form of presentation is illustrated in Fig. 21.1 [11]. These data were derived from groups of recently castrated white or oriental women in whom spinal measurements were performed for 24 months. The patients were randomly allocated to placebo or one of the stated daily doses of conjugated equine oestrogens. It is clear from the mean ($\pm$ SD) values that all groups lost bone apart from the group taking conjugated equine oestrogens 0.6 mg day^{-1}; collectively, the mean percentage loss for these groups was 17.7% over 24 months.

The mean percentage loss in the 0.6 mg day^{-1} group was only 0.26%. the oestrogen dose–response relationships were explored in greater detail, and the data for individual patients are reproduced in Fig. 21.2. Significant spinal loss (defined as more than twice the CV) was seen in two of the six women receiving 0.6 mg day^{-1}. Thus, expression of the results as a mean may conceal a lack of response in some women. Failure to respond may be due to poor compliance but very few studies have commented on this and it is discussed further below. An alternative hypothesis is that the lack of response may reflect the presence of risk factors such as a sedentary lifestyle and/or excessive tobacco or alcohol use in individual women. Whilst the reasons for the lack of response require further elucidation, the clinical implications are of obvious importance.

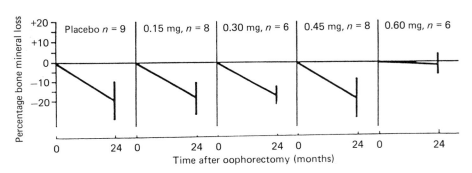

Fig. 21.1. The mean percentage bone mineral loss ($\pm$SD) after 24 months expressed by treatment group, determined by QCT. Zero, placebo; the daily dose of conjugated oestrogens is as stated; n, number of patients. (Adapted and reproduced from Genant et al. [11] with permission.)

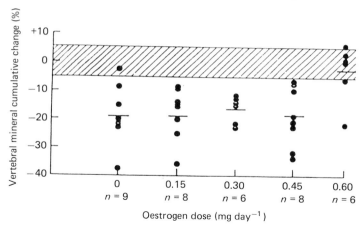

Fig. 22.2. Oestrogen dose–response relationships determined by vertebral mineral measurements for individual women after 24 months of treatment. Zero, placebo; the daily doses of conjugated equine oestrogens are as stated; *n*, number of patients. (Adapted and reproduced from Genant et al. [11] with permission.)

Review of Published Studies

This review is not comprehensive, but has included all the major studies which are representative of the effects of particular oestrogen and/or route of administration at various skeletal sites. All studies included a placebo or untreated "referent" group and adequate details of patients and methods (including the precision in most papers). The studies were of sufficient duration to be meaningful. Differences between the on-treatment and baseline values are shown as percentage changes for the duration of the various studies, and these figures have been calculated if the original report presented absolute values. Because the deleterious effects of alcohol and smoking upon the skeleton have been fully appreciated only relatively recently, the majority of the studies made no comment about matching the treated and control groups for these factors. Compliance, where verified, is referred to in the accompanying text.

Oral Mestranol (Table 21.1)

This was the preparation used by the Glasgow group who studied castrates. Two of the reports are presented from this study, which was initially double-blind and which is the longest, randomised, placebo-controlled investigation worldwide.

The first report [9] gave information on changes in metacarpal mineral content after 5 years of treatment. The percentage changes in the treated and placebo groups have been calculated from the author's original figures; the CV of the method was not stated. This report also included information on the skeletal response when oestrogens were prescribed within 2 months, within 3 years or between 3 and 6 years after oophorectomy. In the placebo group, bone was lost most rapidly in the initial 3-year period after oophorectomy. The data in Table

Table 21.1. Some details of the studies investigating the effects of mestranol on postmenopausal bone mass

Authors	Patient numbers/ treated group	Type of menopause	Duration of study (years)	Skeletal site	Methodology (%CV)	% Change Treated group	Control group
Lindsay et al. [9]	46	Surgical	5	Metacarpal	SPA (NS)	+ 3.8%	− 6.3%
Al-Azzawi et el. [13]	25	Surgical	15	Lumbar Spine Femoral Neck Ward's Triangle Greater Trochanter	DPA (1.7%)	% Difference treated vs placebo 24% 13% 20% 4%	

NS, not stated.

Table 21.2. Some details of the studies investigating the effects of oral conjugated equine oestrogens on postmenopausal bone mass

Authors	Patient numbers/ treated group	Type of menopause	Duration of study (years)	Skeletal site	Methodology (%CV)	% Change Treated group	Control group
Nachtigall et al. [21]	84	Natural	10	Metacarpal	SPA (NS)[a]	+ 8%[b] − 2%[c]	− 9%[b] − 12%[c]
Genant et al. [11]	28	Oophorectomy	2	Spine	QCT (2.8%)	See Figs 21.1 and 21.2	
Lindsay et al [22]	120	Mixed	2	Metacarpal	SPA (NS)	− 8% (0.15)[d] − 5% (0.3) 0 (0.625) 0 (1.25)	− 8%
Ettinger et al. [18]	23	Natural	2	Spine	QCT (NS)	+ 2.3% (0.3+Ca)[e] + 2.5% (0.625)	− 9%

[a]NS, not stated.
[b]Treatment or placebo started within 3 years of menopause.
[c]Treatment or placebo started more than 3 years after menopause.
[d]( ), mg day^{-1} conjugated equine oestrogens.
[e](+Ca) plus calcium supplements.

21.1 relate to those women starting treatment within 3 years of surgery. Compliance was checked carefully, and the mean daily mestranol dose was 0.248 mg

These investigators subsequently reported on bone mineral density in the spine and at three sites in the hip in women continuing in the study for approximately 15 years [13]. Because pretreatment assessments were not available (methods for the spine and hip had not been developed), only the percentage difference in bone density between the groups can be presented. There were significant differences at the spine (24%), the femoral neck (13%) and Ward's triangle (20%); the difference at the greater trochanter (4%) was not significant. The average daily dose of mestranol in this extension phase was 0.26 mg.

Oral Ethinyl Oestradiol

Only scant data are available. Horsman et al.[19] studied 19 women (14 castrates: five after natural menopause) for two or more years. The mineral content of the left distal ulna and radius was determined by SPA. Changes in the mean cortical width and mean cortical cross-sectional area of the second, third and fourth metacarpals were also calculated from plain radiographs. Because of the singular expression of the results it has not been possible to calculate percentage changes at these sites over time. When expressed as mean values postmenopausal bone loss at all sites was prevented by ethinyl oestradiol. Individual responses, however, were very variable. Possible explanations for this variation were not discussed and no comment was made about verification of compliance. Two doses of ethinyl oestradiol (0.25 or 0.5 mg day^{-1}) were prescribed but there was no comment upon dose–response.

Oral Conjugated Equine Oestrogens (Table 21.2)

Data on this preparation are surprisingly sparse. The study by Recker et al. [20] is not reviewed because although the oestrogen-users took 0.625 mg day^{-1} of conjugated equine oestrogens for 21 days each month, they also added methyl-testosterone 5 mg day^{-1} for an identical time. The effects of the latter may have influenced the results.

The study by Nachtigall et al. [21] is unusual: not only was it of long duration (10 years), but it appears to be the only published study performed exclusively on institutionalised postmenopausal women with chronic diseases. This was a double-blind, randomised study and all women had had a natural menopause. Conjugated equine oestrogens were prescribed at a daily dose of 2.5 mg and medroxyprogesterone acetate (Provera: Upjohn Limited) 10 mg day^{-1} was added for 7 days each month. Tratment initiated within 3 years of menopause resulted in an 8% increase in metacarpal mineral density after 10 years; treatment started three or more years after the menopause only conserved bone. There was a 9% decrease in metacarpal bone when placebo was initiated within 3 years of menopause, and a 12% loss when it was started later. Although these differences between the placebo-takers may not be significant, they are at variance with the data of Lindsay et al. [9] who reported greatest bone loss within 3 years of oophorectomy. It is not clear whether the type of menopause is

Table 21.3. Some details of the studies investigating the effects of oral oestradiol on postmenopausal bone mass

Authors	Patient numbers/ treated group	Type of menopause	Duration of study (years)	Skeletal site	Methodology (%CV)	% Change Treated group	Control group
Christiansen et al. [2]	69	Natural	1	Forearm	SPA (1.2%)	+ 1.5% (4)ᵃ + 0.8% (2) 0 (1)	− 2%
Munk-Jensen et al. [24] Continuous E/P	50	Natural	1	Spine Forearm	DPA (1%) SPA (NS)ᵇ	+ 4.9% + 1.0%	− 1.5% − 2.6%
Sequential E/P	50	Natural	1	Spine Forearm	DPA (1%) SPA (NS)	+ 3.9% + 1.1%	− 1.5% − 2.6%

ᵃ( ) mg day^{-1} oestradiol
ᵇNS, not stated.

Table 21.4. Some details of the studies investigating the effects of percutaneous oestradiol on postmenopausal bone mass

Authors	Patient numbers/ treated group	Type of menopause	Duration of study (years)	Skeletal site	Methodology (%CV)	% Change Treated group	Control group
Riis et al. [25]	29	Natural	2	Forearm Proximal Distal Spine	SPA (1%) SPA (1.5%) DPA (4%)	− 0.5% 0 + 5%	− 6% − 7% − 3%
MacIntyre et al. [26]	19	Natural	2	Spine	QCT (2.2%)	− 3.8%	− 10.2%

Table 21.5. Some details of the studies investigating the effects of transdermal oestradiol on postmenopausal bone mass

Authors	Patient numbers/ treated group	Type of menopause	Duration of study (years)	Skeletal site	Methodology (%CV)	% Change Treated group	Control group
Adami et al. [29]	17	Natural	18	Distal forearm	DPA (<1%)	+ 4.3%	− 3.5%

responsible for these differences. There were seven fractures in the control group but none in the oestrogen-users during the study [21].

The data of Genant et al. [11] about the spine have been presented in Fig. 21.1 and 21.2 and have been discussed. These investigators also measured metacarpal and radial bone but did not present the latter results separately because of poor reproducibility.

One of the most widely quoted studies is that of Lindsay et al. [22]. A total of 150 consecutive postmenopausal women were enrolled and 108 completed the study: they were a mixed group who had had either a natural or a surgical menopause. The methodology used was SPA of the metacarpal, and the CV was not stated. Women were randomly allocated to placebo or one of four daily doses of conjugated equine oestrogens, 0.15 mg, 0.3 mg, 0.625 mg or 1.25 mg, and the percentage change over 2 years is as stated. There was no comment as to verification of compliance.

Expression of the results as means showed that conjugated equine oestrogens 0.625 mg and 1.25 mg were equally effective with a zero rate of bone loss over 2 years. However, approximately 9% of women in both these groups lost bone significantly (Lindsay R, personal communication).

Strictly speaking, the study by Ettinger et al. [18] should not be included in this review because of the lack of a valid control group. However, the data are worthy of comment. A total of 73 women within 3 years of the natural menopause were recruited and chose their treatment. The options were no treatment, dietary calcium supplements, or conjugated equine oestrogens 0.3 mg day^{-1} plus calcium supplements; 15 women chose the latter. Eight additional women with low bone mass at the initial screen were advised to take conjugated equine oestrogens 0.625 mg day^{-1}. Some women taking conjugated equine oestrogens added a progestogen for 10 days of each 25-day treatment cycle. Potential confounding factors such as weight, time since menopause, physical activity, tobacco use and parity were recorded and were similar in the groups. This is one of the very few studies to comment upon these factors. Additionally, compliance was carefully checked, Bone mineral content was measured at the lower end of the radius, in the metacarpal and in the spine. Some of the latter results are included in Table 21.2.

Spinal conservation was similar in the groups receiving conjugated equine oestrogens 0.3 mg day^{-1} plus calcium supplements, and conjugated equine oestrogens 0.625 mg day^{-1}. Whether calcium supplements really do allow for a reduction in the oestrogen dose cannot be determined from this study because a group receiving conjugated equine oestrogens 0.3 mg day^{-1} without calcium was not included. Additionally, of the eight women who received conjugated equine oestrogens 0.625 mg day^{-1} two lost more than 3% of spinal bone (which is twice the CV of the method [23]) during the 2-year study period.

Oral Oestradiol (Table 21.3)

Christiansen's group in Copenhagen has made a major contribution to our understanding of the effects of oestrogens on bone: two of their many studies are included, one being on oral oestrogens [2]. A total of 92 women within 5 years of natural menopause were recruited and were randomly allocated to placebo or one of three doses of oral oestradiol (1, 2 or 4 mg daily) each combined with oestriol and with norethisterone acetate 1 mg day^{-1} added for 10 days of each 28-day treatment cycle. The oestradiol 2 mg day^{-1} dose is marketed in the United Kingdom (Trisequens: Novo Nordisk). All women received a calcium supplement of 500 mg day^{-1}. Assessments were performed at 3-monthly intervals for 12 months and 79 women completed the study. Compliance was verified from diary cards and by measurements of serum oestradiol. A dose–response relationship was observed with oestradiol 4 mg day^{-1} exerting greater benefits than 2 mg day^{-1} which, in turn, was better than 1 mg day^{-1}.

The double-blind, randomised, placebo-controlled study by Munk-Jensen et al. [24] is unusual for two reasons. First, active treatment was preceded by a 6-month observation period in which the rate of bone loss was determined and, second, comparisons of two different oestrogen/progestogen formulations were undertaken. In one, oestradiol 2 mg day^{-1} and norethisterone acetate 1 mg day^{-1} were administered continuously in combination (continuous E/P); in the second, norethisterone acetate 1 mg day^{-1} was added sequentially for 10 days each cycle to oestradiol 2 mg day^{-1} given for 22 days and oestradiol 1 mg day^{-1} given for 6 days (sequential E/P).

Of 100 women within 2 years of the natural menopause recruited, 88 completed the study. Verification of compliance was not stated, Spinal bone mineral content was determined by DPA and forearm bone mineral content by SPA: the CV of the latter was not supplied. The mean percentage increase in spinal bone density in the continuous E/P group was 1% greater than that of the sequential E/P group, but this difference was not significant. The correlation coefficient between the forearm and spinal measurements for the cohort during the 6-month observation period prior to active treatment was such that the authors concluded that forearm bone mineral density measurements should not be used as an alternative to spinal measurements when vertebral bone density has to be assessed.

Percutaneous Oestradiol (Table 21.4)

The gel (Oestrogel: Laboratoires Besins-Iscovesco) is not available in the United Kingdom but is widely used in France. Riis et al. [25] studied 29 women within 3 years of the natural menopause and 20 completed the 2-year study. Each day they applied 5 g of percutaneous gel, which contains 3 mg oestradiol. For the second year, natural progesterone (Utrogestan: Laboratoires Besins-Iscovesco) 300 mg day^{-1} was added for 12 days each month. Forearm bone mineral content was measured in the proximal and distal regions by SPA, and spinal bone density was determined by DPA. Compliance appears to have been verified by 3-monthly measurements of plasma oestradiol and oestrone values which, after 12 months, were approximately 650 pmol l^{-1} for both oestrogens. This is well within the premenopausal, proliferative phase range. The percutaneous gel was effective at all sites, and the addition of natural progesterone did not influence bone conservation.

Similar beneficial effects on spinal bone mineral content were observed by MacIntyre et al. [26], who used an identical regimen except that the natural progesterone was added from the commencement of the study. Nineteen women, most within 5 years of the natural menopause, were recruited and 15 completed the study. Both studies confirm that percutaneous oestradiol reduces the rate of spinal bone loss as compared to placebo. Whereas Riis et al. [25] reported a 5% increase after 2 years of active treatment, MacIntyre et al. [26] reported a 3.8% decrease. This difference can be explained only by the dissimilar methods. Whereas QCT assesses only vertebral spongiosa, DPA measures cortical bone as well. Thus, increases in the latter are detected by DPA but not by QCT.

Neither study commented on interpatient variation or gave information on the numbers of women in whom bone conservation was not observed despite good compliance.

Data on lower doses of percutaneous oestradiol are not available.

Transdermal Oestradiol (Table 21.5)

This route of administration is the most recently introduced and, not surprisingly, scant data are available. Although recent publications from the Toulouse group upon the effects of transdermal oestradiol 0.50 mg day^{-1} on spinal bone have included data for a control group [27], the original report [28] did not. Because of the uncertainties over the validity of this control group (and precisely when it was recruited) these reports are not included in this review.

The only controlled study published to date is that of Adami et al. [29]. Seventeen women within 4 years of the natural menopause were recruited and none dropped out. Transdermal oestradiol 0.50 mg day^{-1} was administered in 21 day cycles with medroxyprogesterone acetate 10 mg day^{-1} added for 12 days each cycle. There is no statement regarding compliance. Bone mineral density in the distal forearm was measured after 8 and 18 months when the mean percentage loss in the control group was 3.5%. The mean percentage gain in the treated group was 4.3% which is much higher than that reported by other workers for this site, albeit using different methodology [2,24,25]. The individual results were also presented and six women gained more than 6% bone mineral density during the study. Interestingly, two women lost significant bone mass (more tha twice the CV). The difference between the oestrogen and placebo groups at the end of the study was significant.

Discussion and Conclusions

The most striking aspect of the literature is the paucity of properly designed, controlled studies which have been performed during the last 15 years. This most probably reflects the difficulties with recruiting a study population prepared to undergo long-term assessment. This problem will be overcome as patient awareness of the problems of osteoporosis is heightened and becomes more widespread.

The second problem contributing to the lack of data is the difficulty encountered by doctors with methods which incorporate a radioactive source. Of the two such techniques referred to here, SPA is less expensive and it is relatively easy to produce a low CV ranging around 1%–1.5% which is indicative of good precision and reproducibility. It was employed in eight studies.

However, SPA can provide information only on the appendicular skeleton (metacarpal and wrist) where the response to oestrogens may not reflect that in the spine and hip. Measurements of the latter sites have required DPA but this technique is not easy and it is often difficult to produce reproducible data. This problem should be minimised by DEXA.

Only two studies utilised longitudinal spinal DPA measurements [24,25]. The reported CVs ranged from 1% [24] to 4% [25]. Since the higher figure is similar to the 5% increase and 3% decrease reported in spinal bone in women receiving percutaneous oestradiol or placebo, respectively, for two years [25], this means that very long-term studies will be required unless the CV can be reliably reduced. DPA, like DEXA, possesses the major advantage of determining the status at the hip but there are no prospective data for this site.

QCT is an alternative to DPA in the spine and was employed in three studies [11,18,26]. The technology is much more expensive and the radiation exposure is higher. Furthermore, QCT has been criticised because it appears to overestimate bone loss [30]. Annual rates of loss of spinal bone in untreated women after the natural menopause reported by QCT are approximately 5% [18]; according to DPA this figure is approximately 1.5% [24,25].

What conclusions are justified from the published studies apart from the usual recommendation regarding a need for further research? It is clear that oestrogens influence bone metabolism and reduce the rate of loss: prospective data are available for the metacarpal, distal forearm and spine. However, for many of the individual preparations the data are sparse or non-existent. For example, with conjugated equine oestrogens which have been available for more than 40 years, there are data from two large studies on the metarcapal [21,22]; there are no data on the distal forearm, and there are results from two smaller studies on the spine [11,18]. The former studied 28 castrated women. The latter investigated women after a natural menopause: none took conjugated equine oestrogens 1.25 mg day^{-1} and the eight women who took 0.625 mg day^{-1} all had low bone mass at the pretreatment assessment. With regard to prescribing practices within the United Kingdom, there are no data at any site for some of the more widely prescribed preparations such as Progynova and Cyclo-Progynova (Schering).

Properly conducted dose-ranging studies are few [2,11,22]. Furthermore, few studies have reported the percentage of women not responding to therapy and/or have discussed why this might have occurred. Conjugated equine oestrogens 0.625 mg day^{-1} did not conserve spinal bone in 33% of oophorectomised women (Fig. 21.2) [11], or in 25% of women after natural menopause [18]. With transdermal oestradiol 0.50 mg/day 12% of women lost forearm bone [29]. Generally, verification of compliance has been suboptimal and there are few data on plasma oestradiol concentrations during therapy. There are notable exceptions [25]. However, since plasma oestradiol concentrations have not been correlated with the bone response, no recommendation can be made regarding a minimal plasma level – assuming, of course, that plasma oestradiol concentrations will predict the bone response. Until meaningful data become available, this relationship will remain a hypothesis.

How then should the statement of the Consensus Development Conference [1] be modified? Based on the current information the following statement is justified:

"In study popoulations in which metacarpal mineral content has been measured the minimal effective dose of oral conjugated equine oestrogens is 0.625 mg

day^{-1}: 9% of women lose bone with this dose at this site. In study populations in which spinal bone has been measured the minimal effective dose of oral conjugated oestrogen is 0.625 mg/day: with this dose 33% of castrated women and 25% of women after natural menopause still lose significant bone. It is not known whether a higher dose will be more effective at the spine.

In study populations in which forearm bone mass has been measured the minimal effective dose of oral oestradiol is 2 mg day^{-1}. This dose also conserves spinal bone and it is not known if lower doses are equally effective at this site. The percentage of women not responding at both these sites to oestradiol 2 mg day^{-1} is not known.

In study populations undergoing longitudinal investigations and in which metacarpal mineral content has been measured, mestranol approximately 0.25 mg day^{-1} conserves bone. Cross-sectional data suggest that mestranol 0.26 mg day^{-1} conserves spine and hip bone. The percentage of women not responding to these doses at these sites is not known, nor is it clear whether a lower dose will be equally effective.

There are no prospective data on the effects of oestrogens at the hip.

The reasons why some women fail to respond to exogenous oestrogen therapy are not known."

Acknowledgements. The help of Mrs A. Short in the preparation of this manuscript is much appreciated. The financial assistance of the Imperial Cancer Research Fund Laboratories, Lincolns Inn Fields, London, WC2 to M. I. Whitehead is greatefully acknowledged.

References

1. Consensus Development Conference; Prophylaxis and treatment of osteoporosis. Br Med J 1987; 295:15.
2. Christiansen C, Christensen MS, Larsen N-E, Transbol IB. Pathophysiological mechanisms of estrogen effect on bone metabolism. Dose–response relationships in early postmenopausal women. J Clin Endocrinol Metab 1982; 55:1124–30.
3. Campbell S, Whitehead MI. Potency and hepatocellular effects of oestrogens after oral, percutaneous and subcutaneous administration. In: van Keep PA, Utian W, Vermeulen A, eds. The controversial climacteric. Lancaster, MTP, 1982; 103–25.
4. Powers MS, Schenkel L, Darley PE, Good WR, Balestra JC, Place VA. Pharmacokinetics and pharmacodynamics of transdermal dosage forms of 17 beta-estradiol: comparison with conventional oral estrogens used for hormone replacement. Am J Obstet Gynecol 1985; 152:1099–106.
5. Padwick ML, Endacott J, Whitehead MI. Efficacy, acceptability and metabolic effects of transdermal estradiol in the management of postmenopausal women. Am J Obstet Gynecol 1985; 152:1085–91.
6. Whitehead MI, Lane G, Dyer G, Townsend PT, Collins WP. Oestradiol: the predominant intranuclear oestrogen in the endometrium of oestrogen-treated postmenopausal women. Br J Obstet Gynaecol 1981; 88:914–18.
7. Lindsay R, Hart DM, MacLean A, Garwood J, Clarke AC, Kraszewski A. Bone loss during oestriol therapy in postmenopausal women. Maturitas 1979; 1:279–85.
8. Mashchak CA, Lobo RA, Dozono-Takano R, Eggena P, Nakamura RM, Brenner PF, Mishell DR Jr. Comparison of pharmacodynamic properties of various estrogen formulations. Am J Obstet Gynecol 1982; 144:511–18.
9. Lindsay R, Hart DM, Aitken JM, MacDonald EB, Anderson JB, Clarke AC. Long-term prevention of postmenopausal osteoporosis by oestrogen. Lancet 1976; i:1038–40.
10. Christiansen D, Christensen MS, McNair P, Hagen C, Stocklund KE, Transbol I. Prevention of

early postmenopausal bone loss: controlled 2-year study in 315 normal females. Eur J Clin Invest 1980; 10:273–9.

11. Genant HK, Cann CE, Ettinger B, Gordan GS. Quantitative computed tomography of vertebral spongiosa: a sensitive method for detecting early bone loss after oophorectomy. Ann Intern Med 1982; 97:699–705.

12. Riis BJ, Thomsen K, Strom V, Christiansen C. The effect of percutaneous estradiol and natural progesterone on postmenopausal bone loss. Am J Obstet Gynecol 1987; 156:61–5.

13. Al-Azzawi F, Hart DM, Lindsay R. Long-term effect of oestrogen replacement therapy on bone mass as measured by dual photon absorptiometry. Br Med J 1987; 294:1261–2.

14. Stevenson JC, Whitehead MI. Postmenopausal osteoporosis. Br Med J 1982; 285:585–8.

15. Stevenson JC, Lees B, Devenport M, Cust MP, Gangar KF. Determinants of bone density in normal women: risk factors for future osteoporosis? Br Med J 1989; 298:924–8.

16. Stevenson JC, Banks LM, Spinks TJ et al. Regional and total skeletal measurements in the early postmenopause. J Clin Invest 1987; 80:258–62.

17. Jensen J, Christiansen C, Rodbro P. Cigarette smoking, serum estrogens, and bone loss during hormone replacement therapy early after menopause. N Engl J Med 1985; 313:973–5.

18. Ettinger B, Genant HK, Cann CE. Postmenopausal bone loss is prevented by treatment with low-dosage estrogen with calcium. Ann Intern Med 1987; 106:40–5.

19. Horsman A, Gallagher JC, Simpson M, Nordin BEC. Prospective trial of oestrogen and calcium in postmenopausal women. Br Med J 1977; 2:789–92.

20. Recker RR, Saville PD, Heaney RP. Effect of estrogens and calcium carbonate on bone loss in postmenopausal women. Ann Intern Med 1977; 87:649–55.

21. Nachtigall LE, Nachtigall RH, Nachtigall RD, Beckman EM. Estrogen replacement therapy 1: a 10-year prospective study in the relationship to osteoporosis. Obstet Gynecol 1979; 53:277–81.

22. Lindsay R, Hart DM, Clark DM. The minimum effective dose of estrogen for prevention of postmenopausal bone loss. Obstet Gynecol 1984; 63:759–63.

23. Genant HK, Cann CE, Ettinger B, Gordan GS. Determination of bone mineral loss in the axial and appendicular skeleton of oophorectomised women (Abstract). J Comput Assist Tomogr 1982; 6:216–17.

24. Munk-Jensen N, Nielsen S, Obel EB, Bonne Eriksen P. Reversal of postmenopausal vertebral bone loss by oestrogen and progestogen: a double blind placebo controlled study. Br Med J 1988; 296:1150–2.

25. Riis BJ, Thomsen K, Strom V, Christiansen C. The effects of percutaneous estradiol and natural progesterone on postmenopausal bone loss. Am J Obstet Gynecol 1987; 156:61–5.

26. MacIntyre I, Stevenson JC, Whitehead MI, Wimalawansa SJ, Banks LM, Healy MJR. Calcitonin for prevention of postmenopausal bone loss. Lancet 1988; i:900–2.

27. Ribot C, Pouilles JM, Tremollieres F. Prevention of vertebral bone loss by transdermal 17 beta-estradiol and oral progestin: preliminary report of a 2-year controlled study. In: Whitehead MI, Schenkel L, eds. Transdermal hormone replacement. Carnforth, Parthenon Publishing, 1990; 35–42.

28. Ribot C, Tremollieres F, Pouilles JM, Louvet JP, Peyron R. Transdermal administration of 17 beta-estradiol in postmenopausal women: preliminary results of a longitudinal study. In: Christiansen C, Johansen JS, Riis BJ, eds. Osteoporosis 1987. Copenhagen, Osteopress APS, 1987; 546–8.

29. Adami S, Suppi R, Bertoldo F, Rossini M, Residori M, Maresca V, Lo Cascio F. Transdermal estradiol in the treatment of postmenopausal bone loss. Bone Miner 1989; 7:79–86.

30. Laval-Jeantet AM, Cann CE, Roget B, Daltant P. A post-processing dual energy technique for vertebral CT densitometry. J Comput Assist Tomogr 1984; 8:1164–7.

Chapter 22

Reversal of Bone Loss with Percutaneous Oestrogens

T. Garnett, M. Savvas and J. W. W. Studd

Introduction

It is now accepted that oestrogen replacement therapy after the menopause is effective in preventing the rapid loss of bone which occurs following the cessation of ovarian function [1–4]. Although maintenance of bone mass is sufficient for recently postmenopausal women, it may be inadequate for woman many years past the menopause who have lost a significant proportion of their bone mass. For such women, who have already developed osteoporosis and suffered a fracture, hormone replacement is often not advised as it is considered too late to have any beneficial effect on the skeleton. Nothing will reverse the loss of height and "Dowager's hump" characteristic of the disease, but if it is possible to increase bone density to above the "fracture threshold" oestrogen therapy should be given despite the increased incidence of side effects in patients of this age. The disadvantages of a monthly withdrawal bleed may be an acceptable price to pay if greater bone strength is achieved (Fig. 22.1).

A small increase in bone density over baseline, whether assessed by single or dual photon absorptiometry, dual X-ray or QCT scanners, has been a consistent finding in most prospective studies of the effects of oestrogen replacement therapy on the skeleton over the last 10 years [1–12]. However, such increases have often been dismissed as a transient "hole-filling" phenomenon of doubtful significance. The tendency has been to concentrate on comparisons between treated patients and a control population rather than baseline bone density. If preservation of bone, or slowing down of the rate of loss, is all that is expected

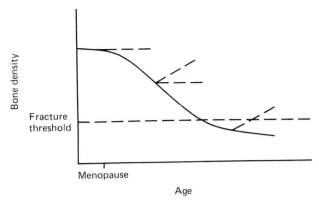

Fig. 22.1. The possible effects of percutaneous oestrogens on bone density in different age groups; ----, effect of treatment.

then a comparison with a control group is required. If, however, an increase in bone density is expected, comparisons with baseline are more important, particularly as, ethically it is increasingly difficult to justify using an untreated control group and thereby deny an effective treatment to an at-risk population.

Reversal of Bone Loss

Reversal of bone loss has been demonstrated in a number of conditions other than postmenopausal osteoporosis. Treasure et al. [13] showed that the osteoporosis characteristic of severe anorexia nervosa returned to normal on return of menstruation. Greenspan et al. [14] and Finkelstein et al. [15] have demonstrated increases in bone density in men with idiopathic hypogonadotrophic hypogonadism when treated with gonadal steroid replacement. More recently a number of studies have confirmed that the bone loss which accompanies the use of analogues of gonodotrophin releasing hormone (GnRH) is reversible on cessation of therapy [16]. Thus the principle of increasing bone density on correction of hormonal imbalances has been established, yet the proposal that postmenopausal bone loss can be reversed with oestrogen replacement therapy has few supporters.

Routes of Administration

Oral oestrogen therapy is the most commonly used form of hormone replacement and most prospective studies to date relate to this route of administration. Lindsay et al. [1] using oral mestranol at a mean dose of 24.8 µg per day and measuring bone density at the third metacarpal by single photon densitometry (SPA) showed a significant increase in bone density over a 5-year follow-up with

Table 22.1. Prospective studies showing an increase in bone density with oral oestrogen therapy

Author	Year	Therapy/dose	No. of patients	Length of follow-up (years)	Menopausal age (years)	Estimated annual % increase	Site of bone measured	Method of assessment	Statistical significance (over whole study)
Munk-Jensen et al. [5]	1988	2 mg Oestradiol	50	1.5	0.5–2.0	6.4%	Lumbar spine	DPA	P<0.01
Christiansen et al. [3]	1980	Trisequens Forte	56	2	0.5–3.0	1.2%	Distal forearm	SPA	P<0.01
Ettinger et al. [4]	1987	Premarin 0.3 mg	15	2	1.0–2.0	1.2%	Lumbar spine	QCT	Not given
Lindsay et al. [1]	1976	Mestranol 24 mg/day	63	5 5 5	0 3 >6	0% ≈0.8% ≈0.8%	Metacarpal Metacarpal Metacarpal	SPA SPA SPA	– P<0.001 P<0.004
Nachtigall et al. [2]	1979	Premarin 2.5 mg	30 37	10	<3 >3	1% 0%	Metacarpal	SPA	
Gallagher et al. [6]	1989	Premarin 0.3 mg 0.6 mg	21 21	2 2	1.5–6.0 1.5–6.0	0.5% 1%	Lumbar Spine	DPA	Not given
Civitelli et al. [7]	1988	Premarin 1.25 mg	10	1	3–7	8.3% 2.6%	Lumbar Femur	DPA DPA	P<0.05 P<0.05

the greatest increase occurring in the first 3 years. Bone density increased at a rate of approximately 1% per year and was not related to menopausal age at the start of therapy.

Nachtigall et al. [2] using Premarin 1.25 mg daily with cyclical progestogens demonstrated a significant increase in bone density of 1% per year measured by SPA at the third metacarpal over a 10-year follow-up. This change was greatest in those within 3 years of the menopause. Similar results using oral hormone replacement therapy have been reported by Christiansen et al. [3] using Trisequens, and measuring at the forearm by SPA. Ettinger et al. [4] using 0.3 mg Premarin showed a 1.2% annual increase in spine bone density measured by quantitative digital radiography.

More recently Munk-Jensen et al. [5] demonstrated a more dramatic increase in spine bone density of 6.5% per year using 2 mg oral oestradiol measured by dual photon absorptiometry (DPA). Civitelli et al. [7] using Premarin 1.25 mg daily demonstrated an increase of 8.3% in bone density at the lumbar spine measured by DPA and 2.6% in the femoral shaft. Gallagher et al. [6] showed a 1% increase in spine bone density in one year after treatment with 0.625 mg of conjugated oestrogen and a 0.5% increase after treatment with 0.3 mg conjugated oestrogen.

It would appear that oral hormone replacement therapy is effective at reversing as well as preventing bone loss after the menopause at a rate which is dependent on the site measured and the dose of oestrogen used. Only two studies have a follow-up period greater than 2 years [1,2] and there was a suggestion in these that the increase in bone density was greatest within the first 3 years of therapy. However, increases were still apparent after 5 and 10 years treatment. Women in these studies were less than 3 years postmenopoausal and may have lost only a small proportion of their initial peak bone density, replacement of which was complete after three years of therapy. Some studies indicate that the effect is only seen in women within 3 years of the menopause [4] but others [7] demonstrated an effect irrespective of menopausal age in patients with severe osteoporosis who had already suffered a vertebral crush fracture (Table 22.1).

Percutaneous Oestrogens

Recently data have become available on the bone-sparing effect of oestradiol patches. Adami et al. [8] demonstrated a 4.3% increase in bone density in women 2–4 years following the menopause after 18 months' treatment compared to a 3% loss in the control group. Patients were treated with Estraderm patches at a dose of 50 µg twice weekly and bone density assessed by dual photon scanning at the lumbar spine. Ribot et al. [9] followed-up a similar group of patients for 2 years and demonstrated an annual increase in bone density of 3% at the lumbar spine. It remains to be seen whether these increases in bone density are continued over a longer period of time.

Percutaneous oestrogen creams (oestrogel), although not widely used in this country, are a common form of hormone replacement therapy in France. Ribot et al. [10] using oestrogel 2.5 g for 20 days in each month demonstrated a 4.7% increase in bone density after treatment for one year. Measurements were taken

Table 22.2. Prospective studies showing an increase in bone density with percutaneous oestrogen therapy

Author	Year	Therapy/ dose	No. of patients	Length of follow-up (years)	Menopausal age (years)	Estimated annual % increase	Site measured	Method of assessment	Statistical significance
Savvas (unpublished)	1989	Implant 75 mg 6/12	25	1	1–15	8.2	Lumbar spine	DPA	P<0.0001
						2.5	Femur		P<0.0001
Hart et al. [12]	1987	Implant 50 mg 6/12	35	2	0–2	4.3%	Lumbar spine	DPA	P<0.001
Ribot et al. [9]	1988	Patch 50 µg	14	2	0.5–3.5	3%	Lumbar spine	DPA	P<0.005
Adami et al. [8]	1989	Patch 50 µg	17	1.5	2–4	3%	Forearm	DPA	P<0.01
Ribot et al. [10]	1987	Cream 1.5 mg/day	40	2	0.5–4.5	4.7%	Lumbar spine	DPA	P<0.002
Riis et al. [11]	1987	Cream 3 mg/day	20	2	0.5–3	4.5%	Lumbar	DPA	Not given

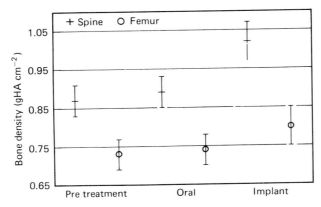

Fig. 22.2. Skeletal effects of oral oestrogen compared with subcutaneous oestrogen and testosterone in postmenopausal women.

at the lumbar spine using dual photon densitometry. In a similar study Riis et al. [11] demonstrated a 4.5% increase in spinal bone density in the first year of a prospective study using cream for 24 days of each calender month.

Oestradiol implants, given at 6-monthly intervals, are a convenient and widely used form of long-term hormone replacement which result in hormone levels which are significantly higher than those achieved by alternative therapies. McKay Hart et al. [12] using 50 mg implants followed-up 19 women within two years of the menopause at 6-monthly intervals for 2 years and demonstrated an increase in bone density of 4.3% per year at the lumbar spine measured by DPA. Savvas et al. [17] have demonstrated the greater bone-sparing effect of hormone implants when compared with oral hormone replacement therapy (Fig. 22.2). In a longitudinal study [18] they have shown a 7.8% increase in bone density at the lumbar spine by dual photon densitometry after just one year of treatment with oestradiol and testosterone (Table 22.2, Fig. 22.3).

Table 22.3. The effects of a 75 mg oestradiol implant on the bone metabolism of postmenopausal women assessed by serial bone biopsies and dual X-ray bone scans

Patient	Age	Menopausal age	Bone biopsy		Bone scan	
			Resorption	Apposition	% Age-matched normal	Increase (% per annum)
1	54	1	↓	↑	88	2.2
2	55	4	↑	↑	99	0.7
3	55	6	→	↑	134	4.9
4	54	7	↓	↑	71	2.2
5	58	9	↓	↓	92	13.8
6	65	10	→	↓	114	10.7
7	49	11	→	↓	86	0.5
8	68	15	↓	↓	103	15.1
Range	49–68	1–15			71–134	0.7–15.1
Mean	(57.2)	(7.8)			(98.3)	(6.25)

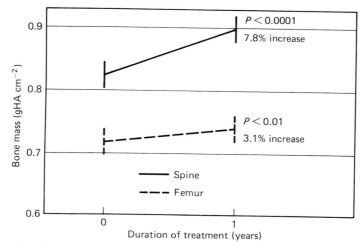

Fig. 22.3. The effects of subcutaneous oestrogens (55 mg six monthly) on bone density at the lumbar spine and femur over one year.

Mechanism of Action

The apparently greater efficacy of implants over other routes of oestrogen therapy in increasing bone density is probably due to the higher serum oestradiol levels achieved with this route of administration. Oral hormone replacement therapy will result in serum oestradiol levels of between one third to a half of the premenopausal levels, which may explain the modest increases in bone density which this mode of therapy achieves [17]. Hormone patches give higher serum oestradiol levels than oral therapy and such studies as there are show a greater increase in bone density in patients treated with patches than with oral therapy [19]. In turn oestrogel cream results in the even higher serum oestradiol levels and the studies available show a 4.7% increase in one year [20].

Hormone implants given on a 6-monthly basis result in serum oestradiol levels at the upper end of the physiological range and these higher serum oestradiol levels may be responsible for the more substantial increases in bone density seen with this form of therapy. The increase in bone density achieved in our prospective implant study was unrelated to age, menopausal age or initial bone density, but was significantly correlated with serum oestradiol levels achieved after one year's treatment (r 0.65, $P<0.02$) (Fig. 22.4). Such a relationship was also demonstrated by Lindsay et al. [21] who showed a correlation between change in metacarpal mineral content in oophorectomised patients and mean circulating oestradiol concentrations, confirming that the endogenous oestrogen in these women helped to control the rate at which bone mineral was lost (Fig. 22.5).

The importance of these observations is that bone can be replaced regardless of menopausal age or the bone density of the patient. Regrettably she has to

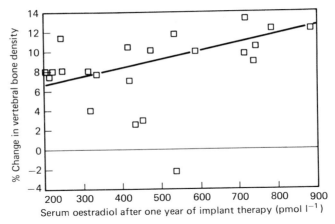

Fig. 22.4. The correlation between the increase in spinal bone density and serum oestradiol levels in postmenopausal women receiving six monthly oestrogen implants (75 mg).

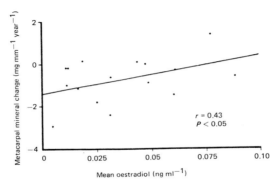

Fig. 22.5. The relationship between the change in metacarpal mineral content in oophorectomised patients and mean circulating oestradiol concentration.

suffer the cyclical complications of oestrogen therapy if she has a uterus and these may be intolerable in the older woman.

The dose-related bone-sparing effect of hormone replacement has been shown in two studies [22,23]. However, both of these studies looked at the minimum dose of oral oestrogen required to maintain bone density using old technology, not at higher oestradiol levels aimed at increasing bone mass. Lindsay et al. [22] showed that 0.625 mg of Premarin could maintain bone density over a two-year period whereas Horsman et al. [23] demonstrated that a dose of 15 μg per day of ethinyloestradiol prevented bone loss, whilst higher doses were capable of increasing bone mass as assessed by metacarpal index.

The manner in which oestradiol leads to an increase in bone density is not clear. Albright et al. [24], nearly 50 years ago, proposed that postmenopausal osteoporosis was a disease of the collagen matrix of bone, rather than calcium metabolism, and made the association between osteoporosis and thin skin.

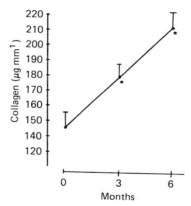

Fig. 22.6. Change in the mean ± SE thigh collagen content in 22 women during a six-month period after a 50 mg oestradiol implant. *P<0.001.

Brincat et al. [25] have demonstrated that skin collagen content and skin thickness can not only be preserved by postmenopausal hormone replacement therapy but that collagen can be replaced at a rate of 30% in one year. If osteoporosis is indeed a disease of collagen matrix it may be that bone collagen is replaced in a similar way (Fig. 22.6). More recently a direct anabolic effect of oestrogens on human osteoblasts has been found in that physiological levels of 17ß-oestradiol stimulated cell proliferation and a twofold increase in collagen mRNA synthesis [26].

It is widely agreed that one of the mechanisms of action of oestrogen replacement therapy is to act as an antiresorptive agent. It has been claimed that a secondary decrease in bone formation after long-term oestrogen administration

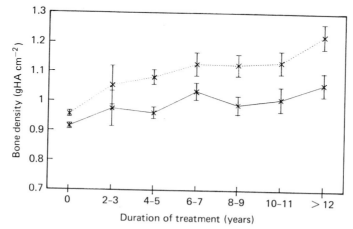

Fig. 22.7. The relationship between bone density at the lumbar spine and femur and duration of therapy with oestradiol implants. ——, Hip; ...., spine.

occurs and suggested that on initiation of treatment oestrogens uncouple the bone resorption and formation processes resulting in a net gain of bone [27]. Subsequently inhibition of bone formation balances this suppression in-bone resorption potentially limiting the capacity of oestrogens to increase bone mineral content in the long-term treatment of postmenopausal osteoporosis. However, few studies have sufficient follow-up to confirm this hypothesis. One would not expect bone density to increase at a rate of 5%–8% per year for the entire duration of therapy and a rapid increase followed by a slower rate of gain is to be expected. One cross-sectional study showed that women who have received oestradiol implants for up to 10 years have significantly better bones than their age-matched counterparts and have failed to show even an age-related loss of bone, but their mean bone density is not above the peak bone density of our reference population (Fig. 22.7) (Garnett and Studd, unpublished data). However, bone density was consistently greater with increasing duration of therapy.

Osteoporosis results from excessive thinning and eventual breaking down of trabecular plates (Fig. 22.8) [28]. Oestrogen replacement therapy at physiological levels may successfully reverse this process in the early stages to re-establish initial peak bone mass. In the later stages of the disease, once the trabeculae have broken down, it is not clear whether re-anastamosis of the seperated plates will ever be possible. Oestrogen is a humoral factor without a directional stimulus and most likely causes recovery in plates which are still intact and thickening of broken down trabecular stumps. If thickening of remaining broken down plates occurs this will result in an increase in bone density which may not be reflected in an increase in bone strength. It is increasing bone strength and decreasing the chances of a fracture, not merely an increase in bone density, which are our primary concern. If the framework on which new bone is being deposited is suboptimal the laying down of new bone

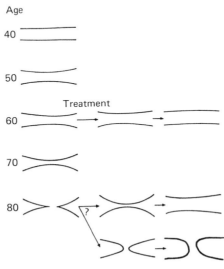

Fig. 22.8. The possible effects of oestrogen therapy in peri- and postmenopausal women.

upon it may not improve bone integrity. With this in mind a longitudinal study has been conducted of postmenopausal patients who will have bone biopsies before and after 6 months of percutaneous treatment (Garnett and Studd, unpublished). Initial results show a wide variation in effect. Resorption, as assessed by the numbers of active multinucleate giant cells in Howship's lacunae shows no consistent pattern. Bone apposition, indicated by active osteoblasts at the site of osteoid mineralisation, appears to be directly related to the menopausal age of the patient. These morphological findings do not correlate with the invariable increases in bone density found by dual X-ray assessment. Serial bone scans may therefore be misleading in their presumptive effect on bone strength in osteoporotic patients. Furthermore, 3%–5% incremental increases in bone density in women who have already lost 60% of their bone mass are of less significance than similar percentage increases in women whose bones are still near peak bone density, as the actual amount of new bone substance deposited will be small.

Conclusion

A small increase in bone density on the initiation of all forms of oestrogen replacement therapy has been a consistent finding since accurate methods of assessing bone density have been available and can no longer be dismissed as a transient effect of doubtful significance. The effects appear to be less with oral therapy than with percutaneous routes of administration and this is likely to be a result of the higher serum oestradiol level achieved with patches, creams and implants. Most studies have not followed-up patients for long enough to demonstrate how long the effect continues and although it would seem to be greatest in the first 3 years of treatment significant increases have been reported to continue after 5–10 years. This cannot continue *ad infinitum* and it is unlikely that bone density will increase beyond original peak bone mass.

In the younger patient, who has not lost a significant amount of bone and whose bone density is still above a theoretical "fracture threshold", the route and dose of oestrogen therapy appear not to be of great importance. For the older woman with established osteoporosis percutaneous therapy resulting in higher oestradiol levels than the premenopausal range would seem to be indicated in an effort to increase bone density above the "fracture threshold". However, increases in bone density in such patients as assessed by scanning techniques may not truly reflect increases in bone strength if the framework upon which bone is being deposited has deteriorated to the extent of trabecular breakdown.

References

1. Lindsay R, Hart DM, Aitken JM, MacDonald EB, Anderson JB, Clark AC. Long-term prevention of postmenopausal osteoporosis by oestrogen. Lancet 1976; ii:1038–9.
2. Nachtigall LE, Nachtigall H, Nachtigall RD, Beckman ME. Estrogen replacement therapy 1: a 10-year prospective study in the relationship to osteoporosis. Obstet Gynecol 1979; 53:277–81.

3. Christiansen C, Christensen S, McNair P, Hagen C. Prevention of early postmenopausal bone loss: controlled 2-year study in 315 normal females. Eur J Clin Invest 1980; 10:273–9.

4. Ettinger B, Genant HK, Cann CE. Post-menopausal bone loss is prevented by treatment with low-dosage estrogen with calcium. Ann Intern Med 1987; 106:40–5.

5. Munk-Jensen N, Nielsen SP, Obel EB, Eriksen PB. Reversal of postmenopausal vertebral bone loss by oestrogen and progestogen: a double-blind placebo controlled study. Br Med J 1988; 296:1150–2.

6. Gallagher JC, Goldgar D, Kable WT. Comparison of estrogen and progestin therapy on cortical and trabecular bone using SPA, DPA and OCT. Sixth international workshop on bone and soft tissue. 1989.

7. Civitelli R, Agunsdei D, Nardi P, Zacchei F, Avioli LV, Gennari C. Effects of one-year treatment with estrogens on bone mass, intestinal calcium absorption, and 25-hydroxyvitamin D-1cx-hydroxylase reserve in postmenopausal osteoporosis. Calcif Tissue Int 1988; 42:77–86.

8. Adami S, Suppi, R, Bertoldo F, Rossini M, Residori M, Maresca V, Lo Cascio V. Transdermal estradiol in the treatment of postmenopausal bone loss. Bone Miner 1989; 7:79–86.

9. Ribot C, Pouilles JM, Tremollieres F. Prevention of postmenopausal bone loss by transdermal 17ß-estradiol: a two year longitudinal study. Proceedings of the XIIth world congress of obstetrics and gynaecology. Rio de Janeiro, Brazil, 1988.

10. Ribot C, Tremollieres F, Pouilles JM, Louvet JP, Peyron R. Transdermal administration of 17ß-estradiol in postmenopausal women: preliminary results of a longitudinal study. In: Christiansen C, Johansen JS, Riss BJ, eds. Osteoporosis. International symposium on osteoporosis, Denmark, 1987.

11. Riis BJ, Thomsen K, Stom V, Christiansen C. The effect of percutaneous estradiol and natural progesterone on postmenopausal bone loss. Am J Obstet Gynecol 1987; 156:61–5.

12. McKay Hart D, Al-Azzawi F, Farish E et al. Effect of ossopan alone, oestradiol implants alone or both therapies combined on bone density and bone biochemistry in oophorectomised women. In: Christiansen C, Johansen JS, Riis BJ, eds. Osteoporosis, International Symposium on Osteoporosis, Denmark, 1987.

13. Treasure J, Russell G, Fogelman I, Muyroy B. Reversal of bone loss in anorexia nervosa. Br Med J 1987; 295:474–5.

14. Greenspan SL, Neer RM, Ridgway EC, Klibanski A. Osteoporosis in men with hyperprolactinemic hypogonadism. Ann Intern Med 1986; 104:777–82.

15. Finkelstein JS, Klibanski A, Neer RM, Doppelt SH, Rosenthal DI, Serge GV, Crowley WF. Increases in bone density during treatment of men with idipoathic hypogonadotropic hypogonadism. J Clin Endocrinol Metab 1989; 69:776–83.

16. Matta WH, Shaw RW, Hesp R, Evans R. Reversible trabecular bone density loss following induced hypo-oestrogenism with the GnRH analogue Buserelin in premenopausal women. Clin Endocrinol 1988; 29:45–51.

17. Savvas M, Studd JWW, Fogelman I, Dooley M, Montgomery J, Murby B. Skeletal effects of oral oestrogen compared with subcutaneous oestrogen and testosterone in postmenopausal women. Br Med J 1988; 297:331–3.

18. Savvas M, Watson NR, Garnett T, Fogelman I, Studd JWW. A prospective study of the effects of oestradiol implants on the bone density of post-menopausal women. Br J Obstet Gynaecol (in press).

19. Powers MS, Schenkel L, Darley PE, Good WR, Balestra JC, Place VA. Pharmacokinetics and pharmacodynamics of transdermal dosage forms of 17ß-estradiol: comparison with conventional oral estrogens used for hormone replacement. Am J Obstet Gynecol 1985; 152:1099.

20. Sitruk-Ware R, de Ligniere B, Basdevant A, Mauvais-Jarvis P. The absorption of percutaneous oestradiol in post-menopausal women. Maturitas 1980; ii:207–11.

21. Lindsay R, Coots JRT, Hart DH. The effect of endogenous oestrogen on plasma and urinary calcium and phosphate in oophorectomised women. Clin Endocrinol 1977; 6:87.

22. Lindsay R, Hart DM, Clark DM. The minimum effective dose of estrogen for prevention of postmenopausal bone loss. Obstet Gynecol 1984; 63:759–63.

23. Horsman A, Jones M, Francis R, Nordin C. The effect of estrogen dose on postmenopausal bone loss. N Engl J Med 1983; 309:1405–7.

24. Albright F, Smith PH, Richardson AM. Postmenopausal osteoporosis, its clinical features. JAMA 1941; 116:2465–74.

25. Brincat M, Versi E, Moniz CF, Magos A. deTrafford J, Studd JWW. Skin collagen changes in postmenopausal women receiving different regimens of estrogen therapy. Obstet Gynecol 1987; 70:123–7.

26. Ernst H, Heath J, Rodan G. Estradiol effects on proliferative messenger ribonucleic acid for collagen and insulin-like growth factor 1, and parathyroid hormone stimulated adenylate cycle activation in osteoblastic cells for caliane and long bones. Endocrinology 1984; 124:825–33.
27. Riggs BL, Melton LJ. Involutional osteoporosis. N Engl J Med 1986; 314:1676–86.
28. Parfitt AM, Mathews CHE, Villanueva AR, Kleerekoper B, Rao DS. Relationships between surface, volume and thickness of iliac trabecular bone in aging and in osteoporosis. J Clin Invest 1983; 72:1396–409.

Discussion

Barlow: With oral therapy we see enormous differences in the individual in plasma levels achieved. One is trying to achieve a certain end point in terms of hormone going into the woman, but in any clinical situation one can never be sure what is delivered, certainly with oral therapy.

Whitehead: We did some of the original plasma profiles on oestrogel in 1979 in patients who as far as we could gauge were compliant and who were applying 5 g of the cream per day, and we showed plasma oestradiol levels which ranged from as little as 200 up to 1100 pmol l^{-1}. There is an enormous range, certainly with cream administration.

There will also be a range of plasma oestradiol values with transdermal application, and there may be enviromental factors with non-oral routes which will influence oestrogen absorption. Higher temperatures, for example, may make the alcohol in the cream evaporate more rapidly, and yet the alcohol is absolutely essential to drive the steroid through the stratum corneum. Certainly with transdermal administration if it is hot, and particularly if it is sticky, there is some preliminary evidence which says that the plasma oestradiol levels that are achieved are lower. Certainly the incidence of breakthrough bleeding with transdermal administration is greater in times when it is hot and sticky.

Kanis: Was fat correction undertaken for the dual photon absorptiometry? How was bone resorption measured on bone biopsies? How was apposition measured on bone biopsies?

Garnett: Dr Fogelman will have to answer the first question because the bone scans in that study were performed at Guy's Hospital.

Fogelman: There is no fat correction.

Garnett: As regards the bone biopsy specimens, these were looked at by Colin Woods at the Nuffield Orthopaedic Centre and the analysis I have given is a very simple analysis in that he simply scanned across the surface of the bone to try and assess the proportion of bone which is undergoing resorption and apposition.

Kanis: So this is the osteoid surface and the eroded surface?

Garnett: Yes. Basically. Which is a very gross way of analysing it.

Kanis: Which is not a way of analysing the apposition, obviously.

Garnett: He would disagree.

Kanis: He would not. He would not disagree.

But it leads me to one of the impressions it would be dangerous for this discussion to give, that is the view that oestrogens are capable of being truly anabolic agents on the skeleton. I accept the thrust of Dr Garnett's thesis, but certainly the changes in bone density that he measures are exaggerated very likely because of changes in body composition, and it is known that oestrogens induce profound changes not only in fat content of the body but also in fat content within the vertebral body, and that this has the effect of exaggerating an effect. Some estimates suggest that up to 50% might be artefactual. If we then suggest that the kinds of changes that are seen, which are of the order of 10%, are entirely consistent with altering bone remodelling. These are the changes that we expect with the pharmacological suppression of bone resorption, with calcitonin, with diphosphonates, with oestrogens, with pharmacological amounts of calcium, with anabolic steroids, it does not matter which agent. The point is that this is an effect which induces a small increment in skeletal calcium and is not the same as inducing a sustained and progressive increase, and so it is wrong to think of oestrogens as being potentially anabolic in that sense.

I accept that they induce a small increment in skeletal mass. This is not associated with the change in architecture and is entirely expected of the inhibition of bone remodelling. This is quite different from the restructuring of the skeleton from an osteoporotic state to a normal state.

Studd: Dr Kanis is speaking with great authority when no one has looked at studies where large levels of increments of the oestradiol increase are produced. That is why we have studies with Professor Boyde and Dr Wood from Oxford, so that we can answer these questions.

Kanis: I accept that the question is valid. I am saying that the changes that have been reported are entirely consistent with other published literature showing the effects of altering bone remodelling.

Fogelman: That is not strictly right. I tend to agree with the thesis, but I was involved with the publication of data which were cross-sectional and showed that with a long-term implant ladies, who were on average aged in their 60th year, had a significantly higher bone density in spine and in femur [1]. They might have been highly selected in some way. They might have been of a higher social class, or goodness know what. But nevertheless, in that cross-sectional study there was a very striking difference between the women who had had long-term implants as opposed to the younger controls, and that has not as yet been explained. But there may have been some bias in that study.

Anderson: That is preventing loss.

Kanis: That is a population study.

I accept the validity of asking the question. I am saying that the data that have been generated do not contribute in any way to answering that question – as yet.

Kanis: The point that I am trying to make is that it would be a mistake for the people to feel – at the current state of knowledge – that oestrogens can replace the bone that has been lost in established osteoporosis.

Garnett: I accept what Dr Kanis is saying, and I agree with what he is saying, but may be equilibrium can be re-established at a different level – and he says himself that there may be increases of between 5% and 10%. If they were accompanied by an increase in bone strength of between 5% and 10%, then that is important and cannot be dismissed as a transient effect. The term transient effect has been used, implying that it will go away after a few years. But it does not.

Kanis: It is the rate of change that is transient.

Garnett: And then a new equilibrium is established.

Kanis: I am not saying that it is pointless to give oestrogens. Do not get me wrong. The impression I got from Dr Garnett's paper was that the inference was that we could replace the skeleton. It is almost a statement that Mr Studd made earlier. The question is valid but the experiments need to be done and as yet it has not been proven.

Garnett: If equilibrium can be re-established, if as it were the thermostat can be re-set at a higher level, there will be a real increase in bone density.

Lindsay: We have to be very careful. United States fluoride studies have demonstrated that increments in bone density cannot necessarily be equated with changes in bone strength. Decrements in bone density can be related to changes in bone strength, but not increments in bone density. So we must be careful of that point.

In a controlled study in patients with established osteoporosis we gave Premarin 0.625 mg/day and compared that with a group who were given calcium alone. The increments in absolute bone mass are approximately the same as those recorded with the higher oestradiol levels, and oestradiol levels in this circumstance are from 200 to 300 pmol ml^{-1}. The problem is that Premarin has other things in it and we do not know the total oestrogenicity, but the changes are consistent throughout all the studies that we have seen prospectively done thus far. There is an increase in the spine of somewhere between 5% and 10% and an increase in cortical bone of much less. The size of the increment is dependent on the remodelling space.

Garnett: Our prospective studies would disagree with that. We compared implant therapy and oral therapy using 2 mg oestradiol valerate and it did not show a significant increase.

Selby: But you were not comparing like with like. A lot of implant work has looked at oestrogen and testosterone.

Garnett: There was no testosterone in the prospective study.

Lindsay: I too agree that the question is worth asking. There is no doubt about that, and it is an important question to ask. But I have yet to be convinced by the data that were presented that the point is proven.

Anderson: Mr Whitehead implied that a mean level is achieved with implants of 600–750 pmol l^{-1} and that that is inevitable. But that is because the implants are being given more frequently than is necessary, or that fits with the biological half-life of the implant. Certainly our experience is that median oestradiol levels can be tailored by adjusting the dose and the frequency of implants.

One of the problems is that one starts off giving the implants too frequently. But if they are maintained at yearly or less intervals, then levels of 200, 300 or even 400 pmol l^{-1} can be achieved, although there is variation between patients. But the levels can be tailored.

Barlow: How would the women be persuaded to tolerate the intervals?

Whitehead: I would accept that totally.

Anderson: But I do not agree. It is not my experience. There is a minority of patients – these are unusual women – who get a tachyphylactic oestradiol problem, but most are maintained asymptomtic at the levels that are usual with the patches.

Whitehead: Our data agree very closely with Mr Barlow's. After a couple of years he was reporting 630 pmol. But that is only 50 mg implanted every 6 months.

Barlow: Six-monthly for 3 years.

Cardozo: But when we give 25 mg every 4 months we maintain levels of 200–400 pmol l^{-1}.

Anderson: Or one can give 50 mg/year. My strategy has always been not to re-implant until the oestradiol level had fallen to <500 pmol l^{-1}, and so we are never in a situation of having given them at 6-monthly intervals and then trying to put the brake on.

We have not published those data, but we have recently done an audit on the median levels and they are well below 500 pmol l^{-1}.

Whitehead: The majority of hospital-based implants that are given in the UK are 50 mg repeated every 6 months.

Anderson: They are giving them far too frequently. In fact, the right dose to achieve a steady-state level at whatever dose one is giving is a year not 6-monthly. If they are being given more frequently, whether it is 50 mg or 100 mg, then because of the very long tail attached to each implant levels are bound to increase progressively.

Whitehead: I would not dispute that but I would agree with Mr Barlow. How does one get the patient not to come back at six or eight months complaining that her symptoms have come back and that she wants another implant.

Anderson: There is a problem with the combined implant because the testosterone implant does last for 6 months, in which case if the symptoms return and she is on the combined implant one should re-give the testosterone. But I do not think it is inevitable. And it is certainly not our experience.

Barlow: These are women who are symptomatic?

Anderson: These are women mostly referred because they cannot tolerate other forms of oestrogen therapy.

Purdie: Can I ask about Mr Whitehead's practical experiences with the combination patch? Did he find that the norethisterone, which can be a pretty nasty hormone, generated many symptomatic problems with premenstrual syndrome, given straight into the systemic circulation as it is?

And may I also ask Dr Selby for his comments on what he thinks might be the effect on the bone of 14 days of norethisterone at daily dose of 0.25 mg delivered over the 24-hour period?

Whitehead: Of the 32 or 33 patients who were initially recruited to the transdermal system, at 18 months one has dropped out because of a treatment problem. Three or four have dropped out because of problems unrelated to treatment, moving house and so on. There has been one clear treatment-related withdrawal.

Selby: In terms of the effect on bone, I would not expect that sort of dose of norethisterone to have any great effect on bone. We have, from Newcastle, some very incomplete data suggesting that if we just give one mini-pill of norethisterone, 350 µg, that has very little effect on biochemical indicators of bone turnover, and I think others have had a similar experience in other systems with that sort of dose of norethisterone.

I would not expect to see any great effect from the norethisterone by itself in that system, but there is still the benefit from the oestrogen.

Stevenson: It was suggested that there is a certain oestradiol level whereby there is no bone loss. Certainly one can look at changes in bone density and plasma oestradiol levels and get a significant correlation, but the correlation is very weak and it really is plus or minus some unknown. There is no set level. It is not true to suggest that one can measure oestradiol levels and that above a certain value there is no reason to worry about the skeleton and that it will always be all right. That is not true at all.

I also believe that there is variation between individuals. The level at which one woman will conserve her skeleton can be completely different from the level at which another woman will conserve her skeleton.

Baird: As I understand it, when women's ovaries fail at the menopause, they get accelerated bone loss, and this is due to lack of secretion of oestrogen from their ovaries. Yet the dose of oestradiol in a 50 mg implant is about two or three times the amount that she would normally produce in full reproductive life through a cycle. So in physiological terms we are giving a pharmacological dose of oestradiol. Is that the intention, and is that what it is necessary to do, or could we give half or a third of that amount to give the amount that the ovaries would normally secrete. Or has this dose just been plucked out of the air?

Studd: It is possible that that is right. It is possible. What are the data from the 25 μg patch on bone? Does that increase bone density?

We have a problem because neither of the chapters which discussed oestrogen levels gave us the mean oestradiol levels that are achieved with oral therapy, with the patch or with the implant data. That might be useful to know.

However, it is a fair assumption that the 25 μg patch works less well on bone than the 50 μg patch and that the effect on bone is correlated with plasma oestradiol levels.

Selby: It certainly does not suppress the biochemical markers of bone resorption as completely as a 50 μg patch.

Baird: A 50 mg implant will release, on average, 300 μg/day oestradiol directly into the circulation. It is like an intramuscular injection. And we are talking about patches which are releasing 25 μg or 50 μg, which is right in the early follicular phase range.

Anderson: But that is not correct. That steady-state release is achieved when the patient has had five or six implants at 6-monthly intervals, but in fact the same sort of median levels can be achieved with a 50 mg oestradiol implant given less frequently. That calculation is based on the assumption that the implant is given every six months.

From Mr Whitehead's data on the patches and investigations by Hilary Critchley and myself, it certainly seems that levels and absorption are highly variable, but the levels we are seeing are around 200 pmol l^{-1}, which would be an average median normal 28-day mean oestradiol level. However, we do not know whether that is what it is actually necessary to achieve.

Whitehead: Because there is no prospective study comparing 50 mg and 25 mg that has been set up as a dose-ranging study.

Anderson: I would suggest that the Estraderm-50 patch gives a reasonable physiological mean oestradiol level.

Whitehead: On our assay system it is 200 pmol l^{-1}, about 55 pg ml^{-1}.

Ross: I am interested in all this talk about oestradiol levels although I do not understand it too well. But what about the differences in sex hormone binding globulin (SHBG) levels with the patches versus oral therapy and how does that impact on free or bioavailable oestradiol levels and what impact therefore might that have on, say, breast or endometrial tissues?

Cust: We did a short-term study looking at SHBG levels with the Estraderm-50 patch and comparing with women who were taking oral oestradiol valerate 2 mg/day both with a cyclical progestogen. During the oestrogen phase of therapy we found no difference in the SHBG levels when they crossed over from a 50 μg patch to 2 mg oestradiol valerate, and we found no difference in the free oestradiol in the two groups.

Anderson: SHBG has a really small effect on the percentage free oestradiol level because of the marked dampening effect of changes in ablumin and the fact that its affinity, certainly compared with testosterone and dihydrotestosterone, is relatively low. And one would be fairly hard-pushed to show any effect of doubling of SHBG on the percentage of free oestradiol.

Selby: I showed slight, but only slight changes in SHBG with 2 mg micronised oestradiol compared with a 50 μg patch and I would not argue with Mr Cust's result.

Ross: What does the SHBG do? Why is it there?

Baird: It is a damper. It has a much greater dampening effect on testosterone.

Boyde: According to animal experimental data, it takes between 200 and 3000 microstrain seen in a bone surface recognised by either the osteocytes or the surface osteoblasts to obtain bone deposition. I do not see how Dr Garnett can speculate that once the trabeculum is broken, the trabecular stumps can thicken up. They could not see any microstrain at all as soon as they become discontinuous, which is one comment.

My other comment is that in the case that people take biopsies to study the processes of remodelling, presumably the wound fills with woven bone. Presumably the woven bone remodels to trabecular bone, and bone grows back again when there was no bone there. Perhaps the bone experts can tell me if it has been followed through in human experimental studies. It has been done ad nauseum in animal models. Is this true also in man?

Kanis: It is true, and the implication for osteoporosis extrapolating literally from that comment is to induce woven bone formation in man, which can certainly be done by fracturing the bones but one is searching for more elegant ways of reproducing that model in women.

Barlow: If we find a dose that makes our patients symptomatically happy and is above the threshold we feel helps bone, does it matter which route we are using to give our oestrogen by if the patient finds it acceptable?

Whitehead: Given the biological variation within an individual, if the dose is bone sparing it does not seem to matter whether it is given orally or transdermally, or percutaneously, or as an implant, from the bone point of view.

Lindsay: The general data would support that.

Anderson: Is it possible that some of the effect seen with oestrogens is due to altered behaviour and physical activity induced by improved wellbeing? Women do generally feel better on oestrogen replacement and that may well be reflected in an alteration in their pattern of activity.

Has anybody looked at exercise assessments?

Brincat: There are studies in female athletes that are now well established and it is quite clear that exercise on its own does not compensate for the lack of oestrogen.

Anderson: But with oestrogen? They were losing weight – I have forgotten who showed that.

Brincat: But even if they exercised enough, it would not compensate for the reduction in oestrogen levels. The studies in women athletes, looking at amenorrhoea etc., are quite conclusive.

Anderson: I am not saying that exercise in the presence of low oestrogen levels is effective, but there may be some additive effect.

Brincat: Yes. It would seem that the oestrogen effect is much bigger than any exercise additive effect.

Whitehead: We did exercise assessments before and during therapy, and in the treated group we did not see any change in the amount of time spent or exercise taken.

Stevenson: It seems that there is only an increase in activity in MPs!

Whitehead: Exercise was not a confounder in this study.

Reference

1. Savvas M, Studd JWW, Fogelman I, Dooley M, Montgomery J, Murby B. Skeletal effects of oral oestrogen compared with subcutaneous oestrogen and testosterone in postmenopausal women. Br Med J 1988; 297:331–3.

Chapter 23

Prevention and Treatment of Osteoporosis

J. C. Stevenson, R. C. Hillard and M. Ellerington

The most serious complication of osteoporosis is fracture. The occurrence of fracture is dependent on a number of factors: these include the frequency of falls, the type of fall involved, the quality of the bone tissue, and most importantly the amount of bone tissue present. As bone tissue is lost the density of the skeleton decreases, reducing its structural integrity. Bone density is directly related to fracture prevalence [1] and incidence [2]. Thus, whilst measures to reduce the chance of falls are clearly important, the prevention of bone loss and maintenance of bone density are the major aims of therapy.

The risk of development of osteoporosis depends primarily on two factors; first, the maximum bone density achieved (peak adult bone density), and second, its subsequent loss.

Peak Adult Bone density

Most studies have clearly shown that peak adult bone density is achieved by the end of [3], or soon after [4–9], linear skeletal growth. There are a number of reasons to suggest that genetic factors are mainly responsible for peak adult bone density. The variance in bone mass is less between monozygotic twins than between dizygotic twins [10]; bone density in adolescent girls correlates with that of their parents [11]; racial differences in bone density [12] are maintained even after geographical translocation; and the daughters of women with osteoporosis have a lower bone density than their peers [13].

Some environmental circumstances may have a significant but lesser influence on peak adult bone density. It is likely, for example, that malnutrition or debility during childhood could prevent the attainment of the genetically pre-ordained peak bone density. Furthermore, factors such as alcohol consumption and cigarette smoking may reduce the peak bone density before the menopause [9]. Pregnancies and oral contraceptive usage can probably be regarded as beneficial to the skeleton [9], but intervals of hypoestrogenic amenorrhoea before the menopause are clearly deleterious.

In terms of prevention of osteoporosis, attention to lifestyle should be emphasised before the menopause, but it seems unlikely that any major benefit could be conferred on the skeleton at this time. Thus treatment of subsequent bone loss after the menopause becomes all important.

Postmenopausal Bone Loss

Loss of ovarian function has the single most important effect on the female skeleton [6,9,14,15] (Figs. 23.1 and 23.2). It results in increased bone turnover with resorption exceeding formation, and the antiresorptive action of oestrogen therapy is well established. Thus oestrogen replacement therapy has become the primary approach for the prevention and treatment of postmenopausal osteoporosis. In the short term, the action of oestrogen causes a modest increase in bone density as the remodelling space is filled in, but in the long term oestrogen appears able to maintain this bone density and hence prevent the increasing risk of fracture [16–23].

Whilst the many benefits of oestrogen therapy, both short and long term, are obvious, there remain a number of women who are either unable or unwilling to

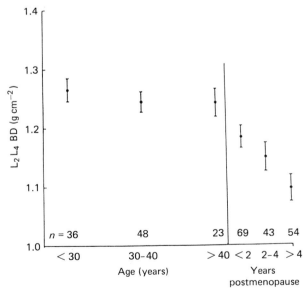

Fig. 23.1. Mean (±SEM) bone density in the lumbar vertebrae in pre- and postmenopausal women. (Reproduced from Stevenson et al. [9] with permission.)

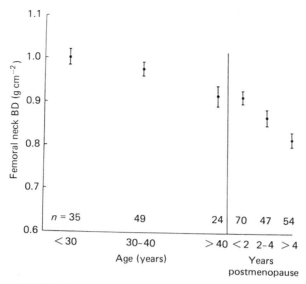

Fig. 23.2. Mean (±SEM) bone density in the femoral neck in pre- and postmenopausal women. (Reproduced from Stevenson et al. [9], with permission.)

take hormone replacement. Furthermore, the advisability of taking oestrogen in the very long term (in excess of ten years) is still the subject of debate. There is thus a place for alternative therapies which also afford skeletal protection, particularly in the older woman.

Prevention and Treatment

Continued loss of bone tissue after the menopause may eventually result in perforation and loss of trabecular elements. This destruction of the micro-anatomical structure of the bone can result in mechanical failure, i.e. fracture. Furthermore, this loss of architecture may eventually render the process virtually irreversible [24]. Thus, although treatment can be initiated at any stage of the disease, the earlier intervention occurs the greater the benefit is likely to be, and prevention of the disease should be the primary aim.

Non-oestrogen drug therapy can be directed along two basic approaches, namely agents which prevent bone resorption and those which stimulate bone formation. To date, the former have been used with greatest effect.

Antiresorptive Agents

Calcitonin is an antiresorptive hormone which has now been used extensively in the treatment of osteoporosis. One early study of women with osteoporotic fractures showed that calcitonin could prevent bone loss and induce small short-term increases in skeletal mass as assessed by total body calcium measurements utilising neutron activation analysis [25]. However, this study used relatively high doses of salmon calcitonin (100 i.u.) administered daily by intramuscular injection. In a study of healthy women in the early postmenopausal period, we were able to show that much lower doses of calcitonin (20 i.u.) given three times per week were as effective as oestrogen in preventing spinal trabecular bone loss [26]. However, a major disadvantage was the route of administration of the calcitonin, by subcutaneous injection. The development of non-invasive administration of calcitonin, by intranasal application, has circumvented this problem, and initial studies have suggested that calcitonin given by this route is effective in both prevention and treatment of osteoporosis [27,28]. The optimal dosage regimen for intranasal calcitonin remains to be determined, and longer-term studies which include effects on fracture rate are awaited.

Another form of antiresorptive therapy, which like calcitonin has proved its worth in the treatment of Paget's disease, is the use of bisphosphonates. These are stable analogues of pyrophosphate which bind to the bone surface and directly inhibit osteoclast action. These compounds have the advantage of being active when administered orally. Preliminary studies of the bisphosphonate, disodium etidronate, in the treatment of women with spinal osteoporosis have demonstrated a small gain in bone density compared with loss in untreated women [29,30]. The etidronate is given as cyclical therapy in courses of two weeks' treatment which are repeated at three-monthly intervals. Newer bisphosphonate compounds have been developed and may well prove very effective in both prevention and treatment of osteoporosis [31]. Further studies are awaited.

Calcium supplementation has been claimed to have an antiresorptive effect and some studies have shown biochemical evidence of a reduction in bone turnover with such therapy [32]. Histological studies, however, have not confirmed a reduction in bone turnover [33]. It is thus unclear whether or not the biochemical effects of calcium supplementation translate into true benefit for osteoporosis prevention, since even extremely large supplements have no measurable effect on bone at the clinically relevant sites of osteoporotic fracture [34]. There is very little evidence for an aetiological role of dietary calcium deficiency in the development of osteoporosis [35–37]. With the customary diet of the United Kingdom population, the daily calcium intake, which is above 400 mg, is not related to hip fracture risk [38]. Furthermore, dietary calcium intake does not influence either the rate of postmenopausal loss or its response to therapy [39,40]. Calcium supplementation cannot be regarded as an effective alternative to the treatments already mentioned.

Similarly, vitamin D and its analogues appear to be without any effect in the management of osteoporosis [41,42].

Stimulation of Bone Formation

Fluoride is a drug which directly stimulates new bone formation. It has been quite widely used and it results in an apparently continuous increase in vertebral bone density. However, it is also a toxic agent, being associated with side effects such as gastrointestinal problems, arthralgia and a "lower limb pain" syndrome: such side effects may occur in up to 40% of patients [43]. A significant proportion of patients show no skeletal response to fluoride therapy [44]. Of more concern, however, is the possibility that increased bone quantity resulting from fluoride therapy is associated with reduced bone quality. Thus an increase in fractures has been reported with fluoride usage [45], and of particular concern is an increase in femoral neck fractures. At the present time, the use of fluoride must be considered with extreme caution.

There is some evidence to suggest that anabolic steroids may stimulate bone formation [46]. There is little doubt that such agents will bring about increases in bone mass [47], although the findings of some studies utilising peripheral bone density measurements may have artificially overestimated such increases because of changes in soft tissue composition induced by these agents [48]. They should be given parenterally to minimise adverse effects on lipid and carbohydrate metabolism. The major clinical side effect appears to be fluid retention, which can prove a significant problem in the older patient in whom cardiovascular function may be impaired.

Physical exercise may have positive effects in increasing bone density [49]. There is a paucity of adequately designed studies on this subject, but some studies (e.g. ref. 50) suggest a positive effect of weight-bearing exercise. Such physical activity does appear to confer a modest benefit in bone density, particularly in the proximal femur [9], and this may perhaps be translated into a reduction in the incidence of hip fracture [38,51]. Much work remains to be done on the type and duration of exercise necessary to increase bone density in the relevant clinical sites, but it is unlikely that such approaches will by themselves provide a realistic alternative to drug therapy. It is clear, for example, that increased physical activity is unable to reverse the bone loss seen with oestrogen deprivation [52,53].

Newer agents which stimulate bone formation, such as parathyroid hormone and certain growth factors, may hold promise for the future, either alone or in combination with antiresorptive agents.

Conclusions

Prevention and treatment of postmenopausal osteoporosis now appears possible. With modern technology, the disease can be detected in its earliest stages and treatment should be instituted as soon as possible before irreversible structural damage can ensue. Hormone replacement therapy remains the mainstay of treatment, but alternative therapies are now becoming available. It seems likely that a major impact on the incidence of fracture could be effected [54], and to this end treatment should be more widely used.

References

1. Melton LJ, Wahner HW, Richelson L, O'Fallon WM, Dunn WL, Riggs BL. Bone density specific fracture risk: a population based study of the relationship between osteoporosis and vertebral fractures. J Nucl Med 1985; 26:24.
2. Melton LJ, Wahner HW, Richelson L, O'Fallon WM, Riggs BL. Osteoporosis and the risk of hip fracture. Am J Epidemiol 1986: 124:254–61.

3. Gilsanz V, Gibbens DT, Carlson M, Boechet MI, Cann CE, Schulz EE. Peak trabecular vertebral density: a comparison of adolescent and adult females. Calcif Tissue Int 1988; 43:260–2.

4. Meema S, Meema HE. Menopausal bone loss and estrogen replacement. Isr J Med Sci 1976; 12:601–6.

5. Riggs BL, Wahner HW, Seeman E et al. Changes in bone mineral density of the proximal femur and spine with aging. J Clin Invest 1982; 70:716–23.

6. Gallagher JC, Goldger D, Moy A. Total body calcium in normal women: effect of age and menopause state. J Bone Miner Res 1987; 2:491:6.

7. Hui SL, Slemenda CW, Johnston CC, Appledorn CR. Effects of age and menopause on vertebral bone density. Bone Miner 1987; 2:141–6.

8. Schaadt O, Bohr H. Different trends of age-related diminution of bone mineral content in the lumbar spine, femoral neck and femoral shaft in women. Calcif Tissue Int 1988; 42:71–6.

9. Stevenson JC, Lees BL, Devenport M, Cust MP, Ganger KF. Determinants of bone density in normal women: risk factors for future osteoporosis? Br Med J 1989; 298:924–8.

10. Smith DM, Nance WE, Kang KW, Christian JC, Johnston CC. Genetic factors in determining bone mass. J Clin Invest 1973; 52:2800–8.

11. Matkovic V, Chesnut C, Genetic factors and acquisition of bone mass. J Bone Miner Res 1987; 2 suppl 1:329.

12. Cohn SH, Abesamis C, Yasamura S, Aloia JF, Zanzi I, Ellis KJ. Comparative skeletal mass and radial bone mineral content in black and white women. Metabolism 1977; 26:171–8.

13. Seeman E, Hopper JL, Bach LA et al. Reduced bone mass in daughters of women with osteoporosis. N Engl J Med 1989; 320:554–8.

14. Richelson LS, Wahner HW, Melton LJ, Riggs BL. Relative contributions of aging and estrogen deficiency to postmenopausal bone loss. N Engl J Med 1984; 311:1273–5.

15. Stevenson JC, Banks LM Spinks TJ et al. Regional and total skeletal measurements in the early postmenopause. J Clin Invest 1987; 80:258–62.

16. Lindsay R, Hart DM, Aitken JM, MacDonald EB, Anderson JB, Clarke AC. Long-term prevention of postmenopausal osteoporosis by oestrogen. Lancet 1976; i:1038–41.

17. Horsman A, Gallagher JC, Simpson M. Nordin BEC. Prospective trial of oestrogen and calcium in postmenopausal women. Br Med J 1977; ii:789–92.

18. Nachtigall LE, Nachtigall RH, Nachtigall RD, Beckman EM. Estrogen replacement therapy. A 10-year prospective study in relationship to osteoporosis. Obstet Gynecol 1979; 53:277–81.

19. Hutchinson TA, Polansky SM, Feinstein A. Postmenopausal oestrogens protect against fractures of hip and distal radius. Lancet 1979; ii:706–9.

20. Lindsay R, Hart DM, Forrest C, Baird C. Prevention of spinal osteoporosis in oophorectomised women. Lancet 1980; ii:1151–4.

21. Weiss NS, Ure CL, Ballard JH, Williams AR, Daling JR. Decreased risk of fractures of the hip and lower forearm with postmenopausal use of estrogen. N Engl J Med 1980; 303:1195–8.

22. Paganini-Hill A, Ross RK, Gerkins VR, Henderson BE, Arthur M, Mack TM. A case-control study of menopausal estrogen therapy and hip fractures. Ann Intern Med 1981; 95:28–31.

23. Christiansen C, Christensen MS, Transbol I. Bone mass in postmenopausal women after withdrawal of oestrogen/gestagen replacement therapy. Lancet 1981; i:459–61.

24. Dempster DW, Shane E, Herbert W, Lindsay R. A simple method for correlative light and scanning electron microscopy of human iliac crest bone biopsies: qualitative observations in normal and osteoporotic subjects. J Bone Miner Res 1986; 1:15–21.

25. Gruber HE, Ivey JL, Baylink DJ et al. Long-term calcitonin therapy in postmenopausal osteoporosis. Metabolism 1984; 33:295–303.

26. MacIntyre I, Stevenson JC, Whitehead MI, Wimalawansa SJ, Banks LM, Healy MJR. Calcitonin for prevention of postmenopausal bone loss. Lancet 1988; ii:1481–3.

27. Reginster JY, Denis D, Albert A et al. 1-year controlled randomised trial of prevention of early postmenopausal bone loss by intranasal calcitonin. Lancet 1987; ii:1481–3.

28. Overgaard K, Riis BJ, Christiansen C, Podenphant J, Johansen JS. Nasal calcitonin for treatment of established osteoporosis. Clin Endocrinol 1989; 30:435–42.

29. Genant HK, Harris ST, Steiger P, Davey PF, Block JE. The effect of etidronate therapy in postmenopausal osteoporotic women: preliminary results. In: Christiansen C, Johansen JS, Riis BJ, eds. Osteoporosis 1987. Copenhagen: Osteopress ApS, 1987:1177–81.

30. Storm T, Thamsborg G, Sorensen OH, Lund B. The effect of etidronate therapy in postmenopausal osteoporotic women: preliminary results. In: Christiansen C, Johansen JS, Riis BJ, eds. Osteoporosis 1987. Copenhagen: Osteopress ApS, 1987:1172–6.

31. Reginster JY, Deroisy R, Denis D et al. Prevention of postmenopausal bone loss by tiludronate. Lancet 1989; ii:1469–71.

32. Horowitz M, Need AG, Philcox JC, Nordin BEC. The effect of calcium supplements on plasma alkaline phosphatase and urinary hydroxyproline in postmenopausal women. Horm Metab Res 1985; 17:311–12.
33. Steiniche T, Hasling C, Charles P, Eriksen EF, Mosekilde L, Melsen F. A randomized study on the effects of estrogen/gestagen or high dose oral calcium on trabecular bone remodeling in postmenopausal osteoporosis. Bone 1989; 10:313–20.
34. Riis B, Thomsen K, Christiansen C. Does calcium supplementation prevent postmenopausal bone loss? N Engl J Med 1987; 316:173–7.
35. Stevenson JC, Osteoporosis: pathogenesis and risk factors. In: Martin TJ, ed. Bailliere's clinical endocrinology and metabolism. Vol 2, no. 1. Metabolic bone disease. London: Bailliere Tindall 1988; 87–101.
36. Kanis JA, Passmore R. Calcium supplementation of the diet. I. Br Med J 1989; 293:137–40.
37. Kanis JA, Passmore R. Calcium supplementation of the diet. II. Br Med J 1989; 293:205–8.
38. Wickham CAC, Walsh K, Cooper C et al. Dietary calcium, physical activity, and the risk of hip fracture: a prospective study. Br Med J 1989; 299:889–92.
39. Riggs BL, Wahner HW, Melton LJ et al. Dietary calcium intake and rate of bone loss in women. J Clin Invest 1987; 80:979–82.
40. Stevenson JC, Whitehead MI, Padwick M et al. Dietary intake of calcium and postmenopausal bone loss. Br Med J 1988; 297:15–17.
41. Nordin BEC, Horsman A, Crilly RG, Marshall DH, Simpson M. Treatment of spinal osteoporosis in postmenopausal women. Br Med J 1980; i:451–4.
42. Ott SM, Chesnut CH. Calcitriol treatment is not effective in postmenopausal osteoporosis. Ann Intern Med 1989; 110:267–74.
43. Riggs BL, Hodgson SF, Muhs J, Wahner HW. Fluoride treatment of osteoporosis: clinical and bone densitometric responses. In: Christiansen C, Johansen JS, Riis BJ, eds. Osteoporosis 1987. Copenhagen: Osteopress ApS, 1987; 817–23.
44. Duursma SA, Glerum JH, Van Dijk A et al. Responders and non-responders after fluoride therapy in osteoporosis. Bone 1987; 8:131–6.
45. Hedlund LR, Gallagher JC. Increased incidence of hip fracture in osteoporotic women treated with sodium fluoride. J Bone Miner Res 1989; 4:223–5.
46. Vaishnav R, Beresford JN, Gallagher JA, Russell RGG. Effects of the anabolic steroid stanozolol on cells derived from human bone. Clin Sci 1988; 74:455–60.
47. Chesnut CH, Treatment of postmenopausal osteoporosis: some current concepts. Scott Med J 1981; 26:72–80.
48. Hassager C, Borg J, Christiansen C. The effect of subcutaneous fat on single-photon ^{125}I absorptiometry measurement of bone mineral content in the distal forearm. In:Christiansen C, Johansen JS, Riis BJ, eds. Osteoporosis 1987. Copenhagen: Osteopress ApS, 1987; 399–401.
49. Stevenson JC, Lees B, Fielding C, Cust MP, Ganger KF, Hillard TC. Exercise and the skeleton. In: Smith R, ed. Osteoporosis 1990. London: Royal College of Physicians, 1990; 119–24.
50. Chow R, Harrison JE, Notarius C. Effect of two randomised exercise programmes on bone mass of healthy women. Br Med J 1987; 295:1441–4.
51. Cooper C, Barker DJP, Wickham C. Physical activity, muscle strength and calcium intake in fracture of the proximal femur in Britain. Br Med J 1988; 287:1443–6.
52. Drinkwater BL, Nilson K. Chesnut CH et al. Bone mineral content of amenorrhoeic and eumenorrhoeic athletes. N Engl J Med 1984; 311:277–81.
53. Lloyd T, Myers C, Buchanan JR, Demers LM. Collegiate women athletes with irregular menses during adolescence have decreased bone density. Obstet Gynecol 1988; 72:639–42.
54. Stevenson JC. Post-menopausal bone loss and osteoporosis. In: Zichella L, Whitehead MI, van Keep PA, eds. The climacteric and beyond, Carnforth, England: Parthenon Publishing, 1988; 125–35.

Chapter 24

Lifestyle, Exercise and Osteoporosis

M. Notelovitz

Introduction

Involutional osteoporosis is incorrectly perceived as a "disease". One clear fact emerges on review of the vast literature on the subject. Bone mass is inversely proportional to osteoporotic-related fractures; the greater the bone mass of individuals, irrespective of age, the less the chance of fracture [1]. Central to the physiological accrual of bone mass are two interrelated processes. The activity of the bone remodelling cycle, and lifestyle factors. These in turn are influenced by the individual's chronological and reproductive age. For example, for a given loading strain the net rate of bone volume change is greater in "growing" than in "mature" bone [2]. This process is influenced by the loss of the modulating effect of oestrogen on the bone remodelling cycle with resulting increased osteoclast activity, deeper resorption cavities and an accelerated rate of bone loss in oestrogen-deprived women [3].

Although genetic [4] and racial [5] factors are primary determinants of skeletal mass, exercise, appropriate nutrition and the avoidance of certain lifestyle practices during the growth phase – the teens and early adult years of women – could result in a greater peak bone mass. This is illustrated hypothetically in Fig. 24.1. The estimated natural lifetime loss in women of 35% of their cortical bone and 50% of their trabecular bone [1] would still result in a postmenopausal bone mass reserve that exceeds the so-called fracture-zone [6]. Therefore, as clinicians, our task is relatively simple: encourage women to accrue as much bone as possible before their menopause by adopting healthy lifestyle practices.

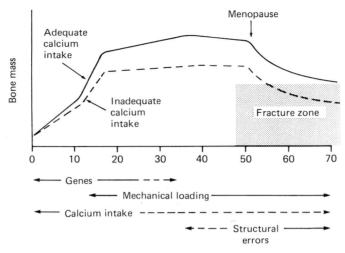

Fig. 24.1.

Exercise: Bone Mass and Strength

Peak bone mass and subsequent bone mineral maintenance is influenced by an interplay between mechanical stress, body composition, nutrition and the individual's endocrine milieu. Each factor influences the other. Exercise is an initiator of the cycle since mechanical loading, muscular activity and gravity stimulate bone cells to begin the genetic process for growth and differentiation. Intermediaries in the process include the generation of piezoelectricity which stimulates cyclic nucleotides, the synthesis of prostaglandins and other matrix-derived bone growth factors. More recently, Bell et al. [7] demonstrated an increase in serum GLA-protein, serum 1,25-dihydroxyvitamin D $(1,25(OH)_2D)$ and urinary cyclic AMP in response to muscle-strengthening exercise, indicative or osteoblast stimulation and increased deposition of skeletal calcium. What is yet to be determined is whether exercise stimulates normal coupling with "old" bone replaced with equal volumes of freshly synthesised and mineralised "new bone", or whether appropriate mechanical loading could actually stimulate osteoblasts to overfill the resorptive cavity. The former situation would maintain the bone mineral content but enhance the bones' mechanical strength; the latter would, in addition, result in bone hypertrophy.

Factors Influencing Exercise and Bone Mass

Gravity and Immobilisation

Bone is lost with bed rest; the estimated loss is 4% during the early phase of bed rest. Three hours a day of quiet standing will restore bone mineral; four hours of walking prevents bone loss associated with 20 hours of bed rest. Bone loss due to immobilisation occurs irrespective of the initial bone mass with all patients ending up with a similar bone mineral content.

Bone needs mechanical stress to maintain its integrity. Basset and Baker [8] postulated that piezoelectricity is generated by the bending force of mechanical stress applied to bone, and that this sets up a negative electrical potential on the concave side of the bone relative to the convex side. This sets in motion a cascade of events eventually ending in the elaboration of bone matrix or osteoid. According to this hypothesis, isometric or horizontal exercise would be less able to restore bone mass resulting from immobilisation – an important point when dealing with bed-ridden or immobilised patients.

Bone remodelling is very sensitive to small changes in cyclic mechanical stress; under experimental conditions, a change of less than 1% of the ultimate strength of a given load applied to bone can result in measurable bone atrophy [2]. These observations have practical applications: osteogenesis is more likely to occur with weight-bearing exercise, and to be effective in the long term, the exercise needs to be sustained. Two clinical studies illustrate these points. Highly trained intercollegiate tennis athletes (weight-bearing) had significantly greater lumbar bone mass (evaluated by dual photon absorptiometry) when compared to age-matched competitive swimmers (non-weight-bearing) [9]. In another study, 13 months of decreased activity in previously exercised women resulted in a reduction in vertebral bone mass from a 6.1% value above pre-existing exercise levels, to a value of 1.1% above the original baseline level [10].

Systemic vs Regional Exercise

Exercise has a systemic and a local effect. The net result – bone mineral maintenance of hypertrophy – might depend on both the type and the frequency of exercise. Female professional tennis players, for example, were found to have greater overall bone mass than age-matched casual tennis players, but in addition had a 28.4% greater cortical thickness in the dominant arm when compared with their own and a control group's non-dominant arm [11]. The same result is seen in the collegiate tennis players and swimmers referred to earlier.

The positive effect of exercise on bone mass may be related to an increase in muscle mass [11]. Studies have shown a relationship between physical activity, psoas muscle mass and lumbar vertebrae ash weight in premenopausal women [12] and in postmenopausal women comparing spine bone mineral content and back extensor muscle strength [13].

These observations have two relevant clinical applications. Tests of muscle strength may correlate with bone mass and serve as a simple non-invasive method of assessing bone mass (? strength); exercises that hypertrophy muscle and increase muscle strength should provide the optimal stimulus to bone mass accrual. Pocock et al. [14] have shown muscle strength in both biceps and quadriceps to be an independent predicter of bone mass in the proximal femur, lumbar spine and forearm. The fact that biceps muscle strength correlates with lumbar bone mineral, again argues for the systemic effect of exercise. Bevier et al. [15] also concluded that grip strength correlated significantly with bone density in elderly women (ages 61–84 years). The role of muscle-strengthening exercises as part of an overall exercise prescription will be discussed later.

Age

Experimentation with animals and clinical experience have shown that a certain amount of mechanical damage serves as a stimulus to bone hypertrophy. However, there is an optimal level beyond which increasing strain levels may have a negative effect [16]. This is especially true for older women.

A few practical points emerge. At present, non-invasive technology that evaluates the structural configuration of trabecular bone is not available, as one has to infer the potential for damage with bone density testing. To screen for latent osteopenia and osteoporosis, all women, before starting meaningful aerobic and/or muscle-strengthenig exercise, should have a bone mineral analysis of their spine and hip using dual photon absorptiometry or dual energy radiography, and, for women over the age of 60, an anteroposterior and lateral X-ray of the spine, to exclude vertebral deformation.

As far as chronological postmenopausal age is concerned, it is never too late to start exercising. Sixteen healthy women with prior Colles' fractures (mean age 61 ± 6 years) participated in an exercise programme that involved walking, running and calisthenics for one hour twice weekly. At the end of 8 months the vertebral bone mineral content (measured by dual photon absorptiometry) had increased by 3%–5%, whereas in an age-matched control group it decreased by 2.7%. The bone mineral content of the distal radius decreased by 3.5% [17]. Smith et al. [18] designed an exercise programme for older women (mean age 81 years) that oriented activity at a level of 1.5–3.0 METs, around a chair (one MET equals the average effort exerted by subjects on a chair at rest). Over a three-year period the exercise group demonstrated a 2.9% increase in midshaft bone mineral content, whereas a matched non-exercise and control group showed a 3.9% decrease in the bone mineral content [18].

From the above it can be concluded that it is never too late to start exercise, but that the programme should be tailored to the age and physical habitus of the patient. In addition, the earlier one starts, the more responsive the bone and the greater the chance of enhancing peak bone mass levels. This point is of considerable importance given the recent documentation of the early loss of trabecular bone in normal premenopausal women. Using single-energy quantitative computer tomography of the lumbar spine, Buchanan et al. [19] reported a progressive decrease of trabecular bone mineral content of the spine with age, in healthy premenopausal women. The respective mean bone densities were: 178 ± 8 mg ml^{-1} in the second decade; 171 ± 6 mg ml^{-1} in the third decade; 158 ± 4 mg ml^{-1} in the fourth decade and 140 ± 12 mg ml^{-1} in the fifth decade. These numbers extrapolate to a 0.73% loss of bone mineral per year. Other studies now suggest that peak bone mass may in fact be reached at 14–19 years of age [20] and not at age 35 years as currently accepted.

Monitoring the Bone Remodelling Response to Exercise

It has become apparent from a number of studies that you can exercise too much. Women marathon runners whose activity was associated with exercise-induced amenorrhoea have reduced lumbar bone mineral (measured by dual photon absorptiometry) with normal or minimally reduced cortical bone - (measured by single photon absorptiometry and radiogrammetry) [21]. This bone loss has been attributed to a deficiency of oestrogen associated with body fat. This has been found by others [22] and "confirmed" by an increase in bone mass after oestrogen levels in the amenorrhoeic runners returned to normal [23,24]. Although an oestrogen-replete state is probably needed for a maximal osteogenic result, the actual cause of exercise-induced osteopenia may be confounded by other factors. Thus, menstruating marathron runners (with obviously intact hypothalamic pituitary–ovarian axis) were also found to lose trabecular bone [25], another study has shown that women with anorexia nervosa (all of whom were amenorrhoeic and obviously hypo-oestrogenic) but who were physically active, had significantly greater bone mass than a similar group of inactive anorectics [26]. Therefore, measuring oestrogen status per se is not a good discriminator of women's responses to exercise.

According to some researchers, physical fitness as measured by maximal oxygen uptake (VO_{2max}) correlates positively with bone mass. Pocock et al. [14] found this relationship for women of all ages (20–75 years; mean age 45 years). Others [27] have shown this to be true only for younger (25–35 years) and not postmenopausal women (55–65 years). Bevier et al. [15] reported that maximal aerobic capacity did not correlate at all with bone density, but their subjects were somewhat older (61–84 years; mean age 70 years).

In the author's experience, testing for aerobic power only shows significant change in response to aerobic exercise, and is therefore of little value in assessing women if, for example, their primary exercise involves muscle-strengthening activities. Therefore it is advocated that in women bone density should be tested regularly using both single and dual photon absorptiometry (or dual energy radiography) both as a prerequisite to the initial exercise prescription and to assess their progress. The latter is most important as a means of ensuring compliance. Densitometry will detect osteopenia in women who are over-exercising prior to their sustaining an injury or developing oligo- or amenorrhoea.

An alternative method of measuring improvement in exercise-induced bone strength is based on an "engineering" rather than a biological principle: measurements of an increase in bone width. Radial expansion of long bones is an important determinant of bone strength. The so-called cross-sectional moment of inertia (CSMI) is what determines a bone's resistance to bending. Increase in the external diameter of the bone brought about by increased formation of periosteal (outer layer) bone can compensate for the inevitable loss in the quality of the bone tissue that occurs with age. A recent study investigated the effects of six months of walking or aerobic dancing on the bone mineral content of 73 early postmenopausal women. The exercising women had a significant increase in the CSMI when compared with the control group. By contrast the bone mineral content of the walking group and the control group decreased over the duration of the study [28]. Unfortunately, there are no practical or standardised tests currently available to measure CSMI, and it is not known whether improvement in the long-bone CSMI will reflect an increase in bone modulus in the vertebrae and femoral neck.

Developing an Exercise Prescription

Combined Treatment: Exercise and Calcium

Exercise is directly associated with the laying down of matrix on the remodelling surface of the trabeculae and cortices of bone. The need for exogenous calcium to meet these increased demands may be a critical factor in maximising exercise-induced osteogenesis.

Chvapil et al. [29] showed that the amount and concentration of collagen in the femurs of adult rats increased with exercise, but that exercise had no effect on the calcium content of the bones. This result may explain why the amenorrhoeic women studied by Drinkwater et al. [21] had lower levels of trabecular but not cortical bone mineral when compared with their eumenorrhoeic controls. Although both groups consumed the currently recommended dietary allowance of 800 mg of elemental calcium per day, the amenorrhoeic women actually required 1500 mg a day to meet the needs of women in low oestrogen states (see later). The need for extra calcium in exercising women has been endorsed by others [30] and is supported by the results of a recent cross-sectional study [31] which showed improved bone mineral accretion in women with a higher intake of calcium and equal energy expenditure. The authors concluded that if their cross-sectional data are confirmed by longitutinal studies, the bone mass accrual from exercise and diet alone could delay the average age of osteoporotic fractures by ten years.

Exercise and Oestrogen

Oestrogen replacement therapy slows the rate of bone loss in postmenopausal women, but does not increase bone mass. The efficacy of long-term use, although associated with a reduced incidence of vertebral and hip fracture, may be compromised by the inhibitory effect of oestrogen on osteoclasts, thereby interfering with the primary initiator of the bone remodelling cycle. Since exercise stimulates osteogenesis, a recent examination has been carried out on the effect of oestrogen replacement therapy plus variable resistance weight training on the bone mineral status of surgically menopausal women (Notelovitz M, Martin D, Tesar R, McKenzie L, unpublished data). Twenty matched surgically menopausal women treated with 0.625 mg of conjugated equine oestrogen daily were studied with nine participating in a closely monitored exercise programme that involved the use of Nautilus muscle-strengthening equipment. After one year, the exercising subgroup increased the bone mineral content of the dorsal and lumbar vertebrae (as measured by total body dual photon absorptiometry) by 8.6% and 8.4% respectively ($P < 0.03$ and $P < 0.04$); the group that received hormonal therapy alone, maintained their axial bone mass. A significant increase of 3.8% ($P < 0.003$) in the appendicular bone mineral content of the radial midshaft of the exercising group was found by single photon absorptiometry. The oestrogen alone treated group had a non-significant decrease in the midshaft bone mineral content. If the results of this ramdomised longitudinal study are confirmed, it will endorse the proposed therapeutic triangle [32]: exercise to stimulate new bone formation; calcium to mineralise the newly formed osteoid and oestrogen to modulate the physiological rate of postmenopausal bone loss. This postulate is indirectly supported by a study of aerobic power in bone mass in pre- and postmenopausal women [27]. Physical fitness in young menstruating women (mean age 31 years) results in an improvement in the vertebral bone density (183 ± 7 mg cm^{-3}) when compared to sedentary controls (163 ± 8 mg cm^{-3}) whereas no difference was found in physically active postmenopausal women (mean age 59 years) and their sedentary controls: 112 ± 5 mg cm^{-3} and 111 ± 5 mg cm^{-3}. This result is consistent with the finding that exercise does not alter bone loss in oophorectomised rats [33] and correlates with exercise-induced amenorrhoea and osteopenia in female athletes [21–24].

Exercise Prescription

Two sets of animal exercise experiments provide guidance regarding an optimal approach to exercise prescription in women. Woo et al. [34] showed that aerobic exercise at an intensity of 65%–80% of maximum heart rate in exercising pigs is osteogenic and ensures an aerobic effect. Lanyan and Rubin [16], in a series of experiments, came to the following conclusions. Increase in bone mass is induced by intermittent strain at or below physiological peak strain. Therefore, one does not need extreme physical activity to produce an osteogenic effect; the remodelling process responds best to changes in the distribution of strain. This suggests that exercises should be diverse and involve different loading situations; strain imposed at fast rates are more effective in inducing new bone formation; and the maximum osteogenic effect requires relatively few repetitions.

Our programme starts with muscle-strengthening exercises concentrating on the large muscle groups: quadriceps, hamstrings, abdominal and back muscles. Patients have to be closely supervised and care taken to establish the individual's repetition maximum. (The maximum weight that can be lifted with one movement = 1 RM). The programme should then be developed to allow for a gradual build-up of muscle strength and endurance [35,36]. The author favours variable resistance exercise machines (versus free weights) and programmes that allow for two sessions (separated by one-minute periods) of 8 to 10 repetition maxima for each of the muscle groups. Three sessions per week are initially devoted to muscle-strengthening exercise and the sessions dropped to two once aerobic fitness has been achieved.

Any aerobic exercise programme – walking on a treadmill, riding a bicycle ergometer, jogging, etc. – must be prescribed after assessment of the individual's cardiovascular fitness. Performance of a graded exercise stress test, together with a study of maximal oxygen uptake allows for the establishment of four parameters necessary for exercise prescription [37]: a definitive measure of the person's physical fitness (VO_{2max}); functioning of the heart at maximal physical stress (EKG); maximum heart rate which allows for an objective level of exercise intensity prescription; and the total exercise time. This procedure provides an indirect method of establishing the muscle strength of the quadriceps and hamstrings – muscles that are essential for effective aerobic exercise. Depending on the patient's initial level of physical fitness, her programme is gradually titrated upwards until she can maintain her heart rate at 70%–80% of her maximal rate for 30 min. She needs to exercise three to four times a week. The aerobic component of the exercise programme should alternate walking on a treadmill, with a Stairmaster, riding a bicycle and using a Nordick rack apparatus. This type of programme meets the following criteria: (a) the exercise is weight-bearing; (b) the activity is diverse, vigorous and not overly repetitive; (c) the programme improves cardiovascular fitness; (d) by its diversity, boredom is reduced to a minimum – an essential ingredient to ensure long-term compliance.

Established Osteoporosis

Inadequate attention is given to the prescription of exercise of women with established osteoporosis, most of whom will present to the physician during their late climacteric. A key issue is to discourage activities that involve flexion of the back. Long-term follow-up of patients with radiologically confirmed osteoporosis revealed recurrent fractures in 16% of women practising back extension exercises, 89% in a flexion programme, 53% in a combined extension and flexion regimen, and 67% in a non-exercising control group [38]. Posture is also important. Avoidance of activities that encourage flexion during sedentary activities, such as sewing, can prevent further stress to already weakened vertebrae [39]. Instruction should also be given to avoid back straining by twisting, lifting and making sudden forceful movements. To remove the strain from the lower back when lifting or reaching lower objects, the large muscles of the legs (i.e. the hamstrings and quadriceps) should be used, by bending the knees and keeping the back vertical during these activities.

Walking is the safest form of exercise for women with osteoporosis. Also safe and effective are group activities such as square dancing, ballroom dancing, and folk dancing, as well as other activities such as riding a three-wheel bike or an exercycle. Swimming is an excellent exercise that allows patients to regain their confidence in being physically active, and at the same time allows them to increase the mobility of their joints. Osteoporotic, or markedly osteopenic, women should be advised to avoid activities such as aerobic (jazz) dance classes that jar the spine and emphasise flexibility. In evaluating these women, care should be taken to test for balance and for orthostatic hypotension and to advise them about practical measures such as the type of shoes they should wear.

Will Exercise Prevent Fractures?

Two articles [30,40] reviewed the published literature on exercise and bone mass and concluded that although numerous studies on the subject have been published, we still do not know the amount or type of exercise that will not only stimulate osteogenesis, but achieve the obvious goal: enhance bone strength and reduce fracture risk. Most of the studies, with one notable exception [41], did not randomise the subjects. Many were cross-sectional evaulations, and no studies extended beyond one year to 18 months. As shown by Dalsky et al. [10], the beneficial effect of exercise on osteogenesis is rapidly lost as the intensity and frequency of exercise diminishes and a sedentary lifestyle is resumed. Other criticisms that were raised include the following. Comparisons were frequently made between highly trained athletes and non-exercising controls, and when recreational athletes were compared with controls, the differences, if present at all, were much less obvious. The site of measurement – the more labile trabecular compartment versus the more stable cortical bone – and the method of bone density testing – radiogrammetry, single and dual photon absorptiometry and computer tomography – added to the numerous variables that have to be controlled for and considered before a consensus can be reached.

One of the major problems involving exercise studies is the difficulty of controlling for everyday influences on the programme, e.g. dietary habits, drug use, and everyday physical activities other than those designated by the programme. Compliance and cost of exercise studies are additional concerns. Short-term studies have a drop-out rate of 25% or more, depending on the demands of the programme. Fortunately, if patients can be kept in an exercise programme beyond three to four months, the drop-out rate decreases considerably. Despite the above, empirical evidence – primarily from personal clinical research and practice – has convinced this author that exercise does indeed serve as a cornerstone to the prevention and treatment of osteoporosis and should be widely prescribed.

Nutrition and Bone Health

In fully mature bone the protein matrix, consisting in the main of collagen embedded in a mucopolysaccharide ground substance, accounts for 35% of the volume of the intercellular material, with mineral occupying most of the remainder. The hydroxyapatite crystals in mineralised bone contain significant amounts of sodium, magnesium, carbonate, and citrate ions, but calcium and phosphorus are the principal minerals. Factors that regulate their supply, absorption, deposition, and withdrawal from bone, underly the importance of nutrition and its role in maintaining bone health.

Absorption and Needs

The amount of calcium in blood, in extracellular fluid, and in the extraosseous cellular compartments accounts for 1% of the total body calcium. The calcium in bone is available to the circulation through an established but ill-understood mechanism involving a pool of readily exchangeable soluble bone calcium. This pool serves as an immediate reservoir for plasma calcium to ensure that a steady state is maintained and to meet the need for calcium in processes as diverse as coagulation of the blood, nerve transmission, cardiac function and muscle contraction.

Skeletal growth during childhood requires the retention of 150 mg of calcium per day; adolescence and early adulthood, when bone growth is maximal, results in 275–500 mg of calcium per day being deposited in bone. During later adult life, when bone growth is replaced by bone maintenance, less calcium is required, but still averages 180 g per year. Translated into recommended daily allowances (RDA) of calcium, infants (less than 1 year) require 540 mg/day; children between 1 and 10 years of age, 800 mg/day; adolescents (11–18 years), 1200 mg/day; and adults (over 18 years), 800 mg/day. More recently, several investigators have shown that whereas these values will allow for certain physiological needs, they are well below the amount of calcium needed to maintain positive bone balance. Heany et al. [42] found that to be in calcium balance, premenopausal women needed 1000 mg/day; women in the perimenopause, 1200 mg/day, and postmenopausal women, 1400 mg/day. This greater requirement for postmenopausal women is due to a combination of less efficient calcium absorption from the gut and poorer calcium reabsorption by the kidneys. Treatment of postmenopausal women with oestrogen results in a better absorptive/reabsorption mechanism, with a resultant decrease in the daily requirement to 1200 mg/day. Based on the present RDA for calcium, the premenopausal requirements for this essential mineral are 25% higher than the RDA, and 75% higher for postmenopausal women. The deficiency of calcium in real terms among the majority of Caucasian postmenopausal women is actually greater. The average intake of calcium by women between the ages of 40 and 65 varies between 450 and 650 mg/day. Thus, the average daily calcium intake should be increased by 100%!

Calcium is absorbed primarily in the small intestine in a gradient that is maximal in the duodenum and proximal jejunum. Absorption of calcium is completed within 4 hours of its intake and is due to a combination of three processes: (1) passive diffusion, (2) binding by transfer to a protein carrier, and (3) active transport. With a low calcium intake, the absorption of calcium is said to become more efficient [43]. The mean absorptive fraction declines from 0.45% at low calcium intakes (200 mg of calcium per day) to approximately 0.15 at intakes above 2000 mg/day. This process is referred to as adaptation and is exhibited to a greater extent in younger than in older persons. Whereas 75% of ingested calcium may be absorbed by children during periods of rapid skeletal growth and remodelling, the value decreases to 30%–50% in adults [44]. Intestinal calcium absorption decreases even more in elderly women (over the age of 70 years), and especially in women with osteoporosis [44].

Despite contrary opinions, calcium is absorbed as efficiently from calcium supplements as it is from food sources known to be rich in calcium, such as dairy products. In carefully performed calcium balance studies, Sheikh et al. [45] were able to establish that it was the amount of available calcium and not the source (milk versus calcium gluconate) that determined whether an individual would achieve calcium balance. The most important point is that the calcium requirement is needed consistently on a daily basis; as with exercise, individuals need to be given the option of meeting this essential daily need by whatever means is convenient, acceptable, and affordable. In a study at The Center for Climacteric Studies (involving 92 women in the 2-year exercise programme to prevent osteoporosis), it was found that initially only 41% of the women met the RDA of calcium and 12%, the desired 1400 mg of calcium required per day. With successive interviews, significant increases in calcium intake were observed. By the fifth interview, at 12 months, 93% of women met the RDA and 82%, the 1400 mg requirement. The desired calcium intake of 1400 mg was met from food sources in 8% of women. Reasons given for not increasing calcium-rich foods include concern for weight gain, lactose intolerance, dislike of certain dairy products, and constipation.

Much is written about the preferred or best type of calcium supplement; basic to the issue, however, is compliance. The fewer tablets (and the least expensive), the more likely it will be that an individual will take the supplement. In this context, three essential points need emphasis:

1. It is only elemental calcium that is available for absorption; calcium carbonate contains 40% of calcium in this form, tribasic calcium phosphate 39%, calcium citrate 24%, calcium lactate 13%, and calcium gluconate 9%. In clinical terms, the availability of calcium from these sources does not differ significantly, but others have suggested that calcium citrate is more bioavailable than calcium

carbonate [46]. The fewer calcium tablets needed to deliver a given amount of calcium, the better the compliance.

2. With the publicity given to the importance of calcium supplementation and osteoporosis prevention, numerous generic products have appeared on the market. Many are not even bioavailable! The disintegration and dissolution times of calcium supplements are critical to calcium absorption and can be tested by placing the tablet in white vinegar. The tablet should dissolve within 30 minutes [47].

3. The timing of calcium supplementation can theoretically maximise its absorption. The division of calcium intake into multiple feedings is less likely to saturate the intestinal absorptive metabolism [44]; calcium also has a diurnal metabolism – it is stored in bone during the day and released during the night [48], when it is needed to provide for the systemic needs of the individual at a time when there is no dietary source. The required amount is taken from the skeleton's soluble calcium pool, by supplementing at night, the drainage from this source of stored calcium may be inhibited or substantially reduced. A further consideration is impaired stomach acid production and its effect on calcium absorption, especially in postmenopausal and elderly women. Recker [49] showed that the fractional absorption of calcium citrate and carbonate were similar in normal subjects, but that significantly less calcium carbonate was absorbed in achlorhydric women. This could be corrected by taking calcium carbonate with a meal.

The author's clinical approach to calcium supplementation is as follows: supplements less than 500 mg/day are taken at night; if greater amounts are needed, a twice daily regimen is prescribed. In older patients, calcium citrate is prescribed, or if calcium carbonate is preferred, it must be taken with a meal.

Factors Affecting Calcium Metabolism

Bone Robbers

The bioavailability of calcium may be influenced by a number of other nutrients and foods. Dietary fibre binds calcium and prevents its absorption. The addition of cellulose [50] and fruits and vegetables [51] high in fibre creates a negative calcium balance by decreasing absorption of dietary calcium. It is probably the uronic acid residues in hemicellulose that account for the complexing of calcium by dietary fibre. Phytic acid, found in bran and the seed coat of beans and grains, can also reduce calcium absorption; the same is true for oxalic acid, found in vegetables such as spinach. Since dietary oxalate in plant food is already precomplexed with calcium, it will have less of an inhibiting effect on the absorption of other dietary calcium than fibre and phytates. Recent research in rats and in humans has suggested that the colon might play an important role in the conservation of dietary calcium. Since the dietary inhibitors of calcium absorption – phytates, oxalate, and fibre – are metabolised by colonic bacteria, it is possible that the calcium found in the small intestine might be released in the colon and made available for absorption. This has been found to be true for individuals who have required small bowel resections.

Lactase Deficiency

Lactase deficiency may lead to calcium deprivation because of the long-term avoidance of dairy products, such as milk. In one of the best-controlled studies, Newcomer et al. [52] found that 27% of women with postmenopausal osteoporosis were lactase deficient, versus 3% of normal women. Although none of the lactase-deficient women were overtly aware of milk intolerance, the intake of both lactose (6.5 g/day, versus 17.0 g/day in controls) and calcium (530 mg/day versus 810 mg/day in controls) was significantly lower. Lactase-deficient individuals not only have a decreased calcium intake, but the associated low lactose intake decreases the absorption of calcium from the gut. Lactase deficiency, per se, inhibits calcium absorption; conversely, the administration of lactose enhances calcium absorption in normal and even in lactase-deficient subjects. A convenient and palatable way of overcoming the problem of lactase deficiency is to advise affected individuals to eat yogurt. Yogurt is manufactured by incubating specialised bacterial organisms with concentrated milk solids. During the process of fermentation, the bacteria produce the lactase enzyme; this allows lactose to be absorbed and with it, calcium. A group of volunteers with a history of lactase deficiency was shown to absorb 50% of the lactose in milk, versus 85% of the lactose in yogurt [53]. This improved absorption was also associated with a decrease in abdominal pain and diarrhoea.

Dietary Protein and Calcium Balance

Excess amounts of protein have been shown to increase the urinary excretion of calcium. Human volunteers given as much as 1600 mg of calcium per day experienced a negative calcium balance of 140 mg/day on a dietary protein intake of 225 g. This negative balance persisted for 48 days without a compensatory increase in the intestinal absorption of calcium or a reduction in the urinary excretion of calcium. If maintained for one year, this could lead to a loss of 4% of the total skeletal calcium.

The RDA of protein for adult men is 56 g/day, but the average man consumes more than 100 g, whereas athletes in training often have intakes in excess of 500 g. In premenopausal women there is a significant inverse relationship between nitrogen intake and calcium balance. A 50% increase in protein is associated with a net calcium loss of 32 mg/day [54]. Administration of protein to normal subjects increases the urinary calcium excretion and may result in a negative calcium balance [42]; the mechanism for this calcium loss may be the sulphur amino acid content of the proteins, which causes a decrease in the renal tubular reabsorption of calcium. This effect is not induced by meats, presumably because of high phosphorus content. Phosphorus decreases urinary calcium excretion. Despite this latter observation, it is pertinent to note that lactoovovegetarians have a slow cortical bone loss, whereas omnivores, such as Eskimos, are rapid cortical bone losers.

Sodium

An excess of dietary sodium in rats is associated with increased secretion of parathyroid hormone (PTH) and loss of bone; a similar feature is noted in humans given more than 2000 mg of sodium (1 teaspoonful) per day [55]. In addition, there is a rise in the fasting urinary excretion of sodium as well as calcium after the menopause. It is not known whether any of these effects are significant or sufficiently long lasting to have a real effect on the development of oesteopenia. It is conceivable that an excess of dietary sodium could play a secondary role in augmenting bone loss.

Vitamin D

Elderly patients and women with osteoporosis absorb calcium less efficiently. This is thought to be due to a deficiency of the activated form of vitamin D, $1,25(OH)_2D_3$ – calcitrol [56], and illustrates the well-known fact that vitamin D is a major factor for the absorption of calcium and for the maintenance of calcium balance.

Because vitamin D is synthesised in the skin in response to solar irradiation, its significance as a nutrient is frequently underestimated. A reduced dietary intake, especially if associated with intestinal malabsorption of fats, could result in the depletion of vitamin D stores in elderly persons not exposed to sunlight. To ensure an adequate intake of vitamin D in elderly women, the author prescribes one multivitamin tablet per day; this provides 400 IU.

Subclinical vitamin D depletion may predispose the elderly to hip fractures as a result of accelerated cortical bone loss associated with secondary hyper-parathyroidism. Despite this, excess amounts of vitamin D may be even more harmful and lead to an increase in urinary calcium excretion and a further loss of cortical bone [57]. An interesting recent hypothesis by McCarthy et al. [58] suggests that 1,25-dihydroxyvitamin D inhibits the proliferation of mega-karyocytes which normally promote collagen synthesis. It is currently recom-mended that dietary and/or supplemental vitamin D should not exceed 1000 IU per day. The role of vitamin D in health and disease has recently been reviewed [59].

Clinical Experience

Until recently, there were no long-term longitudinal studies that showed a decrease in the incidence of osteoporosis-related fractures due to nutritional intervention. Holbrook et al. [60] recently reported that the age-adjusted risk of hip fracture was inversely associated with dietary calcium whether considered as mg/day or as nutrient density, mg per 1000 kcal. In a 14-year prospective follow-up, subjects who had a calcium intake over 765 mg/day had a 60% lower risk of hip fracture when compared with lower intakes. This is very similar to a 50% reduction of hip fractures in a Yugoslavian study comparing high with lower calcium intake villages [61].

The protective effect of calcium is probably determined by the age at which adequate calcium intake occurs and the lifetime exposure to this intake through the pre-, peri- and postmenopausal years. It is further influenced by an oestrogen-replete state, whether the oestrogen is from an endogenous or exogenous source [62,63]. It therefore appears that cross-sectional studies exploring the relationship between calcium use and bone mass will lead to false conclusions if the information is based on the current intake of calcium. It would appear that the dietary threshold between calcium intake and bone protection is about 800 mg/day [60].

Despite comments to the contrary [64], clinical trials of calcium supplementation have shown reduced rates of bone loss. This subject has been reviewed recently [6,65].

The only potential side effect of calcium therapy is renal stones. They rarely develop in women and when they do occur, are found in individuals who lack the enzymes necessary to keep the calcium and urine in solution, and not because of an excessive intake of calcium. Harvey et al. [66] have shown that calcium citrate inhibits calcium oxalate crystallisation and should therefore be the preparation of choice in women at risk of kidney stone formation. In any event, the 24 hour urinary excretion of calcium should be monitored and kept below 300 mg/day; with a high fluid intake, the calcium concentration in urine can be kept at a level incompatible with renal stone formation.

Body Composition

Obesity protects against osteoporosis. A number of composition studies have confirmed this relationship [5,14,15]. Pocock et al. [14] demonstrated that the body mass index (weight/height^2) was a major predictor of bone mass in the lumbar spine, femur and distal forearm. The body mass index is generally thought to be an indication of body fat rather than muscle mass. There is some disagreement on this, however. Bevier et al. [15] have shown that women with increased body fat also have increased lean body mass, and when the latter is controlled for by multiple regression analysis, fat mass did not remain as an independent predictor of spine density.

The predictive effect of obesity, whether it be due to body fat alone or combined with muscle mass, is thought to be due to increased mechanical stress of the excessive weight and the increased synthesis of oestrogen via the conversion of androstenedione into oestrogen in adipocytes [67]. The latter mechanism could explain why regions not normally exposed to weight induced stress such as the distal radius are also positively correlated with increased body mass. The mechanical stress theories are endorsed by loss of the protective effect of obesity following gastric bypass procedure. Krolner et al. [68] found bone loss of bone mineral in the lumbar spine to be closely correlated to the degree of weight loss and hence mechanical stress, since calcium and vitamin D absorption remain normal in these subjects. The loss of bone mass following other surgical procedures, e.g. jejuno-iliostomy, is due to impaired vitamin D metabolism [69].

A neglected area of concern in relation to the prevention of osteoporosis is the damage of behavioural and eating disorders, such as anorexia nervosa [26] and bulimia [70], in adolescents and young adults. As with anorexia nervosa, patients with bulimia often view themselves as being overweight and are preoccupied with their body size and fatness, although studies often show this not to be the case [70]. Menstrual dysfunction occurs in 40% of bulimics, and when present is more likely to result in osteopenia.

The author assesses patients' body composition by using the body mass index as a screen for more precise objective measurements including anthropometrics (skinfold thickness and girth measurements) and more recently, total body dual energy radiography. Showing a distraught adolescent that she does not indeed have increased body fat goes a long way to helping her resolve her psychological and subsequent nutritional problem.

A final caveat. Untreated menopause, especially if naturally premature or surgically induced, frequently overrides the protective effect of obesity with resulting osteopenia. It is our practice to evaluate these patients with bone density testing. Most have subsequently required hormone additive therapy.

Social Habits

Lifestyle and social habits can impact negatively on bone mass accrual and loss. Two common habits – smoking and alcohol use – will be briefly reviewed

Smoking

Cigarette smoking is frequently cited as a risk factor for osteoporosis [71,72]. Smokers are thinner than non-smokers [73], by 5–10 pounds (2.25–4.5 kg) when compared in cross-sectional studies to age and height-matched cohorts, and also have alterations in oestrogen metabolism [74] which results in an earlier menopause and, for those on hormonal therapy, reduced efficacy [72]. A recent study [75], however, concluded that the association of smoking with the reduction in bone mass was independent of age, adiposity and androgen/oestrogen metabolism. Perkins et al. [76] studied the metabolic effects of nicotine and showed that nicotine doubled the energy expenditure of exercise and could explain weight loss by this mechanism as well as the tendency to gain weight when smoking is stopped. The latter is often a deterrent to patients who wish to give up the habit.

One of the more far-reaching consequences of smoking is the observation that this habit may result in reduced peak bone mass [75]. Coupled with an earlier menopause and hence a longer exposure to postmenopausal bone loss and reduced body weight, the stage is set for the early development of osteoporosis. Heavy smoking is a relative contraindication to hormone additive therapy and is confounded by the highly addictive effect of nicotine and the difficulty of quitting. Unfortunately, the statistics in the United States are not encouraging [77]. Over a 20-year period the percentage of women who smoked more than 25 cigarettes a day has increased from 13% (1965) to 23% (1985). Women are also starting to smoke from an earlier age. Of women smokers, currently aged 27 to 28 years 84% started to smoke before the age of 20, compared with 42% now aged 58–67 years. The prevalence of lifetime smoking has also decreased more slowly in women than in men. The relationship between smoking and lung cancer is well known and is well publicised. More needs to be said about the association between smoking and osteoporosis.

Alcohol

Women drink less than men and are more likely to abstain from alcohol, but the number of women who use alcohol and who have alcohol problems has increased considerably since World War II [78]. A US survey of the drinking practices of adult women found the highest rates of alcohol-dependent symptoms were in women aged 21–34 years, and the highest proportion of heavy drinkers in the 35–49-year-old age bracket – ages that are especially vulnerable to the bone remodelling cycle and bone mass accrual.

Women metabolise alchol differently and achieve higher peak alcohol levels than men from equal doses of alcohol per pound of body weight. Although this is partly explained by a higher percentage of body water in men (55%–65%) than in women (45%–55%), a recent study has illustrated another mechanism. Frezza et al. [79] determined that women have decreased gastric alcohol dehydrogenase activity and that this accounts for higher blood levels of alcohol and susceptibility to alcoholism.

Bone loss resulting from alcohol excess may be due to a combination of factors [80]. Poor nutrition, including inadequate intake of calcium and vitamin D, gastrointestinal and pancreatic malfunction, a deficiency of activated vitamin D as a result of liver impairment and a defect in the hydroxylation of the provitamin to its partially activated form. Alcohol inhibits the absorption of calcium from the gut and has been shown to be associated with defective osteoblast activity [81]. This manifests in reduced bone mass. For example, the weight of bones in young alcoholic patients (extrapolated from bone biopsies) is similar to that of postmenopausal patients. This could theoretically result in a markedly reduced peak bone mass. This observation is more obvious in older alcoholics. Spencer et al. [82] demonstrated marked osteopenia in ambulatory relatively young men (31–45 years) and speculated on an aggravation on the condition by associated smoking and the use of aluminium-containig antacids [83]. Even relatively small doses of the latter can lead to a significant calcium loss.

The dose of alcohol that inhibits the bone remodelling cycle – if this is the primary mechanism, as it appears to be in animals – has not yet been established. Given the ready absorbability of alcohol in women, it is fair to conclude that women will be more susceptible than men and need to moderate their intake of alcohol. For the elderly, even greater care is needed since alcohol-induced imbalance could precipitate falls and hip fractures, a major cause of morbidity and death.

Conclusion

If appropriate bone mass will indeed prevent atraumatic fractures (as currently believed), the prevention of osteoporosis becomes a readily obtainable goal. Three prerequisites will have to be met: (a) information about osteoporosis and the recognisable factors responsible for its development needs to be disseminated amongst young adult women; (b) physicians must also be educated about the lifestyle factors that can lead to bone mass accrual and how to prescribe accordingly; (c) patient compliance. This is probably the most difficult objective to meet, primarily because of the asymptomatic nature of developing osteoporosis and the remoteness (to the young adult) of hip fractures and its consequences. In this context, we recently evaluated the value of bone density testing and compliance in a random selected population. These patients were from four medical practices and were contacted by letter. Respondents were sent an educational packet about osteoporosis and were invited six months later to a free seminar. To evaluate the impact of personal contact, subjects were invited to have a free densitometry examination. This was performed using single photon absorptiometry of the radius. Of the original 771 subjects who participated, 378 were screened; a further 132 continued to the final assessment, but declined densitometry testing. Of the women who were screened and found to have a low bone mass 86.4% altered their lifestyle, compared with 68.7% of individuals with normal bone mass and 53.8% of the unscreened population. The most obvious change in all groups was in exercise and diet. In short, demonstrating existing osteopenia had a significant positive effect in making patients aware of the value of altering their lifestyle and maintaining this new pattern of living. By screening for osteopenia and adopting the principles of the previously described therapeutic triangle [32] – physical activity to stimulate new bone formation; good nutrition to mineralise the immature osteoid, and selective hormone use – "the current epidemic of osteoporosis can be stopped, reversed, and with time relegated to history as a medical curiosity" [32].

Acknowledgements. This chapter has been adapted in part from: Notelovitz M. Osteoporosis: screening and exercise. Progr Clin Biol Res 1989; 320:225; and Notelovitz M. Interrelations of exercise and diet on bone metabolism and osteogensis. In: Wynick M, ed. Nutrition and exercise. New York, Wiley, 1986; 203–27.

References

1. Riggs BL, Melton LJ. Involutional osteoporosis. N Engl J Med 1986; 314:1676–84.
2. Carter DR. Mechanical loading histories and cortical bone remodelling. Calcif Tissue Int 1984; 36:519–54.
3. Parfitt AM. Bone remodelling and bone loss: understanding the pathophysiology of osteoporosis. Clin Obstet Gynecol 1987; 30:789–811.
4. Pocock NA, Eisman JA, Hopper JL, Yeates MG, Sambrook PN, Eberl S. Genetic determinants of bone mass in adults: a twin study. J Clin Invest 1987; 80:706–10.
5. DeSimone DP, Stevens, J, Edwards, J, Shary J, Gordon L, Bell NH. Influence of body habitus and race on bone mineral density of the midradius, hip and spine in aging woman. J Bone Miner Res 1989; 4:827–30.
6. Heaney RP. The role of nutrition in prevention and management of osteoporosis. Clin Obstet Gynecol 1987; 50:833–46.
7. Bell NH, Gosden RN, Henry DP, Shary L, Epstein S. The effects of muscle-building exercise on vitamin D and mineral metabolism. J Bone Miner Res 1988; 3:369–73.
8. Basset CA, Baker RD. Generation of electrical potentials by bone in response to mechanical stress. Science 1962; 137:1063–4.
9. Jacobsen PC, Beaver W, Grubb SA, Taft TN, Talmage RV. Bone denisty in women: college athletes and older athletic women. J Orthop Res 1984; 2:328–32.
10. Dalsky GP, Stocke KS, Ehsani AA, Slatopolsky E, Lee WC, Birge SJ. Weight-bearing exercise training and lumbar bone mineral content in post-menopausal women. Ann Intern Med 1988; 108:824–8.
11. Nilsson BE, Westlin NE. Bone density in athletes. Clin Orthop 1971; 77:179–82.
12. Doyle F, Brown J, Lachance C. Relation between bone mass and muscle weight. Lancet 1970; i:391–3.

13. Sinaki M, McPhee MC, Hodgson SF, Merritt JM, Offord KP. Relationship between bone mineral density of the spine and strength of back extensors in healthy postmenopausal women. Mayo Clin Proc 1986; 61:116–22.

14. Pocock N, Eisman J, Gwinn T et al. Muscle strength, physical fitness, and weight but not age predict femoral neck bone mass. J Bone Miner Res 1989; 4:441–8.

15. Bevier WC, Wiswell RA, Pyka G, Kozuk KC, Newhall KM, Marcus R. Relationship of body composition, muscle strength, and aerobic capacity to bone mineral density in older men and women. J Bone Miner Res 1989; 4:421–32.

16. Lanyan LE, Rubin CT. Regulation of bone mass in response to physical activity. In: Dixon AAJ, Russel RGG, Stamp TCP, eds. Osteoporosis, a multidisciplinary problem. London: Royal Society of Medicine London/Academic Press. 1983; 51–61.

17. Krolner B, Toft B, Nielson SP, Trondeveld E. Physical exercise as prophylaxis against involutional vertebral bone loss: a controlled trial. Clin Sci 1983; 64:541–6.

18. Smith E, Reddan W, Smith PE. Physical activity and calcium modalities for bone mineral increase in aged women. Med Sci Sports Exerc 1981; 13:60–4.

19. Buchanan JP, Myers C, Lloyd T, Greer RB. Early vertebral trabecular bone loss in normal premenopausal women. J Bone Miner Res 1988; 3:585–7.

20. Gilsanz V, Gibbens DT, Roe TF et al. Vertebral bone density in children: effect of puberty radiology. 1988; 166:847–50.

21. Drinkwater BL, Nilson K. Chesnut III C, Brenmer WJJ, Shainholz S, Southwood MB. Bone mineral content of amenorrhoeic and eumenorrhoeic athletes. N Engl J Med 1984; 311:277–81.

22. Linnell J, Stager JM, Blue PW, Dyster N, Robertshaw D. Bone mineral content and menstrual regularity in female runners. Med Sci Sports Exerc 1984; 16:373–48.

23. Drinkwater BL, Nilson K, Ott S, Chesnut III C. Bone mineral density after resumption of menses in amenorrhoeic athletes. JAMA 1986; 256:380–1.

24. Lindberg JS, Powell MR, Hunt MM, Ducey DE, Wade CE. Increased vertebral bone mineral in response to reduced exercise in amenorrhoeic runners. West J Med 1987; 146:39–42.

25. Brewer V, Meyer BM, Keele MJ, Upton SJ, Hagan RD. Role of exercise in prevention of involutional bone loss. Med Sci Sports Exerc 1983; 15:445–9.

26. Rigotti NA, Nussbaum SR, Herzog DR, Neer RM. Osteoporosis in women with anorexia nervosa. N Engl J Med 1984; 311:1601–6.

27. Kirk S, Sharp CF, Elbaum N et al. Effect of long-distance running on bone mass in women. J Bone Miner Res 1989; 41:515–22.

28. Yeater RA, Martin RB. Senile osteoporosis: the effect of exercise. Postgrad Med 1984; 75:147–63.

29. Chvapil M, Bartos D, Bartos F. Effect of long-term physical stress on collagen growth in the lung, heart and femur of young and adult rats. Gerontologia 1973; 19:263–8.

30. Dalsky GP. Exercise: its effect on bone mineral content. Clin Obstet Gynecol 1987; 30:820–32.

31. Kanders B, Dempster DW, Lindsay R, Interaction of calcium nutrition and physical activity on bone mass in young women. J Bone Miner Res 1988; 3:145–9.

32. Notelovitz M. Postmenopausal osteoporosis: a practical approach to its prevention. Acta Obstet Gynecol Scand [Suppl] 1986; 134:67–80.

33. Pohlman RL, Darby LA, Lechner AJ. Morphometry and calcium content in appendicular and axial bone of exercise ovariectomized rats. Am J Physiol 1985; 248:R12–R17.

34. Woo SLY, Kuei SC, Amiel D et al. The effects of prolonged physical training on the property of long bone. J Bone Joint Surg 1980; G3A:780–7.

35. Clarke DH. Training for strength. In: Shangold M, Mirken G, eds. Women and exercise, physiology and sports medicine. Philadelphia: FA Davis, 1988; 55–64.

36. Fahey TD. Endurance training. In: Shangold M, Mirken G, eds. Women and exercise, physiology and sports medicine. Philadelphia: FA Davis, 1988; 65–78.

37. Notelovitz M, Fields C, Caramelli K, Dougherty M, Schwartz AL. Cardiorespiratory fitness evaluation in climacteric women: comparison of two methods. Am J Obstet Gynecol 1986; 154:1009–13.

38. Sinaki M, Mikkelsen BA. Postmenopausal spinal osteoporosis: flexion versus extension exercises. Arch Phys Med Rehabil 1984; 65:593–7.

39. Goodman CE. Osteoporosis: protective measures of nutrition and exercise. Geriatrics 1985; 40:59–63.

40. Block JE, Smith R, Black D, Genant HK. Does exercise prevent osteoporosis. JAMA 1987; 257:3115–17.

41. Chow R, Harrison JE, Notarius C. Effect of two randomised exercise programmes on bone mass of healthy postmenopausal women. Br Med J 1987; 295:1441–4.

42. Heany RP, Gallagher JC, Johnstone CC et al. Calcium nutrition and bone health in the elderly. Am J Clin Nutr 1983; 36 (Suppl):986–1013.
43. Heany RP, Ricker RP, Stegman MR, Moy AJ. Calcium absorption in women: relationship to calcium intake, estrogen status and age. J Bone Miner Res 1989; 4:469–75.
44. Avioli LB. Diseases of bone: calcium phosphorus and bone metabolism. In: Beeson PB, McDermott W, Wyngaarden JB, eds. Cecil textbook of medicine. Philadelphia: WB Saunders, 1979; 2225–31.
45. Sheikh MS, Santa Ana CA, Nicar MJ, Schiller LB, Fordtran JS. Gastrointestinal absorption of calcium from milk and calcium salts. N Engl J Med 1987; 317:532–6.
46. Nicar MJ, Pak CYC. Calcium bioavailability from calcium carbonate and calcium citrate. J Clin Endocrinol Metab 1985; 61:391–3.
47. Carr CJ, Shangraw RF. Nutritional and pharmaceutical aspects of calcium supplementation. Am Pharm 1987; S27:149–57.
48. Parfitt AM. Integration of skeletal and mineral homeostasis. In: DeLuca HF, Frost H, Jee W, Johnston, C, Parfitt AM, eds. Osteoporosis: recent advances in pathogenesis and treatment. Baltimore: University Park Press, 1981; 115–26.
49. Recker RR. Calcium absorption and achlorhydria. N Engl J Med 1985; 313:70–3.
50. Slavin JL, Marlett JA. Influence of refined cellulose on human bowel function and calcium and magnesium balance. Am J Nutr 1980; 33:1932–9.
51. Delsay JL, Behall KM, Prather ES. Effect of fiber from foods and vegetables on metabolic responses of human subjects II. Calcium, magnesium, iron and silicon balances. Am J Clin Nutr 1979; 32:1876–80.
52. Newcomer AD, Hodgson SF, McDill DB, Thomas PJ. Lactase deficiency: prevalance in osteoporosis. Ann Intern Med 1978; 89:218–20.
53. Kolars JC, Levitt MD, Aouji M, Saraiano DA. Yogurt – an autodigesting source of lactose. N Engl J Med 1984; 310:1–3.
54. Heany RP, Recker RR. Effects of nitrogen, phosphorus and caffeine on calcium balance in women. J Lab Clin Med 1982; 99:46–55.
55. Kleeman CR, Bohannan J, Bernstein D, Ling S, Maxwell MH. Effect of variations in sodium intake on calcium excretion in normal humans. Proc Soc Exp Biol Med 1964; 115:29–32.
56. Gallagher JC, Riggs BL, Eisman J et al. Intestinal calcium absorption and vitamin D. Metabolites in normal subjects and osteoporotic patients. J Clin Invest 1979; 64:729–36.
57. Nordin BEC, Horsman A, Crilly RG, Marshall DH, Simpson M. Treatment of spinal osteoporosis in postmenopausal women. Br Med J 1980; 280:451–4.
58. McCarthy DM, Hibbins JA, Goldman, JM. A role for 1,25-dihydroxy-vitamin D3 in control of bone marrow collagen deposition. Lancet 1984; i:78–80.
59. Reichel H, Koeffler P, Norman AW. The role of vitamin D. Endocrine system in health and disease. N Engl J Med 1989; 320:980–91.
60. Holbrook TL, Barrett-Connor E, Wingard DL. Dietary calcium and risk of hip fracture: 14-year prospective population study. Lancet 1988; ii:1046–9.
61. Matkovic V, Dostial K, Simonovic I, Buzina R, Brodaree A, Nordin BEC. Bone status and fracture rates in two regions of Yugoslavia. Am J Clin Nutr 1979; 32:540–9.
62. Sandler RB, Slamenda CW, La Porte RE et al. Postmenopausal bone density and milk consumption in childhood and adolescence. Am J Clin Nutr 1985; 42:270–4.
63. Cauley JA, Gutai JP, Kuller LH et al. Endogenous estrogen levels and calcium intakes in postmenopausal women. Relationships with cortical bone measures. JAMA 1988; 260:3150–5.
64. Riis B, Thomsen K, Christiansen C. Does calcium supplementation prevent postmenopausal bone loss? A double-blind controlled clinical study. N Engl J Med 1987; 316:173–7.
65. De Deuxchaisnes CN. The pathogenesis and treatment of involutional osteoporosis. In: Dixon AAJ, Russel RGG, Stamp TCB, eds. Osteoporosis, a multidisciplinary problem. London: Royal Society of Medicine London/Academic Press, 1983; 291–333.
66. Harvey WA, Zobitz MM, Pak CYC. Calcium citrate: reduced propensity for the crystallization of calcium oxalate in urine resulting from induced hypercalciuria of calcium supplementation. J Clin Endocrinol Metab 1985; 61:1223–5.
67. Schindler AE, Ebert A, Friedrich E. Conversion of androstenedione to estrone by human fat tissue. J Clin Endocrinol Metab 1972; 35:627–30.
68. Krolner B, Ranlov PJ, Clemmesen T, Nielsen SP. Bone loss after gastroplasty for morbid obesity: side-effect or adaptive response to weight loss: Lancet 1982; i:956–7.
69. Parfitt AM, Miller MJ, Frame B et al. Metabolic bone disease after intestinal bypass for treatment of obesity. Ann Intern Med 1978; 89:193–9.
70. Howat PM, Varner LM, Hegsted M, Brewer MM, Mills CQ. The effect of bulimia upon diet,

body fat, bone density and blood components. J Am Diet Assoc 1989; 89:929–34.

71. Daniell HW. Osteoporosis of the slender smoker. Arch Intern Med 1976; 136:298–304.

72. Jensen J, Christiansen C, Rodbro P. Cigarette smoking, serum estrogens and bone loss during hormone replacement therapy early after menopause. N Engl J Med 1985; 313:973–5.

73. Rigotti NA. Cigarette smoking and body weight. N Engl J Med 1989; 320:931–3.

74. Baron JA. Smoking and estrogen-related disease. Am J Epidemiol 1984; 119:9–22.

75. Slemender CW, Hui SL, Longcope C, Johnston CC. Cigarette smoking. Obesity and bone mass. J Bone Miner Res 1989; 4:737–41.

76. Perkins KA, Epstein LH, Marks BL, Stiller RL, Jacob RG. The effect of nicotine on energy expenditure during light physical activity. N Engl J Med 1989; 320:898–903.

77. Fielding JE. Smoking and women. Tragedy of the majority. N Engl J Med 1987; 317:1343–6.

78. Blume SB. Women and alcohol. A review. JAMA 1986; 256:1467–70.

79. Frezza M, di Padova C, Pozzato G et al. High blood alcohol levels in women. N Engl J Med 1990; 322:95–9.

80. Saville PD. Changes in bone mass with age and alcoholism. J Bone Joint Surg 1965; 47:492–9.

81. De Vernejoul MC, Bielakoff J, Herve M et al. Evidence for defective osteoblastic function. A role for alcohol and tobacco consumption in osteoporosis in middle-aged men. Clin Orthop 1983; 179:107–15.

82. Spencer H, Rubio N, Rubio E et al. Chronic alcoholism. Frequently overlooked cause of osteoporosis in men. Am J Med 1986; 80:393–7.

83. Spencer H, Kramer L, Norris C, Osis D. Effect of small doses of aluminium containing antacids on calcium and phosphorus metabolism. Am J Clin Nutr 1982; 36:32–40.

Discussion

Barlow: Was there really no trend at all in the calcium against the different countries?

Kanis: There is a highly significant correlation between risk of fracture and calcium intake.

Selby: But that probably also reflects oestrogen use in those countries as well, and if one looks at oestrogen use in those countries there is equally a significant trend.

Kanis: I am not at all suggesting that calcium increases the risk of fracture. All that was suggested was that there is not a strong relationship between calcium intake and the risk of fracture.

Selby: If we were to see the same slide with oestrogen use I think it would demonstrate a very similar picture. Yet if a positive relationship could be shown between oestrogen use in countries and fracture incidence, it would be said to be due to something else.

Kanis: It is a complex area, and perhaps this is not the forum to discuss it, but the arguments centre around what are the requiremetns for normal skeletal health in the average person, and they are a little distinct from the effects of pharmacological doses of calcium.

In terms of normal requirements, I do not believe that there is any good evidence, which I have tried to review as thoroughly as possible, that the kind of recommendations that come out of the United States of a dietary requirement that varies between 800 and 1400 mg/day actually confers an advantage to patients, and there is no evidence that we in the UK are disadvantaged by having an RDA of 400 or 500 mg/day.

Notelovitz: I would agree with that if calcium was being taken by itself, but what if that calcium intake is put together with some other therapeutic modality?

Robert Lindsay has shown that 0.3 mg Premarin did not give a bone mass conserving effect. But if 1500 mg calcium is added to the 0.3 mg Premarin, the effect is similar to 0.62 mg Premarin. This is not conclusive by any means, but we should not discount it.

In terms of making these conclusions about whether or not a population is deprived by a certain amount of calcium, we should not be looking at it purely in relation to the calcium alone. It is calcium plus – whatever.

Kanis: I would agree that there is very good evidence that the pharmacological use of calcium, that is uses of 1–2 g/day, decreases the rate of bone loss. There is very good evidence on prospective reasonably well-controlled studies. What we do not yet know is whether that confers an advantage to the patient in terms of fracture frequency. That is a study that should be done, but unfortunately I do not believe that anybody has the resources to do it. I would urge the Department of Health that this is one of the areas that should be invested in. It is not something that the drug companies are likely to do, and there are other appropriate agents as well.

As a pharmacological tool there may be a role for calcium, but that is quite distinct from what we advise the general population and what we advise the general postmenopausal population.

Fogelman: Dr Notelovitz is in favour of screening perimenopausal women. I am delighted to hear it. I suppose everyone will have to address the question as to whether we are in favour of screening that population, but if we are then other problems arise. What is the definition of abnormal? Should measurements be made at one site?

Notelovitz: We have had a long-term interest in identifying a woman with reduced bone mass because I believe in objective measurement before I prescribe anything. When we started the study we had no alternative other than to use single photon absorptiometry, because that was the only technology available at the time, and that enabled us to develop normative values for the population that we were dealing with and we examined about 1000 patients. Based on that we could get some idea as to what was normal or not in our population group.

At the same time or shortly thereafter we acquired a total body dual photon absorptiometer and we did a correlation between peripheral measurements and total body bone density. We found two things. There was a very close correlation between the far distal bone mineral content of the non-dominant radius and total body bone mineral; our value was 0.8. However, and this second point is important in the understanding of the role of peripheral screening, it did not tell us where that bone mass loss was maximum. but some patients have osteoporosis in the spine, others in the hip, and we just do not know.

Based on that we then began to introduce into clinical practice this protocol of using in low-risk individuals, in non-osteoporotic patients, screening using peripheral measurements, and if we found values that were 80% or less of peak bone mass, we gave them the "diagnosis" of osteopenia, and those were the patients on whom we then did total body dual photon absorptiometry at that time, and now deep dual-energy X-ray densitometry (DEXA).

In three separate studies we have found that by using this methodology of approaching this problem of screening, we can correctly identify as normal bone mass, low bone mass, approximately 83%–86% of the population, which as a screening tool is a reasonable figure to arrive at.

The advantage of this method – and I think we are dealing with a technology that is also evolving, certainly there are various manufacturers that are improving the accuracy and precision of perhipheral measurements – is that the machine can be at the site where the patients visits. The patient who comes to see the primary health care physician for her annual check does not normally come to a menopausal centre or an osteoporosis centre. She comes to see her GP, her gynaecologist, or whoever her primary health care physician is, for her annual check up, and if there is some technique whereby obviously normal and obviously abnormal can be identified and the abnormals referred to a central area, the whole process would be much more cost effective both in terms of the given population for whom screening is needed and also in terms of eventual cost.

Fogelman: The problem is that even if we accept everything Dr Notelovitz is saying, not everybody will be prepared to get 1000 reference controls. So they will look to the experts for some kind of guidance as to what is normal and what is abnormal.

One of the problems is that there in no standardisation of equipment. The different manufacturers will not get together and produce one unit. The figures from one set of equipment do not equate with the figures from somebody else's equipment.

Notelovitz: But when one looks at different studies and looks at whatever technique that they used, and there are two or three other studies, then the difference between the "pre-fracture" group, those patients who on X-ray have osteopenia but no fractures, on a measurement of their bone density is approximately 20%–30% less than peak bone mass.

The figure that we use that seems to work for us is that figure of 20% less than peak bone mass, and other people are using one or two standard deviations below peak bone mass.

Fogelman: But we would have to have a peak bone mass. And how are people to get this?

Notelovitz: That is a value that changes, and that is the problem and I understand it. If the philosophy that I have expounded on is put into operation, decade by decade that value will be different. But at this point in time we have to deal with the population that we have got. The manufacturers or somebody needs to identify women who are normal in all respects and measure their bone mineral content, and then we shall know what the peak value is. They need only measure peak value.

Kanis: There is an EEC initiative to build a standard woman, as it were, that might help in this respect.

Fogelman: We all agree there is a need for this.

Boyde: There is some evidence that formation is coupled to resorption, according to the Frostian hypothesis, in adult skeletal remodelling, but I know of no evidence whatsoever that that is true during the apositional phases of the growing skeleton. And it should be at that stage that extraskeletal deposition should be encouraged, and there that de novo bone formation take place. And that is well known from animal studies.

The spectre of piezoelectricity being involved in the signalling has been raised. Piezoelectricity is a phenomenon which can only be detected in very good non-conductors; it is totally impossible for it to happen in an aqueous environment, and so that actually should not be considered to be the mechanism.

The increased fracture risk reported by Riggs in a fluoride-treated group has been mentioned [1]. This raises the point that the quality and the density of the bone fabric should be monitored. There is a very strong likelihood in the fluoride-treated group that the bone matrix is more densely mineralised. There may not be more of it, and it is also likely that it is of poor quality. One may be fooling oneself by measuring increased bone density because it may be more densely mineralised bone and therefore more brittle, and not really any more of it.

Notelovitz: What Professor Boyde says is perfectly valid, but as clinicians concerned about the fact that the use of sodium fluoride in patients with established osteoporosis might demineralise the hip, we have been using oestrogen together with the sodium fluoride. The information is anecdotal, it is clinical information from day to day practice, but we have seen that we are not losing bone mineral from the hip, we are still seeing the same increase in the spine, but again I do not know what the quality of that spine bone mineral is or whether indeed with time the bone is likely to fracture, and I have no idea.

But all too often we tend to have – if I might use the expression – a simplistic approach to a very complex problem, and it is "only oestrogen", or "only fluoride", or "only calcium", or "only exercise" when in point of fact a multiplicity of treatments are necessary to maximise the end therapeutic goal.

Lindsay: There is a problem with the issue of fluoride effects in the hip. The observational data have now come out in favour of the fact that there is an increased risk of fracture associated with fluoride therapy.

Since total body bone balance tends not to improve overall with fluoride therapy, what Dr Notelovitz might be seeing is the phenomenon Professor Boyde mentioned occurring in the hip; that is improved apparent mineralisation and improved density, which gives one a false sense of security.

Notelovitz: Time will tell. We are doing a study now, double blinded, looking at fluoride by itself against oestrogen.

Kanis: Speaking of the fluoride story, there has been an enormous setback in terms of reporting of the trial from Murray Rigg. It is important to point out that the doses that were used in this study are extremely high and that it is known that the side effects, osteoarticular and gastrointestinal, are dose-related, and against the background of that study the side effects – including extra vertebral fractures – are greater than the benefits. But notwithstanding, there is a 15% decrease in fracture frequency, very similar to the other double-blind studies that have been undertaken. So we need not necessarily discount fluoride completely.

Dr Stevenson showed a heterogeneity of response to calcitonin. This is a very important issue because it raises the question of whether one should be following treatment. To what extent is there heterogeneity of response to oestrogens? We have consistently seen oestrogens prevent bone loss. Does it do that in all patients and do we as physicians have a responsibility to monitor in whatever way we can the effects of treatment when we are giving oestrogens for bone loss?

Stevenson: That was the point I was trying to bring across. Looking at all the published data that give the raw value, 0.625 mg oestrogen will prevent bone loss for a group, but there will always be some individuals who will lose bone density from the spinal trabecular bone or from the hip or whatever, and it varies from study to study. But it is never 100%.

I believe that to monitor an individual, serial bone density measurements need to be taken to monitor any treatment. No-one can infer that they are doing good from oestradiol levels, from urinary calcium excretion, from anything else. If one wants to know that if one is preserving bone, one must measure bone in that site. And for an individual that is the only way to be absolutely sure that the treatment is working.

Anderson: Returning to the question of exercise, what is the effect of immobilisation with, for example, spinal fractures and pain, or indeed what influence in individual cases may episodes of enforced immobilisation have on the development or perpetuation of oesteoporosis?

Notelovitz: It has a marked negative effect. A healthy male who is put to bed will lose 4% of bone mass within a month.

Anderson: What percentage of the problem is due to that, particularly in the patient who, say, has had one wedge fracture with minimal trauma? Does the immobilisation tip them into a steep slope of rapid deterioration?

Notelovitz: I do not know the answer to that. Maybe the bone experts do.

Anderson: Because if that does happen, then in fact prompt treatment of such patients with something that arrests bone resorption temporarily early in the stage of their disease might well be more important than we give credit for.

Notelovitz: Yes. That is very important.

Lindsay: It is clear that if patients with osteoporosis are put to bed, they will get worse. The argument is that they should be mobilised as quickly as possible. The problem in mobilisation is that if stresses are then created on a repairing fracture, that might worsen the fracture. There are remarkably few data on the natural history of osteporosis per se, and the best data probably go back to Elias

Jones' study in Calcified Tissue, which showed that patients with spinal osteoporosis vertebral crush fracture syndrome had a rate of loss that was parallel to rates of loss seen immediately after oophorectomy, despite these people being 10–20 years older. So there may be a subpopulation in whom bone loss is not more rapid after menopause, but in whom it probably continues for a longer period of time.

Notelovitz: Those are the patients that I use calcitonin on very freely because it has an analgesic effect as well. And those are the patients that I do use braces for for a limited period of time, to get them up and about as quickly as possible.

Reference

1. Riggs BL, Hodgson SF, Muhs J, Wahner HW. Fluoride treatment of osteoporosis: clinical and bone densitometric responses. In: Christiansen C, Johansen JS, Riis BJ, eds. Osteoporosis. Copenhagen: Osteopress ApS, 1987; 817–23.

Section V
HRT and the Community

Chapter 25

Premenopausal Hormone Therapy

J. O. Drife

Introduction

In the context of discussions on hormone replacement after the menopause, the title "Premenopausal hormone therapy" may seem a contradiction in terms. It may appear illogical to administer exogenous oestrogen while a woman's ovaries are still producing endogenous hormones. Premenopausal hormone therapy, however, is in widespread use. Millions of young women take sex steroids in the form of the combined oral contraceptive (COC), which abolishes ovarian function through its action on the hypothalamus. Hypothalamic amenorrhoea could also be produced by analogues of gonadotrophin-releasing hormone but these are unsuitable as contraceptives because they cause menopausal symptoms. The COC produces reversible ovarian failure but simultaneously provides hormone replacement.

The COC has important beneficial effects on health [1], but it has adverse effects on the risk of cardiovascular disease and these risks appear to rise with age [2]. Among women who smoke, the COC is contraindicated after the age of 35 because of the risk of cardiovascular disease. Non-obese normotensive non-smokers have been recommended to stop the COC after the age of 45 (though it is now suggested that they can continue until the menopause). However, exogenous sex steroids given as postmenopausal hormone replacement therapy (HRT) to older women apparently protect against cardiovascular disease [3].

This paradox deserves scrutiny for two reasons. First, doctors and women will remain unhappy about the safety of HRT until the perceived difference in risks between the COC and HRT can be fully explained. Second, older premeno-pausal women may request hormonal treatment, either for contraception or because of symptoms. We need to have a clear idea about the indications and contraindications for exogenous sex steroids in this age group, and about whether the best formulation for these women is the COC or HRT.

Physiology

The menopause is defined as a woman's last period, but the cessation of endometrial shedding is only one aspect of ovarian failure. Ovarian function does not cease suddenly, but begins to alter before the menopause and continues for some time after the menopause itself [4]. Metcalf [5], in a longitudinal study of New Zealand women passing through the menopause, found three patterns of hormone excretion. (1) Premenopausal women (age 40–51 years) had regular periods and hormone patterns similar to those seen in fertile young women. (2) Women in the menopausal transition (age 40–55 years) had irregular periods with erratic hormone fluctuations: before the menopause there were episodes of high gonadotrophin secretion and low urinary oestrogens, and for six months after the menopause hormone patterns were similar to the anovulatory cycles of the menopausal transition. (3) Older women (age 57–67 years) had senescent ovaries with unvarying high gonadotrophins and low oestrogen levels.

Thus a woman before the menopause may be exposed to low oestrogen levels for several weeks at a time, or conversely to persistent elevation of oestrogen levels unopposed by progesterone. Interestingly, of the 31 women studied by Metcalf [5], in four cases the last cycle before the menopause was "ovulatory", as defined by a rise in urinary pregnanediol.

According to Coope [6], symptoms of oestrogen deficiency, and depression in particular, may precede the menopause itself. A woman may ask for HRT because of these symptoms, or she may still be troubled by the premenstrual syndrome and ask whether continuous hormone therapy would control this problem. Some well-informed women may be concerned about the risks attached to prolonged unopposed oestrogen excretion in the premenopausal years. These risks, together with the risk of unwanted pregnancy, could be reduced by taking the COC right up till the menopause if it were otherwise safe to do so.

Risks of COCS

The main concerns regarding the safety of COCs are about cardiovascular disease and cancer.

Cardiovascular Disease

COCs cause a three- to sixfold increase in the risk of venous thromboembolism. This is probably an oestrogen effect, and the excess risk disappears quickly when COCs are stopped. The overall risk of haemorrhagic stroke is doubled in COC-users and the risk of thrombotic stroke is increased severalfold. The risk of myocardial infarction is related to age and smoking, which is why COCs are contraindicated over the age of 35 in smokers, but not necessarily in non-smokers. COCs cause a slight increase in blood pressure [2]. It is well recognised, however, that our knowledge about the cardiovascular risks of the COC is based on studies involving older high-dose COCs, and that firm data on modern low-dose pills are scanty.

Cancer

COCs protect against benign breast lumps, endometrial cancer, uterine fibroids and epithelial cancer of the ovary [1]. On the other hand, there is some evidence that early use of COCs may increase breast cancer risk and that prolonged use generally may increase cervical cancer risk, though these data are certainly not conclusive [7].

Comparison with HRT

The effects of HRT on the risk of cardiovascular disease and cancer are fully discussed elsewhere in this volume, but can be briefly summarised by saying that unopposed oestrogen therapy now appears to offer some protection against cardiovascular disease, and appears in most studies to have no effect on the risk of breast cancer, though there is some concern over prolonged use [8]. This picture is different from the overall perception of the risks of the COC, and the difference could be explained in a variety of ways. It could be due to differences in formulation between COCs and HRT – in the dosage, the type of steroids, or the duration of their use. There might be differences in the distribution and binding of hormones before and after the menopause. Finally, ageing could make a difference to the way the end-organs respond to sex steroids.

Dosage and Formulation

Modern COCs contain 30–35 μg of ethinyloestradiol because this has been thought to be the minimum dosage which will suppress gonadotrophin secretion. Older COCs contained higher doses of ethinyloestradiol and as mentioned above most data on the side effects of COCs came from studies on higher-dose pills. Two COCs contained only 20 μg of ethinyloestradiol; one, Loestrin, has norethisterone as its progestogen and has a higher failure rate than standard 30 μg COCs. The other, Mercilon, contains the more potent progestogen deso-gestrel and is claimed to have a low failure rate similar to that of standard COCs. In spite of this low oestrogen dosage, however, the amount of ethinyloestradiol in these two COCs is still double that recommended for HRT. The greater safety of HRT compared with COCs may, therefore, be due to the fact that relatively small doses of oestrogen are adequate to suppress climacteric symptoms.

The difference in dosage is less marked for progestogens, however. The daily dose of progestogen in proprietary packs of combined HRT is in the same range as in COCs. Indeed, HRT formulations may include 250 µg of levonorgestrel or up to 1.5 mg of norethisterone daily – doses which are higher than the daily progestogen doses in some COCs. The total monthly exposure to progestogen, however, is lower with HRT preparations than with the COC because the duration of exposure is shorter – progestogens being taken for only 7–12 days per month. This aspect is discussed more fully below.

Potency

Unlike COCs, different brands of HRT contain different oestrogens with competing claims regarding safety and acceptability. The *British National Formulary* states that "ethinyloestradiol is the oestrogen of choice for most conditions. The natural (as opposed to synthetic) oestrogens have not been shown to have any advantages." This view is not shared by the manufacturers of "natural" oestrogens, who can with justification point out that most of the research on long-term safety of HRT has involved conjugated equine oestrogens, and that the reassuring results of these studies cannot necessarily be extrapolated to other types of oestrogen.

Different oestrogens vary in potency but comparisons are difficult because much depends on which end-organ is used as a test system [9–11]. For example, a large difference in potency between the effects of two oestrogens on the endometrium may not accurately reflect their relative effects on plasma lipids. Only a limited number of end-organs have been used to test potency, and we lack information on the relative effects of different oestrogens on less accessible tissues such as breast or bone.

Formulation

As mentioned above, COCs and HRT differ in the duration of hormone administration. With COCs a woman takes oestrogen and progestogen simultaneously for 21 days and then takes no steroids for seven days. With proprietary regimens of HRT she is exposed to oestrogen either continuously or for 21 days per month, and this is opposed by progestogen for only 7–12 days of each month. The reason for the relatively short courses of progestogen is to reduce progestogen exposure to the minimum necesary to protect the endometrium. Since progestogen appears to reduce the beneficial effects of oestrogen on the cardiovascular system, this seems a wise policy.

Nevertheless, there are theoretical disadvantages to a regimen of unopposed oestrogen followed by progestogen. In some end-organs, such as the endometrium, unopposed oestrogen causes synthesis of progestogen receptors, and progestogen inhibits further synthesis of oestrogen receptors. therefore a progestogen may have a greater effect after a course of unopposed oestrogen than if it had been administered simultaneously with the oestrogen. The endometrium of COC-users does not undergo full secretory change because there is no interval of oestrogen priming before exposure to progestogen.

This could be important in mammary tissue. Epidemiological studies have been broadly reassuring about the effect of HRT on breast cancer incidence, but most of these studies have concentrated on the effect of unopposed oestrogen treatment. Little information is available on opposed regimens of HRT, though the recent study by Bergkvist et al. [8] (discussed in Chapter 14) raises the possibility – based on a small number of cases – that opposed HRT regimens may have an adverse effect on breast cancer risk. Some workers have suggested that the addition of progestogen to HRT regimens should reduce the risk of breast cancer just as they do for endometrial cancer [12–14], but the evidence for this is far from conclusive [15]. Indeed, the response of mammary tissue to the normal menstrual cycle does not support this idea.

During the normal menstrual cycle the breasts tend to enlarge in the second half of the cycle [16,17], when progesterone is present in the circulation. They do not swell in response to unopposed oestrogen. Blood flow in the breast also increases in the second half of the normal cycle [18]. Studies of breast biopsies from premenopausal women have shown that in the second half of the cycle there are increases in the number of mitoses in mammary glandular tissue [19] and in the incorporation of labelled DNA precursors into the nuclei of the glandular cells [20–23]. This suggests that cellular proliferation in the mammary gland is initiated by progesterone rather than by oestrogen. However, it is likely that both hormones are involved: studies of the hormone requirements for lactation have shown that various hormones are involved in maturing the gland during pregnancy.

There have been few studies of the response of mammary tissue to COCs [24]. Enlargement of the breast occurs in contraceptive-controlled cycles just as in normal cycles [16], but breast biopsies do not show excessive activity in mammary glandular tissue from COC users [22].

Route of Administration

Both COCs and HRT are administered orally in the majority of cases, but HRT can be given by implants or by transdermal patches. These routes of administration avoid the first-pass metabolism in the liver, but there is as yet no epidemiological evidence to confirm that this increases the safety of the preparations [25].

Distribution and Binding

It is well recognised that differences in body weight and composition between different individuals mean that when a standard COC is administered there may be widely differing blood levels of steroids [26]. However, it seems unlikely that these individual variations will have a consistent effect in making HRT more or less dangerous than the COC. It has been claimed that as a woman ages there is a steady decrease in the level of circulating sex-hormone binding globulin (SHBG), thus leading to a steady incrase in the level of free sex-hormone in the circulation [6]. However, the menopause does not change SHBG levels [27] and, according to Maruyama et al. [28], levels of SHBG increase with age.

Endogenous Hormones

Another difference between the COC and HRT is that the COC inhibits ovarian activity, but the levels of steroid in HRT are inadequate to provide reliable ovarian suppression through feedback at a hypothalamic level. This is why HRT preparations are unsuitable as contraceptives. If HRT is given before the menopause, ovarian activity is likely to continue and the woman will be exposed to a mixture of endogenous and exogenous steroids. This may not necessarily be harmful to her, but it will cause difficulties in the interpretation of epidemiological data on premenopausal HRT.

End-organ Responsiveness and Ageing

Finally, differences in the response to COCs and HRT may be due not to differences in the hormonal stimulus but to differences in the innate capacity of the end-organs to respond to hormones. Hormone-responsive tissues may respond differently at different ages. For example, although the endometrium retains its ability to synthesise specific proteins after the menopause [29], the effect of ageing of the endometrium is seen with in vitro fertilisation [30]. Implantation rates of apparently healthy embryos are lower in women over the age of 40 than in younger women. Since adequate numbers of embryos were implanted and circulating hormone levels were normal, the reduction in implantation rates seems to be due to ageing of the endometrium.

Ageing may also affect the breast. The stromal tissue of the breast of a young girl at puberty is extremely sensitive to oestrogen, and breast enlargement is the first sign of increasing oestrogen production at puberty [31]. It is not known whether this sensitivity is maintained throughout reproductive life, but there is evidence that the breast becomes less sensitive to hormone changes as it ages, and there is a slight diminution of the size of glandular elements in the breast [32,33].

A woman's lifetime risk of breast cancer is influenced by both her age at menarche and her age at the menopause. Early menarche and late menopause both increase the risk of subsequent breast cancer [34]. Thus the longer the breast is exposed to endogenous ovarian activity, the greater is the risk of cancer. However, a reduction of only two years in the age of menarche – from 13 to 11 years – can double the incidence of subsequent breast cancer, whereas at the other end of reproductive life doubling the incidence of subsequent breast cancer requires a 20-year increase in the age at menopause, from 40 to 60 years. This suggests that the breast may be more susceptible to the adverse effects of hormones at a young age than at an older age [35].

Thus the same exogenous hormonal stimulus could be harmful at one stage of a woman's life and harmless later on. This possibility is reflected in current concerns about a possible link between COCs and breast cancer: there is still some concern that COC use early in life may have a harmful effect on the incidence of breast cancer [36], but all studies have been reassuring that COC use later in the reproductive years – after age 25 years or after the first pregnancy – does not increase the risk of breast cancer.

Conclusion

Epidemiological studies have shown that the risks and benefits of the COC may not be the same as the risks and benefits of HRT. The difference is most clearly seen with respect to cardiovascular disease, the risk of which is increased by COCs but diminished by HRT. These differences may be explained by dosage, but the difference in dosage between HRT and modern low-dose oral contraceptives is not large. It may be that the risks of modern low-dose COCs are much less than we currently believe from out-of-date epidemiological data based on studies of older COCs. It is also possible that the differences between COCs and HRT can be partly explained by differences in end-organ responsiveness due to ageing. We should be cautious about figures on differences in potency between oestrogens because these depend on which organ-system is used to test potency. A very important question regarding the difference between HRT and COCs relates to the duration of progestogen exposure: current proprietary regimens of HRT involve unopposed oestrogen followed by progestogen, thus, mimicking the natural cycle, which is known to be stimulatory to the breast. Further research is now needed to discover whether long courses of progestogen (as in the COC) or short courses (as in HRT) are safer, particularly for the breast.

References

1. Drife JO. The benefits of combined oral contraceptives. Br J Obstet Gynaecol 1989; 96:1255–8.
2. Drife JO. Complications of combined oral contraception. In: Filshie M, Guillebaud J, eds. Contraception: science and practice. London: Butterworths, 1989; 39–51.
3. Hunt K, Vessey M. Long-term effects of postmenopausal hormone therapy. Br J Hosp Med 1987; 38:450–60.
4. Richardson SJ, Senikas V, Nelson JF. Follicular depletion during the menopausal transition: evidence for accelerated loss and ultimate exhaustion. J Clin Endocrinol Metab 1987; 65:1231–7.
5. Metcalf MG. The approach of the menopause: a New Zealand study. NZ Med J 1988; 101:103–6.
6. Coope J. Hormone replacement therapy. Exeter: Royal College of General Practitioners, 1989.
7. Vessey MP. Oral contraception and cancer. In: Felshie M, Guillebaud J, eds. Contraception; science and practice. London: Butterworths, 1989; 52–68.
8. Bergkvist L, Adami H-O, Persson I, Hoover R, Schairer C. The risk of breast cancer after estrogen and estrogen–progestin replacement. N Engl J Med 1989; 321:293–7.
9. Hammond CB, Maxson WS. Estrogen replacement therapy. Clin Obstet Gynecol 1986; 29:407–30.
10. Mandel FP, Geola FL, Lu JKH, Eggena P, Sambhi M, Hershman JH, Judd HL. Biologic effects of various doses of ethinyl estradiol in postmenopausal women. Obstet Gynecol 1982; 59:673–9.
11. Young RL, Goldzieher JW. Current status of postmenopausal oestrogen therapy. Drugs 1987; 33:95–106.
12. Mauvais-Jarvis P. Effects on the breast of drugs used in fertility regulation. Human Reprod 1987; 2:159–62.

13. Gambrell RD, Maier RC, Sanders BI. Decreased incidence of breast cancer in postmenopausal estrogen–progestogen users. Obstet Gynecol 1983; 63:435–43.
14. Metcalf MG, Mackenzie JA. Menstrual cycle and exposure to oestrogens unopposed by progesterone: relevance to studies on breast cancer incidence. J Endocrinol 1985; 194:137–41.
15. Barrett-Connor E. Postmenopausal estrogen replacement and breast cancer. N Engl J Med 1989; 321:319–20.
16. Milligan D, Drife JO, Short RV. Changes in breast volume during the normal menstrual cycle and after oral contraceptives. Br Med J 1975; iv:494–6.
17. Malini S, Smith EO, Goldzieher JW. Measurement of breast volume by ultrasound during normal menstrual cycles and with oral contraceptive use. Obstet Gynecol 1985; 66:538–41.
18. Pickles VR. Blood-flow estimations as indices of mammary activity. J Obstet Gynaecol Br Emp 1959; 60:301–11.
19. Anderson TJ, Ferguson DJP, Raab GM. Cell turnover in the "resting" human breast: influence of parity, contraceptive pill, age and laterality. Br J Cancer 1981; 44:117–81.
20. Masters JRW, Drife JO, Scarisbrick JJ. Cyclic variations of DNA synthesis in human breast epithelium. Natl Cancer Inst 1977; 58:1263–5.
21. Drife JO. Breast modifications during the menstrual cycle. Int J Gynaecol Obstet 1989; Suppl 1:19–24.
22. Going JJ, Anderson TJ, Battersby S, MacIntyre CCA. Proliferative and secretory activity in human breast during natural and artificial menstrual cycles. Am J Pathol 1988; 130:193–204.
23. Meyer JS, Connor RE. Cell proliferation in fibrocystic disease and postmenopausal breast ducts measured by thymidine labelling. Cancer 1982; 50:746–51.
24. Longman SM, Buehring GC. Oral contraceptives and breast cancer: in vitro effect of contraceptive steroids on human mammary cell growth. Cancer 1987; 59:281–7.
25. Anonymous. Patch up the menopause. Lancet 1988; i:861–2.
26. Back DJ, Breckenridge AM, Crawford FE, MacIver M, Orme ML'E, Rowe PH. Interindividual variation and drug interactions with hormonal steroid contraceptives. Drugs 1981; 21:46–61.
27. Longcope C, Hui SL, Johnston CC. Free estradiol, free testosterone, and sex hormone-binding globulin in perimenopausal women. J Clin Endocrinol Metab 1987; 64:513–18.
28. Maruyama Y, Aoki N, Suzuki Y, Sinohara H, Yamamoto T. Variation with age in the levels of sex-steroid-binding plasma protein as determined by radioimmunoassay. Acta Endocrinol 1984; 106:428–31.
29. Seppala M, Alfthan H, Vartiainen E, Stenman U-H. The postmenopausal uterus: the effect of hormone replacement therapy on the serum levels of secretory endometrial protein PP14/beta-lactoglobulin homologue. Human Reprod 1987; 2:741–3.
30. Edwards RG, Steptoe PC. Current status of in-vitro fertilisation and implantation of human embryos. Lancet 1983; ii:1265–9.
31. Drife JO. Breast development in puberty. Ann NY Acad Sci 1986; 464:58–65.
32. Drife JO. The normal mammary gland. MD Thesis, University of Edinburgh 1981.
33. Short RV, Drife JO. The aetiology of mammary cancer in man and animals. Symp Zool Soc London 1977; 41:211–300.
34. Pike MC, Ross RK. Breast cancer. Br Med Bull 1984; 40:351–4.
35. Pike MS, Krailo MD, Henderson BE, Casagrande JT, Hoel DG. "Hormonal" risk factors, "breast tissue age" and the age-incidence of breast cancer. Nature 1983; 303:767–70.
36. Drife JO. The contraceptive pill and breast cancer in young women. Br Med J 1989; 298:1269–70.

Discussion

Persson: Referring to the safety of COCs on breast tissue, I thought that Anderson [1] had shown that with combined COCs there is an increased rate of mitosis. But Dr Drife says the opposite.

Drife: We did not have many cases but we certainly found a diminution in thymidine uptake and I do not think Anderson found a substantial increase in mitotic rate with COCs.

Vessey: My recollection of Anderson's later work is that the pattern that he saw for labelled thymidine uptake (which he substituted – if that is the right term – for his histological method) was a similar cyclical pattern generally in non-OC users and in OC users [2]. But he was concerned that there was a difference between nulliparae and parous women. As I recollect, OCs had a more prominent effect in the nulliparous women, which was one of the ways he tried to integrate the "early OC use – breast cancer" issue with breast activity.

Drife: We started on this work before Anderson and our hypothesis was that cyclical activity was seen only after first pregnancy, leading to the suggestion that the progestogen receptors were not well developed before first pregnancy [3]. Recently, however, Anderson reported that activity increases in the luteal phase of the cycle in both nulliparous and parous women, and that the nulliparous breast is very responsive to COC use, whereas the parous breast is almost unaffected [4].

Studd: We have been using oestrogens to treat premenstrual syndrom (PMS) on the principle that we can stop the cyclical symptoms if we stop ovulation, in just this age group. We might start with a 200 µg oestrogen patch decreasing it stepwise to 100 µg, or oestradiol in a 100 mg pellet decreasing to 50 mg, and all of those doses cause anovulation, and are contraceptive and treat the PMS. So this is another possiblity.

We have discussed how these climacteric depressive symptoms start before the menopause and bone loss starts before the menopause, and it is another option.

We know this therapy stops ovulation but that tells us nothing about long-term contraception and acceptability. That can be studied with great detail. Although I would support the view that the OC age be extended, this therapy is also another option for patients who do have symptoms, particular PMS.

Vessey: The notion that we might extend OCs upwards is quite well founded. Risk seems to be much lower. I am aware that the Obstetrics and Gynaecology Committee of the FDA has suggested that that should be the case although it has yet to be approved by the FDA itself.

It is interesting that both in the US and the UK, because of the lower age restriction that was imposed following the Royal College of General Practitioners' paper in 1977, there is hardly any use now in women aged over 35 or aged over 40 and it will be difficult to test the hypothesis for a long time to come.

I have mentioned that we studied all deaths for cardiovascular disease in a case-controlled study in women up to age 40 for the years 1986–88. We stopped at age 40 because the level of use of COCs by women aged over 40 was about 3% and it was not worth trying to study that age group. So as far as cardiovascular risk is concerned that must remain a speculation for another unspecified number of years, while that recommendation filters through again.

Drife: It may not simply be the recommendations of the profession but also the preference of women. There is an instinctive dislike of the idea of being on a medication for more than a decade and women may simply not want to do it even if they are reassured that it is safe.

Ross: There are a fair number of published data on breast cancer risk for use during the perimenopausal period, or at least during the 40–50 years age range. My recollection of those data is that they are fairly consistent in showing a fairly marked increment in risk, certainly larger than the kinds of risk we see with HRT, given that those are related to the older higher-dose pills. I am wondering if those published data give Dr Drife pause for thought in making that recommendation.

Drife: I have the opposite impression. My understanding of the literature is that all the worry about the COCs is in young women either before age 25 or before first pregnancy and that there is consistency in showing no risk in the older woman.

Vessey: I must support Professor Ross here. This is an issue that Malcolm Pike has written about a fair bit.

There is not much information on breast cancer risk in relation to the use of OCs by women in the 45–54 age group, or even the 40–49 age group. The numbers of studies that include a significant amount of exposure in that age group are really quite small. Malcolm Pike has gathered them together and has suggested that there are anxieties at both ends of the life span, i.e., the very early use and the perimenopausal use of OCs.

Ross: The rationale being that it is periods of anovulatory cycles that increase risk.

Vessey: It is true that in the case-controlled study [5] which we did between 1969 and 1980, the one group in which we found an elevated risk was that late 40–44 year-old usage group. And another classic paper, another frightening paper, was the one that published by Jick et al. [6] in which he had assembled a group of women who were using OCs very late and in which he had a relative risk of breast cancer of about 2.0 or 3.0. I know that Malcolm Pike has pulled this literature together.

Drife: His conclusion was that the results are based on small numbers and are inconclusive [7].

Persson: The meeting last year in London I believe came to the conclusion that there were no data to say that there was an increased risk after age 45 years. The worry was among those aged <35 years with a grey area between 35 and 44 years. That was my impression of the conclusions at that meeting.

Vessey: The problem is that there are just so few data. Because for the last 10 or 15 years OCs have not been substantially used in that age group, there are very few studies that have that late exposure, and on the whole they were not a subject of major discussion at the RSM meeting. I think we must leave the question open.

Hart: One point that may not have been stressed enough is that contraception is perhaps the biggest worry of the premenopausal woman with menopausal symptoms coming for treatment: "Would I fall pregnant on this therapy?" Most of the cyclical preparations are not contraceptive, and a consensus report should maybe address itself slightly to that.

The second point is that if we go for OCs later rather than HRT earlier, what of the large number of women who have been sterilised and who do not need the OC for contraception? But a lot of women do have symptoms before they become amenorrhoeic, so there is a large call for treatment of menopausal symptoms before the actual menopause. Bone loss starts before the menopause, and I would not be too happy to have the profession thinking that the consensus of this meeting was that HRT should not be used until the periods have ceased completely.

To move on from that, does anyone know of any good work done on the control of menopausal symptoms – psychological, vasomotor and somatic – by oral contraceptives? I know of no references. It may well work very nicely but I am not aware of any work on this. So have we got good evidence for saying "Use the pill rather than HRT"?

The final point is that control of bleeding is more difficult in women who have not yet become totally amenorrhoeic, so while for patients who are some years past the menopause combined continuous oestrogen with pro-gestogen may well give them symptom control and no bleeding, there can be a lot of difficulties with trying combined continuous treatment with people who are still having some periods.

Drife: My first remit was to try to find published literature on the control of symptoms before the menopause, either with the pill or with HRT regimens. There appears to me to be very little published; in fact there appears to be nothing published.

Selby: Anecdotally as an endocrinologist, a woman is quite often with very early ovarian failure, say in her 20s, it is socially more acceptable for her to take OCs rather than a preparation that we would normally consider using in menopausal age women, and they appear to get symptom control with that. But I do not know of any controlled studies that have looked at it.

Baird: It would be absolutely extraordinary if flushes were not relieved by giving mestranol 35 µg.

Cardozo: If ovarian function in premenopausal women is to be suppressed by using very low dose COCs, are there no worries that they might develop premenopausal osteoporosis? All the long-term use of OCs has been 30 µg and above. If we are now advocating the use of preparations which have 20 µg of oestrogen, are we not worried that if this is used for 20 or 30 years osteoporosis might be brought forward rather than pushed back?

Drife: The amount we are giving would be the same as HRT. So if we say that HRT would prevent osteoporosis, it follows that these preparations will do so as well.

Cardozo: But HRT prevents osteoporosis in women in an older age group. We do not know that it would prevent osteoporosis in women in a younger age group.

Lindsay: I think the evidence suggests that 20 µg will be enough. But it would be nice to have some prospective controlled data looking at it, just for safety's sake.

There is a mixture of evidence about the use of OCs and effects on bone mass in younger ovulating women. Some studies suggest that there is an associated small increase in bone mass, and other studies suggest that there is essentially no change. But there is certainly no evidence of a decline in bone mass. Most of the work was done with OCs containing 30–35 μg oestrogen.

Fogelman: Some of the data show no loss, some a slight gain. There is a mix of data. But no one has shown actual losses.

Purdie: There was a paper from the Leeds Group [8] that showed that 30 μg of ethinyloestradiol was protective, but it was not given in combination with progestogen.

References

1. Anderson TJ, Ferguson DJP, Raab GM. Cell turnover in the "resting" human breast: influence of parity, contraceptive pill, age and laterality. Br J Cancer 1982; 46:376–82.
2. Going JJ, Anderson TJ, Battersby S, MacIntyre CCA. Proliferative and secretory activity in human breast during natural and artificial menstrual cycle. Am J Pathol 1988; 130:193–204.
3. Drife JO. Breast cancer, pregnancy and the pill. Br Med J 1981; 283:778–9.
4. Anderson TJ, Battersby S, King RJB, McPherson K, Going JJ. Oral contraceptive use influences resting breast proliferation. Hum Pathol 1989; 20:1139–44.
5. Vessey MP, Baron J, Doll R, McPherson K, Yeates D. Oral contraceptives and breast cancer: final report of an epidemiological study. Br J Cancer 1983; 47:455–62.
6. Jick H, Walker NM, Watkins RN et al. Oral contraceptives and breast cancer. Am J Epidemiol 1980; 112:577–85.
7. Pike MC, Chilvers C. Oral contraceptives and breast cancer: the current controversy. J R Soc Health 1985; 105:5–10.
8. Horsman A, Jones M, Francis R, Nordin C. The effect of estrogen loss on postmenopausal bone loss. N Engl J Med 1983; 309:1405–7.

Chapter 26

Hormone Replacement Therapy in the Menopause: Risks, Benefits and Costs

M. Roche and M. Vessey

Introduction

The use of hormone replacement therapy (HRT) for the relief of menopausal symptoms and the prevention of osteoporotic fractures has been advocated for some time. More recently, it has been suggested that HRT may lead to a reduction in heart disease and stroke. These benefits have to be weighed against the possibility of an increased risk of endometrial cancer and breast cancer. For individual women and their doctors, a careful assessment of the evidence on the balance of risks and benefits is of great importance. For a health service with limited resources, the health benefits for individuals must be weighed against the resource costs and compared with the benefits which might be gained from spending the money on other health care programmes.

In the United States the use of HRT is already recognised as a major health issue, with large numbers of postmenopausal women taking HRT, often for long periods of time. The situation in Britain is very different, with much lower levels of use and, in particular, with very little long-term use.

Two American studies, published in the early 1980s have looked at the cost effectiveness of HRT [1,2]. The 1980 study by Weinstein [1] considered the cost effectiveness of unopposed oestrogen therapy. Weinstein concluded that oestrogen replacement therapy is relatively cost effective in women with prior hysterectomy or with evidence of osteoporosis within 10 years of menopause. In women with a uterus and without osteoporosis, cost effectiveness depends on whether the woman has symptoms and, if so, on the value given to the relief of symptoms.

The 1983 study by Weinstein and Schiff [2] was a comparison of the cost effectiveness of unopposed oestrogen therapy with combined oestrogen and progestogen therapy (since the mid-1970s, often prescribed as an alternative to oestrogen alone for women with a uterus). The authors concluded that the costs of endometrial monitoring and treatment of endometrial morbidity (including cancer) were eliminated by combined therapy and that this more than offset the higher drug costs. Neither study included assumptions about the effect of HRT on heart disease or stroke.

The purpose of the present chapter is to update the analysis (using a similar but simpler approach) to include assumptions about the effects of HRT on heart disease and stroke and to look at costs of treatment in the British context. Some preliminary findings are presented.

Methods

The approach taken is to look at two hypothetical treatment cohorts compared with an untreated control cohort. Three consequences of treatment with HRT are considered: mortality and morbidity induced or prevented by HRT and net health care costs per patient.

Treatment Options

Treatment is evaluated in two hypothetical cohorts. The first cohort consists of 1 000 000 women entering the menopause at age 50 years having had a hysterectomy. It is assumed that these women are treated for 15 years till the age of 65, with 100% compliance throughout the period of treatment. The second cohort consists of 1 000 000 women entering the menopause at age 50 years with an intact uterus and likewise receiving HRT (with 100% compliance) for 15 years from age 50 to 65.

Mortality and Morbidity Rates

For the untreated control group it is assumed that current population mortality and morbidity rates apply – which seems reasonable given the low levels of long-term use of HRT and the fact that the effects of interest are related to long-term use. Mortality rates for breast cancer, ischaemic heart disease and cerebro-vascular disease are taken from national mortality statistics [3]. National mortality data are thought to provide a considerable underestimate of mortality associated with fractured neck of femur, so instead a case fatality rate of 10% is applied to the annual hospital admission rate. Hospital admission data are used as a proxy for morbidity in this study. Hospital admission rates have been obtained from data for England for the year 1985 published in the Hospital Inpatient Enquiry (HIPE) [5].

For the treatment cohorts, best estimates of elevation or reduction in relative risk are derived from a review of the epidemiological literature.

Costs

Only certain health service costs are considered in this analysis. Three component costs are identified: cost of the drug itself, monitoring costs and costs (or savings) of treatment for breast cancer, fractured neck of femur, heart disease and stroke. Treatment costs (i.e. per hospital admission) are estimated using an approximation based on average acute inpatient cost per day [4] multiplied by mean length of stay for each condition from HIPE [5]. All future costs have been discounted at 5% per annum.

Data and Assumptions

Treatment

For the cohort of women without a uterus, treatment is assumed to consist of 15 years of Premarin (0.625 mg conjugated oestrogen) daily, at an annual drug cost of £11.00. Premarin has been chosen because the great majority of epidemiologial studies currently available concern the use of this drug. In addition, it is assumed that all women will be seen on two extra occasions each year by their GP to monitor the treatment, at an estimated cost of £5.80 per visit [6] – giving a total annual cost of £22.60.

It is assumed that, because of the well-established increased risk of endometrial cancer with unopposed oestrogen therapy, the cohort of women with a uterus will be treated with combined oestrogen and progestogen therapy (Prempack-C; 0.625 mg conjugated oestrogen daily and 75 μg levonorgestrel for 10 days each cycle). The drug cost for this regimen is £45.00 per year, giving a total annual cost of £56.60.

Endometrial Cancer

The evidence connecting oestrogen only therapy with an increased risk of endometrial cancer is compelling. A review of the topic [7] cited 20 case-control studies, all but one of which showed an increased risk. Most studies confirm that the risk appears to be related to the duration of use, with roughly a 4–8-fold increase in risk after 5 years of use.

In contrast, there is little epidemiological evidence on the effect of combined therapy on endometrial cancer risk. However, clinical research on the effect of progestogen on the endometrium shows that it reverses the action of unopposed oestrogen. In addition, a recent Swedish cohort study [8] supports the contention that the addition of a progestogen eliminates the increased risk of endometrial cancer.

For the present purpose it is, therefore assumed that women taking combined therapy will not be at increased risk of devloping endometrial cancer.

Breast Cancer

The evidence on the effect of oestrogen only therapy on breast cancer remains controversial. It is fairly well established that there is no excess risk with short-term use. With long-term use of 10 years or more there is evidence from several studies of a modest increase in risk. A review article by Henderson et al. [9] quotes eight case control studies using healthy controls, all but one of which showed an increased risk of breast cancer with long-term oestrogen use (with relative risks ranging from 1.3 to 2.0). The largest and one of the best designed of these studies, conducted by Brinton et al. [10] showed an increased risk of 30% after 10 years and 50% after 20 years. Two important issues remain unresolved: the duration of increased risk after cessation of therapy and the case fatality rates for HRT-induced cancers.

In addition, the question of the effect of combined therapy on breast cancer risk remains unanswered. It has been postulated by some that, as for endo-metrial cancer, the increased risk associated with oestrogen use might be reversed by the addition of a progestogen [11]. Others have suggested, on the basis of a review of the role of endogenous and exogenous hormones in the aetiology of breast cancer, that the addition of a progestogen might actually increase the risk above that of unopposed oestrogen [12]. There have, so far, been few epidemiological studies addressing this issue. A recent Swedish cohort study [13], however, concluded that long-term oestrogen use (in this cohort mostly oestradiol) is associated with an increased breast cancer risk, and that this increase in risk is not prevented and may even be made worse by the addition of a progestogen.

For the purpose of this analysis, it is assumed that the use of HRT (both oestrogen-only and combined therapy) is associated with an increased risk of developing breast cancer. The risk is assumed to increase by 30% after 10 years of use and 50% after 15 years of use and is assumed to remain elevated after treatment is discontinued. Case fatality rates are assumed to be the same as for an untreated population. Each hospital admission for treatment of breast cancer is costed at £1200.

Osteoporotic Fractures

There is convincing evidence that oestrogen replacement therapy is effective in preventing the development of osteoporosis [14,15] and reducing the risk of associated fractures of the hip and wrist [16,17]. Weiss et al. [16] suggested a reduction of about 50%–60% after 5 years of use. There is once again a lack of epidemiological evidence on the effect of combined therapy. However, clinical research on the effect of progestogen on bone mineral content has suggested that combined therapy is as effective as unopposed oestrogen [18]. The major unresolved issue is the duration of effect after cessation of treatment.

Only hip fractures are included in this analysis. It is assumed that there is a 20% reduction in risk during the first 5 years of treatment and a 60% reduction after 5 years – this is assumed to apply equally to oestrogen-only and combined therapy. The risk is assumed to remain reduced for as many years after the cessation of treatment as treatment was administered. Each hospital admission for fractured neck of femur is costed at £2800.

Ischaemic Heart Disease

The question of the effect of HRT on the risk of developing heart disease remains unsettled. However, most community based case control studies have shown a protective effect. Three large well-conducted prospective studies have also shown a protective effect on mortality from ischaemic heart disease [19–21]. For example, the Nurses Health Study [20] of over 32 000 postmenopausal women showed a 50% reduction in the risk of both fatal and non-fatal heart disease in women who had ever used oestrogen replacement therapy. There is inconclusive evidence on the duration of effect after cessation of treatment.

There have been few epidemiological studies of the effect of combined therapy. However, it is assumed that the beneficial effect of oestrogen is at least partially due to its favourable action on serum lipids. This action is known to be reduced or reversed by the administration of progestogens and it therefore seems highly likely that the beneficial effect will also be reduced.

For this study, it is assumed that for oestrogen only therapy the risk of developing heart disease is reduced by 25% after 5 years of use and by 50% after 10 years of use. For combined therapy the risk is assumed to be reduced by 12% after 5 years of use and by 25% after 10 years of use. For both forms of therapy the risk is assumed to remain reduced after the cessation of therapy for a period equal to the period of treatment. A hospital admission for treatment of ischaemic heart disease is costed at £1200.

Cerebrovascular Disease

While there is a considerable body of work on the effect of HRT on heart disease, there have been few studies of the effect on cerebrovascular disease. A recent study by Paganini-Hill et al. [22] showed a 50% reduction in stroke mortality in women taking oestrogen therapy – a similar result to the findings reported for ischaemic heart disease.

For the present analysis, the assumptions made about the effect on stroke are exactly the same as those for heart disease. Each hospital admission for treatment of stroke is costed at £6500.

Results

Deaths and Hospital Admissions

Applying these assumptions to the two treatment cohorts and comparing their mortality and morbidity experience to that of the untreated control group has enabled the calculation of numbers of deaths and hospital admissions induced or prevented by each treatment strategy.

Table 26.1 shows the effect on overall mortality. Both treatment strategies led to an overall reduction in deaths during the period of observation, with oestrogen only therapy showing over twice the benefit of combined therapy.

Table 26.2 shows the deaths and hospital admissions for breast cancer induced by both treatment strategies. Allowing for differences in the base populations, both strategies would cause an extra 10 000 deaths and about an extra 30 000 hospital admissions due to breast cancer.

On the benefit side, Table 26.3 shows the predicted impact on deaths and hospital admissions due to fractured neck of femur. Both strategies would prevent about 2000 deaths and 22 000 hospital admissions due to fractured neck of femur.

Table 26.1. Deaths from all causes (thousands)

	Age group (years)			
	50–59	60–69	70–79	Total[a]
No HRT	53	130	268	452
ORT 50–65[b]	−2	−18	+2	−19
O + P 50–65[c]	−1	−7	+2	−7

[a]Total may differ slightly from the sum of the columns, due to rounding.
[b]Oestrogen replacement therapy: Premarin (0.625 mg conjugated oestrogen) taken from age 50 till 65.
[c]Combined oestrogen and progestogen therapy: Prempak-C (0.625 mg conjugated oestrogen daily and 75 µg levonorgestrel for 10 days each cycle) taken from age 50 till 65.

Table 26.2. Breast cancer (ICD9:174): deaths and hospital admissions (thousands)

50–59 years		60–69 years		70–79 years		Total	
D[a]	A	D	A	D	A	D	A
No HRT							
8	35	10	37	11	29	30	100
ORT 50–65							
0	0	+4	+15	+6	+16	+10	+31
O + P 50–60							
0	0	+4	+15	+6	+15	+10	+30

[a]D, deaths, A, admissions. See Table 26.1 for other abbreviations.

Table 26.3. Fractured neck of femur (ICD9:820+821): deaths and hospital admissions (thousands)

50–59 years		60–69 years		70–79 years		Total	
D	A	D	A	D	A	D	A
No HRT							
0	5	1	13	4	37	5	54
ORT 50–65							
0	−2	−1	−7	−1	−12	−2	−22
O + P 50–65							
0	−2	−1	−8	−1	−13	−2	−22

See Table 26.1 for abbreviations.

Table 26.4 shows the predicted benefit from a reduction in deaths and hospital admissions due to ischaemic heart disease. Treatment with unopposed oestrogen would lead to 23 000 fewer deaths and 41 000 fewer hospital admissions compared with 12 000 fewer deaths and 21 000 fewer admissions with combined therapy.

Table 26.4. Ischaemic heart disease (ICD9:410–414): deaths and hospital admissions (thousands)

50–59 years		60–69 years		70–79 years		Total	
D	A	D	A	D	A	D	A
No HRT							
9	33	32	58	76	75	117	166
ORT 50–65							
−2	−5	−16	−29	−6	−7	−23	−41
O + P 50–65							
−1	−2	−8	−14	−3	−4	−11	−21

See Table 26.1 for abbreviations.

Table 26.5. Cerebrovascular disease (ICD9:430–438): deaths and hospital admissions (thousands)

50–59 years		60–69 years		70–79 years		Total	
D	A	D	A	D	A	D	A
No HRT							
3	15	12	34	41	76	57	125
ORT 50–65							
−1	−2	−6	−17	−3	−6	−9	−25
O + P 50–65							
0	−1	−3	−8	−1	−3	−5	−13

See Table 26.1 for abbreviations.

Table 26.6. Summary of costs used in the analysis

Drug treatment
Oestrogen only (Premarin): £11.00 per year
Oestrogen + progestogen (Prempak-C): £45.00 per year

Monitoring
Two extra GP visits per year at £5.80 per visit

Treatment costs based on average acute inpatient cost per day × mean length of stay for each condition

Breast cancer	£1 200
Ischaemic heart disease	£1 200
Cerebrovascular disease	£6 500
Fractured neck of femur	£2 800

The predicted impact on stroke is shown in Table 26.5. Unopposed oestrogen therapy would lead to 9000 fewer deaths and 25 000 fewer hospital admissions, and combined therapy to roughly half this reduction.

Health Care Costs

Table 26.6 summarises the costs used in this analysis. These figures have been used to calculate an average net cost per woman treated from 50 till 65 years and followed-up for 30 years. Table 26.7 shows the results. For oestrogen-only

Table 26.7. Average cost per woman treated for 15 years and followed-up until age 79 years

	ORT (£)	O + P (£)
Direct costs Drug	110	453
Monitoring	117	117
Indirect costs Breast cancer	13	13
Ischaemic heart disease	(18)	(9)
Cerebrovascular disease	(65)	(33)
Fractured neck of femur	(20)	(20)
Total cost		
	137	521

Figures in brackets in are savings.
All costs are discounted at 5% per annum.

therapy there is a predicted net cost of £137, with cerebrovascular disease providing the most substantial saving. For combined therapy, drug costs are higher and savings from prevention of heart disease and, especially, stroke are lower, leading to a net cost to the health service for each woman treated of £521.

Sensitivity Analysis

A single sensitivity analysis, looking at a shorter period of treatment (10 years as opposed to 15), has been conduced for illustrative purposes. All the assumptions about disease risks are left unchanged. The impact of this shorter period of treatment on health care costs is summarised in Table 26.8. The most striking difference between these results and those for 15 years of treatment is that the savings due to the beneficial effect on heart attacks and strokes are markedly reduced and this effect is more significant for unopposed oestrogen therapy where the savings were initially greater. Indeed, there is now a net cost of £103 to the health service for 10 years of oestrogen therapy (compared to a saving of £141 for 15 years treatment) and a marginal increase from £366 to £395 for 10 instead of 15 years of combined therapy.

Table 26.8. Average cost per woman treated for 10 years and followed-up until age 79 years

	ORT (£)	O + P (£)
Direct costs Drug	83	342
Monitoring	88	88
Indirect costs Breast cancer	9	9
Ischaemic heart disease	(11)	(6)
Cerebrovascular disease	(35)	(18)
Fractured neck of femur	(7)	(7)
Total cost		
	127	408

Figures in brackets in are savings.
All costs are discounted at 5% per annum.

Discussion

From this analysis it would seem that the benefits in terms of reduced mortality and treatment costs are greater for women without a uterus receiving oestrogen only therapy than for women with a uterus receiving combined therapy. Indeed a net cost to the health service of only £137 per women is suggested if hysterectomised women are treated with oestrogen therapy. By the age of 50 years up to 20% of the female population of England will have had a hysterectomy [23] and thus a strategy aimed at this group alone would have major public health implications.

However, there are clearly many uncertainties about the assumptions and costs used in this study. It would be possible to perform a large number of sensitivity analyses allowing for different sets of assumptions and arriving at different answers. For example, assumptions about different periods of treatment (e.g. 10 or 20 years) or different compliance rates (a compliance rate of below 100% would be more realistic) could have been made (see Table 26.8). This analysis has looked at only two subgroups of the total population of menopausal women, namely those with and without a uterus. It would be possible to divide the population in other ways, for example, between women with and without menopausal symptoms or women at high or low risk of developing osteoporosis.

While the evidence concerning endometrial cancer and osteoporotic fractures is convincing, there is a need for further research to clarify the effect of HRT on breast cancer, heart disease and stroke. Even for osteoporotic fractures, more information is needed on the duration of effect after the cessation of treatment. Furthermore, the effects of long-term combined oestrogen and progestogen therapy are largely unknown.

Also omitted from this study is a consideration of non-health service costs and of the effect of HRT on quality of life. Menopausal symptoms are known to be very common and for many women the relief of these symptoms will count as a major and immediate benefit of HRT.

However, in spite of these limitations, a study such as this provides a framework for the systematic evaluation of the risks, benefits and costs of HRT. All assumptions are made explicit and can therefore be discussed and contested.

Update

Further work is now planned to expand and improve on the original study. The health care costs used in the study were crude approximations only, and it is intended to derive more precise costings of hospital admissions for different procedures and conditions. Techniques of life-table analysis will be used to calculate life-years saved and a quality of life measure will be incorporated into the analysis. The effect of different periods of treatment, different rates of compliance with treatment and different arrangements for follow-up of women receiving treatment will be studied. Allowing for these variables, the relative cost effectiveness of treating women with and without menopausal symptoms and with and without a uterus will be considered. In addition, the impact on the cost effectiveness equation of an osteoporosis screening programme will be studied.

Acknowledgement. This paper is a modified and corrected version of work that has appeared in Osteoporosis, Smith R, ed. London, Royal College of Physicians, and is reproduced with kind permission of the publishers.

References

1. Weinstein MC. Estrogen use in postmenopausal women – costs, risks and benefits. N Engl J Med 1980; 303:308–16.
2. Weinstein MC, Schiff I. Cost-effectiveness of hormone replacement therapy in the menopause. Obstet Gynecol Surv 1983; 38:445–55.
3. Office of Population Censuses and Surveys. 1986 Mortality statistics: cause. London: HMSO, 1988.
4. Department of Health and Social Security and Welsh Office. Health Service Costing Returns: year ended 31st March 1987. London: DHSS, 1988.
5. Department of Health and Social Security and Office of Population Censuses and Surveys. 1985 Hospital Inpatient Enquiry. London: HMSO, 1987.
6. Marinker M. The referral system. J R Coll Gen Pract 1988; 38:487–90.
7. Hunt K, Vessey M. Long term effects of postmenopausal hormone therapy. Br J Hosp Med 1987; 38:450–60.
8. Persson I, Adami H-O, Bergkvist L, Lindgren A, Pettersson B, Hoover R, Schairer C. Risk of endometrial cancer after treatment with oestrogens alone or in conjunction with progestogens: results of a prospective study. Br Med J 1989; 298:147–51.
9. Henderson BE, Pike MC, Ross RK, Mack TM, Lobo RA. Re-evaluating the role of progestogen therapy after the menopause. Fertil Steril 1988; 49 (suppl.):9S–15S.
10. Brinton LA, Hoover R, Fraumeni JF Jr. Menopausal oestrogen and breast cancer risk: an expanded case-control study. Br J Cancer 1986; 54:825–32.
11. Gambrell RD Jr. Proposal to decrease the risk and improve the prognosis of breast cancer. Am J Obstet Gynecol 1984; 150:119–32.
12. Key TJ, Pike MC. The role of oestrogens and progestagens in the epidemiology and prevention of breast cancer. Eur J Cancer Clin Oncol 1988; 24:29–43.
13. Bergkvist L, Adami H-O, Persson I, Hoover R, Schairer C. The risk of breast cancer after estrogen and estrogen–progestin replacement. N Engl J Med 1989; 321:293–7.
14. Lindsay R, Hart DM, Aitken JM, MacDonald EB, Anderson JB, Clarke AC. Long term prevention of postmenopausal osteoporosis by oestrogen: evidence for an increased bone mass after delayed onset of oestrogen treatment. Lancet 1976; i:1038–41.
15. Horsman A, Gallagher JC, Simpson M, Nordin BEC. Prospective trial of oestrogen and calcium in post-menopausal women. Br Med J 1977; ii:789–92.
16. Weiss NS, Ure CL, Ballard JH, Williams AR, Daling JR. Decreased risk of fractures of hip and lower forearm with postmenopausal use of estrogen. N Engl J Med 1980; 303:1195–8.
17. Paganini-Hill A, Ross RK, Gerkins VR, Henderson BE, Arthur M, Mack TM. A case-control study of menopausal estrogen therapy and hip fractures. Ann Intern Med 1981; 95:28–31.
18. Christiansen C, Christensen MS, Transbol TB. Bone mass in postmenopausal women after withdrawal of oestrogen/gestagen replacement therapy. Lancet 1981; i:459–61.
19. Bush TL, Cowan LD, Barret-Connor E. Estrogen use and all cause mortality: preliminary results from the Lipid Research Clinics Program follow-up study. JAMA 1983; 249:903–6.
20. Stampfer MJ, Willett WC, Colditz GA, Rosner B, Speizer FE, Hennekens CH. A prospective study of postmenopausal estrogen therapy and coronary heart disease. N Engl J Med 1985; 313:1044–9.
21. Henderson BE, Ross RK, Paganini-Hill A, Mack TM. Estrogen use and cardiovascular disease. Am J Obstet Gynecol 1986; 154:1181–6.
22. Paganini-Hill A, Ross RK, Henderson BE. Postmenopausal oestrogen treatment and stroke: a prospective study. Br Med J 1988; 297:519–22.
23. Coulter A, McPherson K, Vessey M. Do British women undergo too many or too few hysterectomies? Soc Sci Med 1988; 27:987–94.

Chapter 27

Should HRT be Recommended in the Community?

D. H. Barlow

Introduction

Previous chapters have examined the efficacy and safety of hormone replacement therapy (HRT) and we must now consider whether widespread treatment of our community is appropriate. Because doctors have always been free to offer HRT to women the question for us is not whether an individual doctor should use the drug but whether there should be "national policy" on this matter. Examples of the application of national policies on health include immunisation policy, cervical cancer screening and recently the decision to advise breast cancer screening by mammography. Without adequate resources the application of national policy can be rather fragmented, as has been the case with cervical cancer screening. If there were to be a major expansion of HRT use it would be essential that this would be undertaken in general practice, since there is not a nationwide network of specialist clinics which could undertake the work of advising, treating and monitoring the women and I cannot envisage new resources to set up such a network. If large-scale treatment is to be based in general practice, it would be of great importance to have the willing collaboration of GPs, and their agreement that widespread and reasonably long-term treatment is advisable. Despite the recent growth in the prescription of HRT by GPs, I believe many remain unconvinced that large-scale longer-term treatment is advisable.

The Community Picture

It is clear that a sizeable proportion of menopausal women experience symptoms which make them seek help from their GPs. In a community study of more than

400 women in Glasgow aged 40 to 60 years we found that 42% of women after a natural menopause, 57% of those hysterectomised and 76% of those oophorectomised had felt in need of help for menopausal symptoms [1]. Despite Glasgow being relatively well served with menopause clinics (it has three) we found that these made a negligible contribution, having seen only 1% of the women. That study was carried out in 1983, before the current publicity on osteoporosis prevention. We found that only 4% of the women who had had a natural menopause were current HRT users. In the most "at risk" group (the oophorectomised women) 27% were current HRT users. It might be argued that, being from 1983, these relatively low rates do not reflect recent practice but a recent study from London general practices on more than 3000 women found HRT use in only 10% of all women studied and in only 30% of oophorectomised women [2].

In the Glasgow population there was a clear preference to avoid the long-term use of HRT, and thus the percentage of women who had ever been exposed to some HRT was much higher than the figures for current use. For the women who had had a natural menopause, "ever use" was 15%. After oophorectomy it was 46% (Table 27.1) [1]. Table 27.2 shows that only 2% of the women received HRT for more than three years and that these women were almost exclusively from the oophorectomised group, of whom 21% did receive more than three years treatment. The relatively short duration of treatment might be understandable if the women remained well after cessation of therapy but it was found that 74% of those no longer on treatment remained symptomatic at the time of the study. This leads to the conclusion that the doctors, the women or both had a reluctance to continue with HRT even in the face of symptoms.

Table 27.1. Use of HRT in 424 Glasgow women surveyed in the community

	No. of patients	Current use (%)	Past use (%)	Ever use (%)
Premenopause	175	5.1	3.4	8.5
Postmenopause	188	3.7	11.7	15.4
Hysterectomy	28	10.7	17.9	28.6
Hysterectomy BSO[a]	33	27.3	18.2	45.5
Total	424	6.6	9.2	15.8

BSO, bilateral salpingo-oophorectomy

Table 27.2. Duration of use of HRT in 424 women surveyed in the community

	No. of patients	2 years	2–3 years	3 years
Current use				
Premenopause	175	7	2	0
Postmenopause	188	2	2	3 (1.6%)
Hysterectomy	28	1	2	0
Hysterectomy BSO[a]	33	1	1	7 (21.2%)
Total	424	11	7	10 (2.4%)
Past use				
Total	424	33	4	2 (0.4%)

Attitudes to HRT

Attitudes among doctors about HRT use vary considerably. Negative attitudes include:

Not interfering with a "natural" process
Alleviating symptoms is simply postponing problems
The risks are too high or are too ill-defined
Since the doctor is not sure how best to monitor treatment it is easiest to avoid it.

It would be wrong, however, to attribute non-use of HRT entirely to doctor's reluctance. Compliance with prescribed HRT is reported to be well short of complete. Women's reasons for non-compliance or reluctance to start HRT will include:

A wish to avoid taking "hormones" as something "not natural"
A fear that the treatment might cause cancer
The occurrence of side effects
The dislike of continuing to menstruate

In the Massachusetts Women's Health Survey of 2500 women prescribed HRT 20% stopped within nine months, 10% took it only intermittently and 20%–30% did not use the prescription [3]. Similarly in the recent large breast cancer study from Sweden, 9% of the women studied in the subgroup analysis reported having not taken the HRT which had been prescribed [4].

The Current GP View

In an effort to understand better the nature of the interaction between the woman and her GP, we studied, over a six month period, all menopause-related consultations taking place with women aged 40 to 69 years. We had the detailed age/sex register for each practice so the consultations could be related to the background population. Overall, 416 women consulted on 572 occasions and represented between 6% and 15% of all eligible women in the practices. The peak consulting rate was at 45 to 49 years with 8% of that group having at least one consultation in the six months. As might have been predicted, flushing was the commonest complaint being involved in 68% of consultations but psychological symptoms (52%) and vaginal dryness (45%) were also commonly discussed. Osteoporosis was discussed with 25% of the women but as can be seen in Table 27.3 there was a progressive increase in interest up to 60 years of age. Very few women, however, discussed this as the only issue, implying that most were also suffering with menopausal symptoms.

Local general practitioner opinion has been tested in relation to a number of HRT issues by means of a questionnaire presented at occasions where GPs were attending lectures on topics other than menopause issues. A 100% response was achieved and some revealing replies were obtained. There was no consistent pattern but some doctors clearly expressed negative views: 28% agreed with the

Table 27.3. Number and percentage of women (aged 40–69 years) consulting nine group practices in Oxford to discuss osteoporosis over a 6-month period

Age group (years)	Osteoporosis discussed	Osteoporosis only
40–44	5/35 (15%)	0
45–49	27/140 (19%)	2
50–54	34/125 (27%)	4
55–59	27/75 (36%)	4
60–64	4/24 (17%)	0
65–69	6/16 (38%)	2
	103	12

proposition that "only symptomatic women should consider using HRT"; 23% did "not favour long courses of HRT"; 27% agreed that for flushing they "usually try non-hormonal medication before turning to HRT", but despite these relatively negative views only 9% agreed that they "prefer to avoid prescribing HRT if possible".

Constraints

When considering a recommendation that HRT be used widely and for long periods it is important to reflect on the constraints within which such a policy would have to function. It must be acceptable to the general practitioners who would carry out the recommendation; it must also be acceptable to women and it should not meet with too much opposition from the pundits who have ready access to the printed and broadcast media. The media can have a real effect on public confidence in HRT by publicising reports on long-term risks in sensationalist terms, perhaps without reference to the body of literature preceding the study being publicised. Financial resources are limited so we can be asked to establish that long-term HRT is an effective use of resources. The other constraint which should not be ignored is the need to accumulate data on the long-term effects of HRT in women who take current "opposed" regimes.

Objectives

If an effective policy is to be developed the objectives should be clearly defined. These should be:

1. The relief of the menopausal syndrome
2. A reduction in rates of osteoporotic fractures
3. A reduction in coronary artery disease
4. A reduction in the incidence of stroke

With these objectives in mind we must decide on the optimal duration of therapy. In relation to relieving the menopausal syndrome this will be an individual decision between the doctor and the woman but the other objectives require long-term treatment. In determining the optimal duration of treatment the aim should be to balance a number of factors which are differently affected by duration of treatment. These are:

1. Maximise beneficial effects
2. Minimise risks
3. Maximise compliance
4. Maximise cost-benefit ratio
5. Minimise adverse comment, since this can easily affect patient confidence.

It is likely that maximum compliance and minimum adverse comment would be ensured if the treatment duration were short whereas the calculations of Professor Vessey's group imply that 15 years might be optimal for cost-effectiveness. To test the appropriate treatment duration for maximum benefit and minimum risk the available evidence must be considered.

For How Long Should We Treat?

The studies of fractures show that five or more years of treatment will yield favourable reductions in risk although it is not clear whether this benefit to bone is sustained into very old age when femoral neck fracture is a particular problem. For example with more than five years of HRT Weiss et al. [5] reported a risk ratio of 0.38; Kreiger et al. [6] an odds ratio of 0.4; and Paganini-Hill et al. [7] a risk ratio of 0.14 with oophorectomised women. The large prospective studies of cardiovascular disease mostly indicate a valuable reduction in risk ratios of death from myocardial infarction, in the range 0.3–0.6 [8–11]. Duration of use is not always reported but again it looks as if five years of HRT provide significant benefit. As far as stroke risk is concerned, the data of Paganini-Hill et al. [12] suggest a relative risk of 0.55 with up to 8 years of treatment and only a slight further reduction with longer use (RR = 0.50). These data suggest that about five to ten years of HRT beyond the menopause should provide substantial benefit, at least based on unopposed oestrogen treatment.

Table 27.4. Comparison of the relative risk of breast cancer in HRT users by duration of use

Reference	Duration (years)					
	1	1–4	5–9	10–14	15–19	20+
Kaufman et al. [14]	0.9	0.9	0.7	1.7	–	–
Brinton et al. [15]	0.9	0.9	1.1	1.3	1.2	1.5
Wingo et al. [16]	1.0	1.1	1.1	0.8	1.3	1.8
Bergkvist et al. [4]	0.7	1.1	1.3	1.7[a]	–	–

[a]Lower confidence interval greater than 1.0

The effect of duration of use on risk principally relates to endometrial and breast cancers. The current use of progestogens has essentially eliminated the endometrial cancer risk [13] so, assuming that opposed therapy is favoured, we are left with the complex question of breast cancer risk, which has been discussed in detail in earlier chapters. In general most studies show little overall increased risk (Table 27.4) but beyond ten years' treatment the relative risk tends to rise [4,14–16]. In some studies the lower confidence-limit exceeded 1.0 with longer-term treatment [4,17] and in some there has been an elevation of risk even with the relatively short-term treatment of 3 years [11,18]. Again a recommendation of five to ten years may be the appropriate duration to recommend to women who want the long-term benefits of HRT without undue risk. With the current data on breast cancer it is important that the women are aware of the balance of risk to be considered and that those with higher risk of breast cancer assess the matter carefully.

Treatment Strategy

These studies rely heavily on evidence from unopposed oestrogen therapy, and when opposed regime data can be examined we may wish to reappraise these recommendations. I am aware that opting for endometrial safety by proposing opposed oestrogen regimens may result in some reduction in the cardiovascular benefit but the use of those progestogen regimens with the least effect on lipids will minimise this tendency. To adopt a policy of unopposed oestrogen HRT on a wide scale in the UK would have serious cost implications since NHS gynaecology services do not have spare capacity to undertake large-scale endometrial monitoring and most GPs do not wish to take on this task. Thus a realistic HRT service for the UK would be GP based, using opposed oestrogen therapy without routine endometrial biopsy, but with gynaecology clinic support for endometrial biopsy after abnormal bleeding, with set guidelines for referral. Breast self-examination should be encouraged and when the national breast screening programme is in place these women should make use of it.

If the programme were to be adopted it would be important to provide targets to test the application of the policy. I have chosen three imaginary targets for duration of treatment as an example (Table 27.5). The first is a minimum acceptable standard which might easily be achieved and which would be an increase in long-term HRT use for many doctors. The second is a higher target which might be what we realistically hope the programme could achieve. Third, there could also be a guideline for what could be regarded as "excellent" delivery of HRT to the population, which would be achieved by a few doctors.

Table 27.5. Possible targets for HRT use in a hypothetical national HRT policy

	1–2 years	2–5 years	6–9 years	11–15 years
Minimum acceptable	30%	20%	15%	10%
Achievable	60%	50%	30%	20%
Excellent	80%	75%	50%	30%

Target Groups

If there are to be recommendations about HRT, these can be aimed at specific groups of women: i.e. symptomatic women, women with premature oestrogen deficiency, hysterectomised women, women at high fracture risk, healthy women seeking HRT and healthy women in general.

Examples of suggested recommendations are as follows:

Symptomatic women
Treat with confidence
Individualise duration
"Benign" progestogen favoured if uterus present

Premature oestrogen deficiency
Treat with confidence
Encourage treatment until "50"
"Benign" progestogen if uterus present

Hysterectomised women
Potential benefits of long-term treatment maximised
More cost-effective
No progestogen
Encourage long-term therapy

High fracture risk
Difficult to identify but if suspected encourage treatment
Long-term HRT
"Benign" progestogen if uterus present

Women who seek long-term HRT
Ensure adequate counselling
Provide long-term therapy
"Benign" progestogen if uterus present
Discuss policy on continuing at intervals

Other healthy women
Make information available
Address anxieties about treatment
Offer access to HRT if desired

Are These Policies Practicable?

Large-scale and relatively long-term treatment is feasible only if women and doctors want it. The evidence for its application to all of the above groups, except the last, is strong. Only with more data can we be sure about the relevance of HRT to relatively uninterested healthy women. The other groups constitute a large number of largely untreated women who could benefit significantly. The GP survey referred to above suggests that at least some GPs are now prepared to treat more widely. I found that 77% agreed that "the health benefits of HRT exceed the risks" and none disagreed. Similarly, 57% agreed that "HRT is cost effective in the long term". As far as long-term HRT is concerned, 23% "do not favour long courses of HRT (5 or more years)" but 67% were "happy to use long courses of HRT if the woman wishes it". It would, therefore, appear that there is a group of GPs who would be prepared to be involved in more widespread treatment and perhaps with their support the compliance rates could be improved. This chance of improved compliance is particularly relevant for the hysterectomy cases, who are estimated to constitute about 20% of women of the age range under consideration [19].

Suggestions

I suggest that a consensus statement on the use of HRT can be produced, with guidelines on screening, monitoring, etc., but it would be much more valuable if the Department of Health were prepared to issue guidelines recommending HRT for the special target groups discussed above, in publications such as the *British National Formulary* and other policy documents. It is clear that we need data on progestogen-opposed regimens and even longer-term follow-up, but while we wait another generation of women is passing the point where help can be given to greatest effect. A large GP-based national prospective study with adequate funding is now possible. It could be based on the healthy women who wish HRT, and if it is adequately controlled, some of the elusive answers might eventually emerge.

References

1. Barlow DH, Grosset KA, Hart H, Hart DM. A study of the experience of Glasgow women in the climacteric years. Br J Obstet Gynaecol 1989; 96:1192–7.
2. Spector T. Use of oestrogen replacement therapy in high risk groups in the United Kingdom. Br Med J 1989; 299:1434–5.
3. Ravnikar VA. Compliance with hormone therapy. Am J Obstet Gynecol 1987; 156:1322–4.
4. Bergvist L, Hans-Olov A, Persson I, Hoover R, Schairer C. The risk of breast cancer after estrogen and estrogen–progestin replacement. N Engl J Med 1989; 321:293–7.
5. Weiss NR, Ure BL, Ballard JH, Williams AR, Darling DR. Decreased risk of fractures of the hip and lower forearm with postmenopausal use of estrogen. N Engl J Med 1980; 303:1195–8
6. Kreiger N, Kelsey JL, Holford TR, O'Connell T. An epidemiological study of hip fracture in postmenopausal women. Am J Epidemiol 1982;116:141–8.
7. Paganini-Hill A, Ross RK, Gerkins VR, Henderson BE, Arthur M, Mack TM. Menopausal estrogen therapy and hip fractures. Ann Intern Med 1981; 95:28–31.
8. Bush TL, Cowan LD, Barrett-Connor E et al. Estrogen use and all-cause mortality. JAMA 1983; 249:903–6.
9. Stampfer MJ, Willett WC, Colditz GA, Rosner B, Speizer FE, Hennekens C. A prospective study of postmenopausal estrogen therapy and coronary artery disease. N Eng J Med 1985; 313:1044–9.
10. Henderson BE, Paganini-Hill A, Ross RK. Estrogen replacement therapy and protection from acute myocardial infarction. Am J Obstet Gynecol 1988; 159:312–17.
11. Hunt K, Vessey MP, McPherson K, Coleman M. Long-term surveillance of mortality and cancer incidence in women receiving hormone replacement therapy. Br J Obstet Gynaecol 1987; 94:620–35.
12. Paganini-Hill A, Ross RK, Henderson BE. Postmenopausal oestrogen treatment and stroke: a prospective study. Br Med J 1988; 297:519–22.
13. Persson I, Adami H-O, Bergkvist L, Lindgren A, Pettersson B, Hoover R, Schairer C. Risk of endometrial cancer after treatment with oestrogens alone or in conjunction with progestogens: results of a prospective study. Br Med J 1989; 298:147–51.
14. Kaufman DW, Miller DR, Rosenberg L et al. Non-contraceptive estrogen use; the risk of breast cancer. JAMA 1984; 252:63–7.

15. Brinton LA, Hoover R, Fraumeni JF. Menopausal oestrogens and breast cancer risk: an expanded case-control study. Br J Cancer 1986; 54:825–32.
16. Wingo PA, Layde PM, Lee NC, Rubin G, Ory HW. The risk of breast cancer in postmenopausal women who have used estrogen replacement therapy. JAMA 1987; 257:209–15.
17. Ewertz M. Influence of non-contraceptive exogenous and endogenous sex hormones on breast cancer risk in Denmark. Int J Cancer 1988; 42:832–8.
18. Mills PK, Beeson WL, Phillips RL, Fraser GE. Prospective study of exogenous hormone use and breast cancer risk in Seventh Day Adventists. Cancer 1989; 64:591–7.
19. Coulter A, MacPherson K, Vessey MP. Do British women undergo too many or too few hysterectomies? Social Sci Med 1988; 27:987–94.

Discussion

Drife: Was the questionnaire administered before or after Dr Barlow had spoken about HRT or was there no direct connection? Had he spoken at the meeting?

Barlow: These meetings are monthly or bi-monthly social gatherings of GPs with a meal followed by a speaker. This study was done while they were having coffee at the end of the meal in both cases and before the lecture in both cases. I knew it was important that they had not had any discussion. Because it was anonymous their names were not put on the questionnaire, but looking around the room it was clear that we got a 100% response rate. That 100% response rate is an important element because I am sure that many of those who receive postal questionnaires throw them away.

Vessey: Obviously that is something of a selected group. We get about a 70% response from general practitioners. Nonetheless, I thought their responses were very interesting.

Lindsay: All the analyses that I see about cost-effectiveness leave us with a cohort of people who are alive. I have two questions about that. First, what happens to them? Presumably they die sometime. What do they die from? Second, should we be adding the costs of what happens to them into the analysis?

Vessey: It is an extremely good point. The analysis that we have done is valid up to age 79, but what we have done in this analysis, partly for simplicity and partly because it is difficult to speculate what happens further on, is that we have ignored what happens beyond age 79 in the survivors. There are more people surviving into their 80s in the treated group who will die from something, and they presumably will die from more or less the same distribution of causes as the general population and there will be costs associated with those additional deaths in comparison with the untreated women who may have died earlier and who may have had costs associated with their deaths. So to that extent this must be regarded as an incomplete analysis.

In further analyses we shall be considering the survival curves and some of the traditional measures like years of life saved and we will also have to make assumptions about what happens in the oldest age groups. But certainly 30 years from now there would be an increased proportion of survivors, and they would cost money.

This is one of the problems with all preventive strategies. If death is in fact postponed and people are preserved to an older age, they may then be very expensive to look after in old age.

The one answer that I would offer as somebody who is interested in preventive medicine, is that much so-called curative clinical medicine has the same objectives. It is aimed at increasing survival. Clearly if a patient aged 65 is admitted with peritonitis from a ruptured appendix it is very cheap to let him die, but if he gets surgery he may then live to be 85 and cost the state an unspecified amount. There is this difficulty. But I fully accept Dr Lindsay's criticism of this analysis. We cut it off at 79.

Meade: I thought Professor Vessey's analysis extremely interesting and clearly presented. Of course some of the lives that are saved will be saved before age 79.

Vessey: Some 19 000.

Meade: I am thinking of a study that my colleague, Joy Townsend did of a very similar nature, to look at the implications of people stopping smoking. She found that although there were savings to the Health Service associated with people stopping smoking they were not very great because most of the diseases associated with smoking kill off sufferers pretty quickly and so they do not involve a lot of expenditure. But what really was impressive was the increase not only in the medical costs of the survivors, but particularly in the social security entitlement that they could draw. So what emerged from that, and what I suspect may emerge from Professor Vessey's analysis, is that there may be good news for the Department of Health, or for Premarin, but there may be very bad news for the Department of Social Security and the Treasury when it comes to the overall balance. And we do have to look at whose pocket the money is either going into or coming out of.

My second point concerns the great interest I have in and the importance I would attach to Professor Vessey's sensitivity analyses. He showed us what the picture is when he makes the assumptins he so clearly set out, and he made it clear that that was one starting set of assumptions which can be varied quite considerably. There are two assumptions about which I would be interested to hear Professor Vessey comment.

First, it will come as no surprise that I feel that the benefits to vascular disease that he assumes might be overestimates, and second, particularly in the Premarin analysis, the savings due to stroke could be much less if the effect is much smaller.

The other point about the sensitivity analyses that might have an effect on outcome is compliance. He has assumed 100% compliance, which is likely to be an overestimate. I think he said he had one example of a sensitivity analysis and if it was available it might be useful to look at it.

Vessey: I agree with everything that Dr Meade says. Certainly one thing is certain: that on the basis of those assumptions which I showed, there is clearly a gain in mortality terms and in morbidity terms, at least hospital morbidity, so on the basis of those assumptions there certainly would be a net saving of life and there would be a gain in years of life.

The cost data I agree are vastly more tenuous, for all the reasons that Dr Meade has described, and certainly the results would be very sensitive to the assumptions that are made.

For this sensitivity analysis, if we assumed that instead of women being treated for 15 years they were treated for only 10 years, then fewer lives are saved without a great change in costs. That may seem paradoxical but it is attributable to the complex interplay of assumed risks.

Roche: There is still a reduction in mortality, but less so than for 15 years. But there is less of a reduction from stroke, heart disease and fractured neck of femur.

Barlow: Beyond 10 years what increases is the adverse publicity from the pundits, because the breast cancer question gets worse and worse as we follow it. And that adverse publicity would be enough to ruin any treatment policy.

Edwards: To leave out the other fractures destroys the story about the benefits of using HRT to prevent osteoporosis. While the hip fracture question is serious and it is the one we have statistics about, for the group of women from 50 or younger than 50, particularly the women who have vertebral fractures, the human costs are great and the costs to the country in GP visits, the cost of hospital referrals, the cost of X-rays, the cost of pain-killers for those who are not diagnosed (which must be huge) and the costs of losing experienced women from the workforce at that time are not insignificant.

I would be interested to know when Professor Vessey intends to do that study.

Vessey: The Colles' fractures we felt fairly comfortable with because they would not feature very strongly. We have been looking, as I said, at inpatient hospital costs.

About the crush fractures of the vertebral column: it is very difficult to get at any reasonable kind of Health Service usage data for that kind of event. I would not underrate the costs in terms of pain and in terms of GP visits. Dr Roche scoured the literature thoroughly and this is a difficult one to get at, in terms of Health Service costs – real data as opposed to guesses.

Edwards: The costs at the GP end will be quite high, but there will not be many figures at all.

Vessey: It is staggeringly difficult. Is the pain due to osteoporosis, or is it due to any one of numerous other causes? And there is now a strong policy of discouraging GPs from taking X-rays of the back. I know that X-rays are not much use in diagnosing osteoporosis, other than end-stage osteoporosis, but it is tricky.

Edwards: The problem is that almost all the women who are eventually diagnosed as having osteoporosis, those who are on our lists, have spent years and years being fobbed off with pain-killers and antidepressants before they were properly diagnosed.

Stevenson: One of the major costs in the analysis is the treatment.

Baird: And those are the cheapest prescriptions.

Stevenson: I would suggest that if I approached Wyeth and Ayerst and offer them 1 million prescriptions per year for the next 15 years, then I would be able to get the treatment at half that price at least. There could be a large saving there.

If these 1 million women had been selected because they were at a very high risk rather than average risk, would that not then make quite a clear saving overall? Obviously extra costs would have to be added in for an initial selection and screening process, but then the savings would be much greater. Could that be done?

Vessey: This is one of the things that the Department of Health has asked us to look at and something that we will be discussing with the bone experts, to see if we can focus on the high-risk groups.

On the other hand, if the breast cancer risk really turns out to be quite small, perhaps smaller than we have assumed here, and if the benefits in terms of cardiovascular disease are really substantial, perhaps even more substantial than here, the notion of screening for higher-risk groups might become even less important because the overall benefit might outweigh any notion of focusing the therapy on high-risk groups for osteoporosis.

Kanis: We do not know the size of the problem in regard to vertebral fractures in the UK. The estimates of vertebral fracture prevalence from different surveys in different parts of the world depend on how vertebral fracture is classified, but there is a sixfold difference in apparent prevalence. We assume that there are not sixfold differences in people. Of radiographically diagnosed vertebral fracture – again this is a very soft figure – symptoms may occur in 40% or even less.

We see a referral population which is highly biased and selective and we do not know the size of the problem. The overall hospital costs are trivial. The overall general practice costs today I believe are trivial, but that is not to say that they should be trivial.

But could Professor Vessey be overestimating his costs in the sense that a component of those costs is the cost of treating breast cancer, cardiovascular illness, stroke, etc.? If he were to take a cut-off up to a certain age rather than to the lifetime, then he is costing breast cancer and so forth. But all these women will die from something and will cost, and many of them will die in hospital and will require hospital treatment. So that cost is deferred rather than incurred. The distribution of those costs and the time might well be spread but he may be doing himself a disservice in saying that this is not cost-effective.

Vessey: Dr Lindsay made a similar point. It does need further exploration. For instance, a reduction in the risk of stroke – stroke is an enormously expensive disease whereas some other diseases, say cancer of the pancreas, are probably not very expensive. Everybody has got to die and the exact nature of the diseases that are traded off is very important in relation to costs. This analysis does not grapple with that problem beyond age 79 and it probably does not grapple with the problem completely up to age 79.

Roche: In economic terms there certainly are benefits in deferring costs. It depends how great they are eventually. If the costs are much magnified then the benefits might be reduced. But the reason for discounting future costs is that people and nations like to defer costs if they can.

Studd: Dr Barlow twice mentioned people living longer and drawing pensions, and it is absolutely true. Brian Henderson tells me that the data from the Leisure World study show an extra 4 or 5 years of life. They may be quality years, but they are certainly expensive years as regards non-earning dependent life.

It does not make too much sense to speak about targeting groups, premature menopause groups, hysterectomy groups or whatever, or those that are informed and ask for it. That is like saying that those that are informed can have pure water but the rest must drink from the village pond. I do not quite understand that.

Conclusions and Recommendations

Conclusions

1. Postmenopausal osteoporosis is one of a number of disorders caused by oestrogen deficiency.
2. The amount of bone tissue after the menopause is a function of peak bone mass (which is determined by genetic factors and lifestyle) and subsequent bone loss after the menopause.
3. Peak bone mass is achieved in the premenopausal years and there is evidence that some bone loss may occur at some sites before the menopause, though the clinical relevance of this is not yet certain.
4. Hip fractures in the elderly are the result of skeletal weakness combined with extraskeletal factors such as an increased number of falls and poor balance and reflexes.
5. The absolute number of hip fractures is rising due to the greater number of elderly people and an increase in the age-specific incidence of the fracture.
6. Hip fractures cause considerable mortality, reduced mobility and increased dependency, and the hospital costs alone are currently estimated to be £165 million per year in the UK.
7. The prevalence of vertebral osteoporosis in the UK is unknown and the magnitude of the problem is probably underestimated. Physicians treating osteoporosis see spinal crush fractures as a major problem. Women are as concerned about loss of height and poor body image as they are about hip fractures.
8. There is good evidence that further bone loss can be prevented at any stage of osteoporosis but it is questionable whether skeletal architecture and competence can be restored once lost. Therefore, the emphasis must be on prevention of bone loss by early intervention.
9. Bone density measurements currently provide the single best estimate of the risk of subsequent fracture. Their role as a screening tool needs evaluation.
10. Oestrogen is the most effective method currently available for prevention of bone loss in women, though other modalities are available. Oestrogen and other antiresorptive agents may be appropriate for the treatment of many patients with established osteoporosis.
11. Women with premature menopause – natural or surgical – are at high risk of osteoporosis but many have never had oestrogen replacement therapy.
12. Equivalent doses of oestrogen given by any route are equally effective in preventing osteoporosis.
13. Depressed mood can occur before the menopause and may be improved with oestrogen therapy in some women.
14. Oestrogen therapy raises the sensory threshold of the bladder and therefore improves symptoms of frequency, nocturia, urgency and dysuria. There is some evidence that oestrogens prevent recurrent cystitis, but HRT cannot be recommended as a treatment for genuine stress incontinence.

15. There is evidence that there may be a duration-dependent increased risk of breast cancer with HRT. There is no evidence that progestogens protect against this risk.
16. Oestrogen therapy increases the incidence of endometrial hyperplasia and carcinoma. This excess risk is significantly reduced or eliminated by cyclical progestogen.
17. Apart from withdrawal bleeding, the addition of a cyclical progestogen may result in symptoms such as dysmenorrhoea and premenstrual syndrome.
18. Oestrogens confer some protection against ischaemic heart disease and stroke but it is not known whether the addition of cyclical progestogen diminishes this effect.
19. Combined oral contraceptive data cannot be applied directly to HRT.
20. Women who are receiving oestrogen treatment after hysterectomy will not require additional progestogen.
21. Treated hypertension is not a contraindication to HRT.
22. Risk–benefit analyses incorporating reasonable assumptions about the effects of HRT on different organ systems lead to the conclusion that there is an overall beneficial effect of treatment on morbidity and mortality.

Recommendations

1. HRT is of proven efficacy in preventing bone loss. Its use in Britain is low at present and it should be more readily available.
2. Certain groups of women should be considered especially for treatment: symptomatic women, those with premature menopause (natural or surgical) and those at high risk for osteoporosis.
3. More information should be made available to asymptomatic women to allow them to make an informed choice about HRT.
4. Women taking HRT should be encouraged to participate in available breast screening programmes.
5. Non-invasive measurement of bone mass may be useful in clinical decision-making about initiation of HRT for prevention of osteoporosis, and these techniques should be made more readily available.
6. Studies are required to establish the place of bone density measurements in screening programmes to detect women at high risk of osteoporosis.
7. In order to have an effect on osteoporosis, HRT must be continued for more than two years. Studies are required to determine the optimum duration of treatment.
8. There is a need for continuing evaluation of the long-term effects of HRT.
9. The Health Service provision for the prevention and treatment of osteoporosis is less than the current demand, which is increasing. Bone disease and osteoporosis overlap with many specialties, but urgent consideration should be given to the increasing need for physicians and gynaecologists who have training in bone disease and HRT.

Subject Index